Pathobiology of the Parathyroid and Thyroid Glands

UNITED STATES AND CANADIAN ACADEMY OF PATHOLOGY, INC.

Pathobiology of the Parathyroid and Thyroid Glands

EDITED BY

VIRGINIA D. LiVOLSI, M.D.

*Professor and Director,
Section of Surgical Pathology
University of Pennsylvania Medical Center
Department of Pathology and Laboratory Medicine
Philadelphia, Pennsylvania*

and

RONALD A. DeLELLIS, M.D.

*Professor of Pathology
Tufts University School of Medicine
and Senior Pathologist
New England Medical Center Hospital
Boston, Massachusetts*

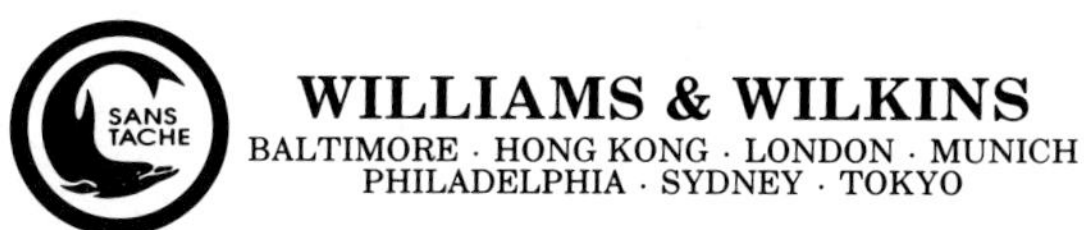

WILLIAMS & WILKINS
BALTIMORE · HONG KONG · LONDON · MUNICH
PHILADELPHIA · SYDNEY · TOKYO

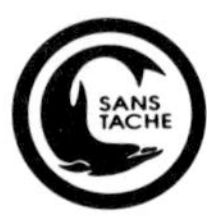

Publisher: Deanna F. Gemmill
Associate Publisher: Carole E. Pippin
Copy Editor: Maryalice Ditzler
Designer: Dan Pfisterer

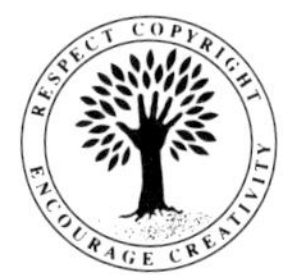

Printed in the United States of America

Library of Congress Cataloging-in-Publication Data

Pathobiology of the parathyroid and thyroid glands / edited by
   Virginia A. LiVolsi, Ronald A. DeLellis.
      p. cm.—(Monographs in pathology; no. 35)
   Based on a course held at the annual meeting of the United States and Canadian
Academy of Pathology, March 18, 1992.
   Includes bibliographical references and index.
   ISBN 0-683-04817-1
   1. Thyroid gland—Pathophysiology—Congresses. 2. Parathyroid gland—Patho-
physiology—Congresses. 3. Thyroid gland—Cancer—Congresses. I. Livolsi, Virginia
A. II. DeLellis, Ronald A. III. Series.
   [DNLM: 1. Parathyroid Diseases—pathology—congresses. 2. Parathyroid
Glands—pathology—congresses. 3. Thyroid Diseases—pathology—congresses. 4.
Thyroid Gland—pathology—congresses. W1 MO568H no. 35 / WK 300 P297 1992]
RC655.49.P38   1993
616.4′3071—dc20
DNLM/DLC
for Library of Congress   92-48313
                                                                             CIP

Foreword

Drs. Virginia LiVolsi and Ronald DeLellis assembled a distinguished faculty for the Long Course of the 1992 Annual Meeting of the U.S. and Canadian Academy of Pathology. Thereupon they became co-editors for this 35th issue in the series, "Monographs in Pathology." In this manner, they perpetuate and embellish the educational content of the oral presentations. Members of the faculty have expanded and enriched the text of their individual presentations while maintaining a balanced content of scholarly and utilitarian information.

The Academy wishes to express its sincere gratitude to Drs. LiVolsi and DeLellis and to their associates who are centrally responsible for the production of this volume. The assistance of Williams & Wilkins and its staff is gratefully acknowledged.

F. STEPHEN VOGEL, M.D.
Series Editor

Preface

This monograph presents the United States and Canadian Academy of Pathology's Long Course on "Pathobiology of the Parathyroid and Thyroid Glands." This course, held at the Annual Meeting of the Academy on March 18, 1992, in Atlanta, represents an update on the pathobiology of the thyroid (after an almost 30-year hiatus since the last long course on this topic which was organized by Drs. J. B. Hazard and D. E. Smith). It also marks the first time that the Academy has included a discussion about parathyroid pathology in the Long Course.

The past three decades have witnessed a remarkable series of advances in our understanding of the thyroid and parathyroid glands. This monograph is not intended to be a comprehensive text on the pathology of these two endocrine organs, but rather its purpose is to bring together recent concepts and diagnostic interpretations of important facets of the pathobiology of the thyroid and parathyroid glands.

The first chapter, by Drs. Charles Capen and Thomas Rosol, reviews the biochemistry, molecular biology, and pathophysiology of the parathyroid glands. It also includes a discussion of the newly identified parathyroid hormone-related protein, its mechanism of action, and its relationship to malignancy associated with hypercalcemia. In the second chapter, Dr. J. Aidan Carney discusses the pathology of hyperparathyroidism. With recollections of the history of the disorder, he provides an overview of hyperparathyroidism and brings it into modern times in the context of intraoperative techniques for the diagnosis of uniglandular versus multiglandular disease. Dr. Carney stresses the importance of intraoperative cooperation between pathologists and surgeons in the appropriate diagnosis and therapy of primary hyperparathyroidism.

Chapter 3, by Dr. Stephen Baylin and his colleagues, reviews the physiology of the thyroid C-cell and its major hormone, calcitonin. The molecular genetic aspects of multiple endocrine neoplasia type II are discussed in light of the relevant pathologic findings in this syndrome. Dr. Ronald DeLellis, in Chapter 4, provides an overview of the pathology and immunohistochemistry of medullary thyroid carcinoma. He reviews the historical milestones in the pathologic analysis and assessment of familial medullary thyroid carcinoma and its precursor lesion, C-cell hyperplasia.

In Chapter 5, Drs. Terry Davies and David Kendler provide new insights into the genetic aspects of autoimmune thyroid disease. The immunopathologic changes are correlated with the clinical presentations and the genetic aspect of Graves' disease and Hashimoto's thyroiditis.

In Chapter 6, Dr. Virginia LiVolsi reviews follicular and Hürthle cell lesions of the thyroid with an emphasis on nodules and neoplasms and the criteria for the differential diagnosis of these lesions and their mimics. The histologic changes, which can occur following fine needle aspiration biopsy of such lesions, are discussed and illustrated. In Chapter 7, Dr. Juan Rosai describes the pathology of papillary thyroid carcinoma and its numerous variants, particularly as they relate to clinical behavior.

In the final Chapter, Dr. Barbara Atkinson summarizes the utility of fine needle aspiration cytology and the criteria used in the assessment of thyroid lesions, emphasizing the problematical area of the common follicular lesions of the thyroid.

The editors wish to express their gratitude to the Academy for the invitation to organize and co-chair this Long Course, to the USCAP Education Committee members, and their liaison, Dr. Milton Feingold for useful advice and guidance, to Dr. Nathan Kaufman for encouragement and support, to Mr. James Crimmins and the staff of the USCAP for planning of the local arrangements, and to Dr. F. Stephen Vogel for his help and guidance in bringing the manuscript to completion. Finally, the editors wish to thank the contributors for not only their outstanding presentations at the long course itself, but also for their timely submission of the completed manuscripts.

RONALD A. DeLELLIS, M.D.
VIRGINIA A. LiVOLSI, M.D.

Contributors

BARBARA F. ATKINSON, M.D.
Professor and Chairman, Department of Pathology and Laboratory Medicine, Medical College of Pennsylvania, Philadelphia, Pennsylvania

DOUGLAS W. BALL, M.D.
Instructor in Medicine, Department of Medicine, Johns Hopkins Medical Institutions, Baltimore, Maryland

STEPHEN B. BAYLIN, M.D.
Professor of Oncology and Medicine, Oncology Center and Department of Medicine, Johns Hopkins Medical Institutions, Baltimore, Maryland

CHARLES C. CAPEN, D.V.M., PH.D.
Professor and Chairman, Department of Veterinary Pathobiology, Ohio State University, Columbus, Ohio

J. AIDAN CARNEY, M.D.
Professor of Pathology, Department of Laboratory Medicine and Pathology, Mayo Medical School, Rochester, Minnesota

TERRY F. DAVIES, M.D.
Director, Division of Endocrinology and Metabolism, and Professor of Medicine, The Mount Sinai Medical Center, New York, New York

ANDRÉE C. DE BUSTROS, M.D.
Assistant Professor of Medicine, Department of Medicine, Johns Hopkins Medical Institutions, Baltimore, Maryland

RONALD A. DeLELLIS, M.D.
Professor of Pathology, Tufts University School of Medicine and Senior Pathologist, New England Medical Center Hospital, Boston, Massachusetts

DAVID L. KENDLER, M.D.
Associate in Medicine, Division of Endocrinology and Metabolism, Department of Medicine, The Mount Sinai Medical Center, New York, New York

VIRGINIA A. LiVOLSI, M.D.
Professor and Director, Section of Surgical Pathology, Department of Pathology and Laboratory Medicine, University of Pennsylvania Medical Center, Philadelphia, Pennsylvania

BARRY D. NELKIN, Ph.D.
Associate Professor of Oncology, Oncology Center, Johns Hopkins Medical Institutions, Baltimore, Maryland

JUAN ROSAI, M.D.
Chairman, Department of Pathology, Memorial Sloan-Kettering Cancer Center, and Professor of Pathology, Cornell University Medical School, New York, New York

THOMAS J. ROSOL, D.V.M., Ph.D.
Associate Professor, Department of Veterinary Pathobiology, The Ohio State University, Columbus, Ohio

Contents

Chapter 1

Pathobiology of Parathyroid Hormone and Parathyroid Hormone-Related Protein: Introduction and Evolving Concepts

CHARLES C. CAPEN and THOMAS J. ROSOL

Calcium plays a key role in many fundamental biologic processes and also is an essential structural component of the skeleton. These processes include neuromuscular excitability, membrane permeability, muscle contraction, enzyme activity, hormone release, and blood coagulation, among others. The precise control of calcium in extracellular fluids is vital to health. To maintain a constant concentration of calcium, despite marked variations in intake and excretion, endocrine control mechanisms have evolved that consist primarily of the interactions of three major hormones—parathyroid hormone (PTH), calcitonin, and cholecalciferol (vitamin D).

The objective of this chapter is to summarize recent advances in the understanding of the pathobiology of parathyroid glands and the secretion of parathyroid hormone, and the evolving concepts associated with the production of PTH-related protein (PTHrP) by cancer cells. The physiologic role of this new hormone in a variety of normal tissues is another exciting chapter in the endocrinology of the calcium-regulating hormones.

PARATHYROID HORMONE

FUNCTIONAL CYTOLOGY

Parathyroid glands are composed of chief cells which are concerned with the biosynthesis of one hormone (Fig. 1.1). Chief cells have a normal secretory cycle with the majority being in the inactive stage under steady-state conditions. In response to a low calcium ion signal, chief cells enter the active phase with synthesis and packaging of a "batch" of hormone. After secretion of parathyroid hormone, the chief cell involutes back to the resting (inactive) phase. In response to long-term stimulation, chief cells undergo a sequence of morphologic changes culminating in the formation of water-clear cells. Conversely, long-term suppression by elevated blood calcium ion results in parathyroid glands with predominantly inactive and atrophic chief cells. Mitochondrion-rich oxyphil cells form

1

in parathyroid glands of humans and certain animal species with advancing age. Synthetic and secretory organelles are largely crowded out by the proliferation of mitochondria in the cytoplasm, suggesting that oxyphil cells are not actively involved in the biosynthesis of parathyroid hormone.

Chief cells that are interpreted to be in an inactive (resting or involuted) stage of their secretory cycle predominate in the parathyroid glands under normal conditions. Inactive chief cells are cuboidal and have uncomplicated interdigitations between contiguous cells. The relatively electron-transparent cytoplasm contains poorly developed organelles and infrequent secretory granules. The cytoplasm often has either numerous lipid bodies and lipofuscin granules or aggregations of glycogen particles. Chief cells in the active stage of the secretory cycle occur less frequently in the parathyroid glands of most species. The cytoplasm of active chief cells has an increased electron density due to the close proximity of organelles and secretory granules, increased density of the cytoplasmic matrix, and loss of glycogen particles and lipid bodies.

Another cell type in the parathyroid glands of certain animal species and human beings is the oxyphil cell (Fig. 1.1). These cells are absent from the parathyroid glands of the rat, chicken, and many species of lower animals. Oxyphil cells are observed either singly or in small groups interspersed between chief cells. They are larger than chief cells and their abundant cytoplasmic area is filled with numerous large, often bizarre-shaped, mitochondria. Glycogen particles and free ribosomes are interspersed between the mitochondria. Granular endoplasmic reticulum, Golgi apparatuses, and secretory granules are poorly developed in oxyphil cells of normal parathyroid glands, suggesting that oxyphil

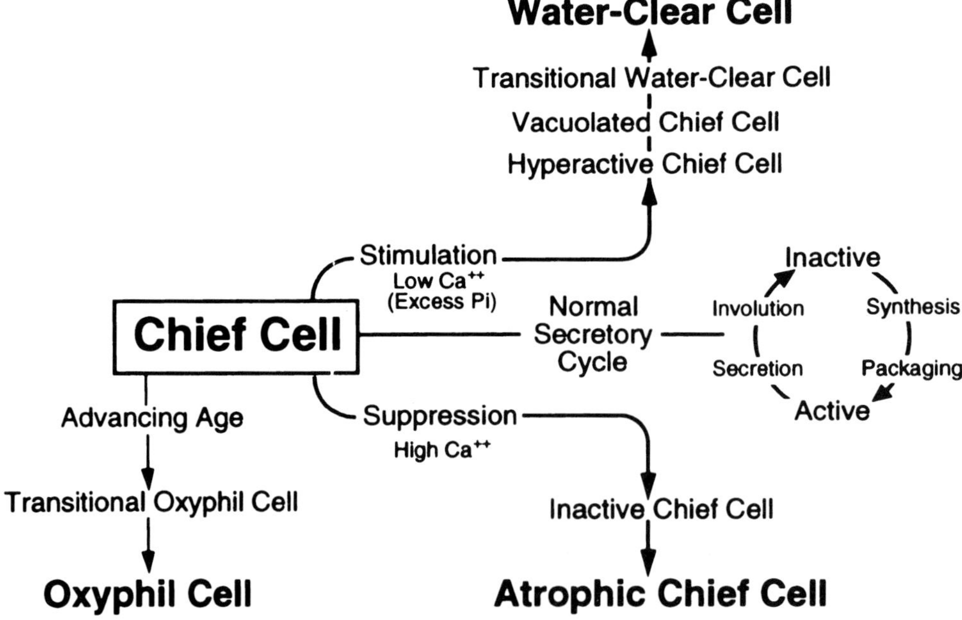

FIG. 1.1.   Functional cytology of parathyroid gland under normal and pathologic conditions.

cells do not have an active function in the biosynthesis of parathyroid hormone. Oxyphil cells have been shown histochemically to have a higher oxidative and hydrolytic enzyme activity than chief cells associated with the marked increase in mitochondria.

Cells are observed with cytoplasmic characteristics intermediate between those of chief and oxyphil cells. These transitional oxyphil cells have numerous mitochondria, but other organelles are present including rough endoplasmic reticulum, Golgi apparatuses, and secretory granules. The significance of oxyphil cells in the pathophysiology of the parathyroid glands has not been elucidated completely. They are not altered in response to either short-term hypocalcemia or hypercalcemia in animals, but both oxyphil cells and transitional forms may be increased in response to long-term stimulation of human parathyroid glands. Therefore, oxyphil cells do not appear to be degenerate chief cells as previously suggested, but rather are derived from chief cells as the result of aging or some other metabolic derangement.

BIOSYNTHESIS BY CHIEF CELLS

Parathyroid chief cells in humans and many animal species store relatively small amounts of preformed hormone but respond quickly to variations in need for hormone by changing their rate of synthesis. Parathyroid hormone, like many peptide hormones, is first synthesized as a larger biosynthetic precursor molecule that undergoes post-translational processing in chief cells. Preproparathyroid hormone (preproPTH) is the initial translation product synthesized on ribosomes of the rough endoplasmic reticulum in chief cells. It is composed of 115 amino acids and contains a hydrophobic signal or leader sequence of 25 amino acid residues that facilitates the penetration and subsequent vectorial discharge of the nascent peptide into the cisternal space of the rough endoplasmic reticulum.[96] PreproPTH is rapidly converted within 1 min or less of its synthesis to proparathyroid hormone (proPTH) by the proteolytic cleavage of 25 amino acids from the NH_2-terminal end of the molecule.[57] The intermediate precursor, proPTH, is composed of 90 amino acids and moves within membranous channels of the rough endoplasmic reticulum to the Golgi apparatus (Fig. 1.2). Enzymes within membranes of the Golgi apparatus cleave a hexapeptide from the NH_2-terminal (biologically active) end of the molecule forming active PTH (Fig. 1.2). Active PTH is packaged into membrane-limited, macromolecular aggregates in the Golgi apparatus for subsequent storage in chief cells. Under certain conditions of increased demand (*i.e.*, low calcium ion concentration in extracellular fluid compartment), PTH may be released directly from chief cells without being packaged into secretion granules by a process termed "bypass secretion."

Although the principal form of active PTH secreted from chief cells is a straight chain peptide of 84 amino acids (molecular weight 9500), the molecule is rapidly cleaved into amino- and carboxy-terminal fragments in the peripheral circulation and especially in the liver. The purpose of this fragmentation is uncertain since the biologically active amino-terminal fragment is no more active than the entire PTH molecule (1–84). The plasma half-life of the NH_2-terminal fragment is considerably shorter than that of the biologically inactive carboxy-

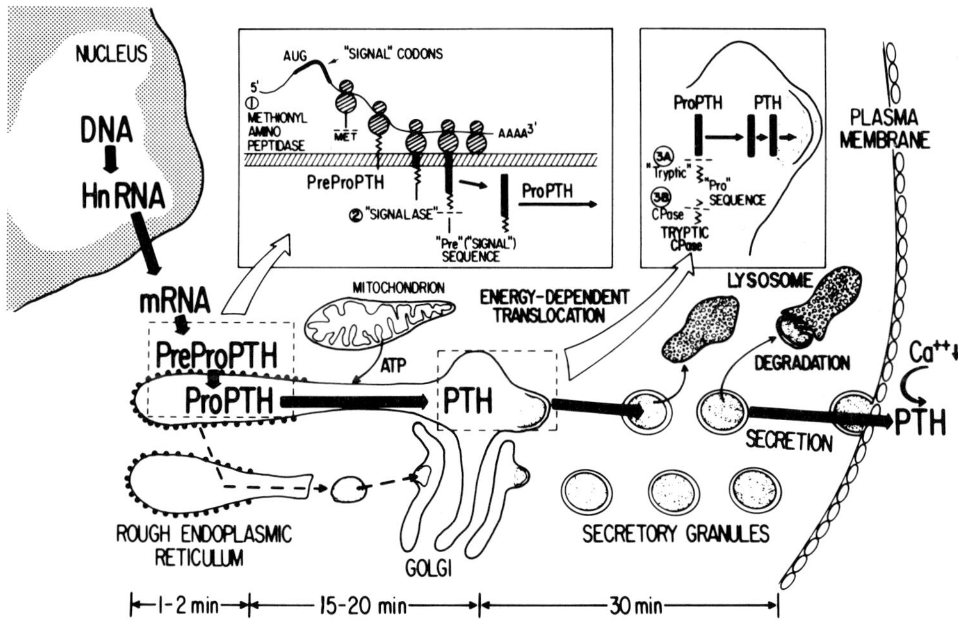

Fig. 1.2.   Subcellular compartmentalization, transport, and cleavage of precursors of parathyroid hormone (*PTH*). Preproparathyroid hormone (*preproPTH*) is the initial translation product from ribosomes of the rough endoplasmic reticulum, which is rapidly converted to proparathyroid hormone (*proPTH*). The hydrophobic sequence on the NH_2-terminal end of the preproPTH facilitates penetration of the leading portion of the nascent peptide into the lumen of the endoplasmic reticulum. ProPTH is transported to the Golgi apparatus where it is converted enzymatically by a carboxypeptidase (*CPase*) to biologically active PTH. A major portion of the biosynthetic precursors and active PTH is degraded by lysosomal enzymes and is not secreted by chief cells under normal conditions. Parathyroid secretory protein may function as a binding protein for PTH during intracellular storage in secretion granules and be released with PTH into the extracellular space. (Reprinted by permission from Habener, J. F., and Potts, J. T., Jr. Biosynthesis of parathyroid hormone, part 1. *N. Engl. J. Med.* 299:580, 635, 1978.)

terminal fragment of parathyroid hormone. The COOH-terminal and other portions of the PTH molecule are degraded primarily in the kidney and tend to accumulate with chronic renal disease. The immunoheterogeneity caused by the multiple circulating fragments of PTH created significant problems in the development and application of highly specific radioimmunoassays to diagnostic problems in human patients and experimental animals.[54]

CONTROL OF SECRETION

Secretory cells in the parathyroid gland store small amounts of preformed hormone but are capable of responding to minor fluctuations in calcium concentration by rapidly altering the rate of hormonal secretion and more slowly by altering the rate of hormonal synthesis.[163] In contrast to most endocrine organs that are under complex controls involving both long and short feedback loops, the parathyroid glands have a unique feedback controlled by the concentration of calcium (and to a lesser extent magnesium) ion in serum. If the blood calcium is elevated by the intravenous infusion of calcium, there is a rapid and pronounced reduction in circulating levels of immunoreactive parathyroid hormone (iPTH). Conversely, if the blood calcium is lowered by EDTA (ethylenediaminetetraacetic acid), there is a brisk and substantial increase in iPTH levels.

The concentration of blood phosphorus has no direct regulatory influence on the synthesis and secretion of PTH; however, several disease conditions with hyperphosphatemia in both animals and man are associated clinically with secondary hyperparathyroidism. An elevated blood phosphorus level may lead indirectly to parathyroid stimulation by virtue of its ability to lower blood calcium. If the blood phosphorus is elevated significantly by an infusion of phosphate and calcium administered simultaneously in amounts to prevent the accompanying reduction of blood calcium, plasma iPTH levels remain within the normal range. Magnesium ion has an effect on parathyroid secretion rate similar to that of calcium, but its effect is not equipotent to that of calcium.[114] The more potent effects of calcium ion in the control of PTH secretion, together with its preponderance over magnesium in the extracellular fluid, suggests a secondary role for magnesium ion in parathyroid control.

Calcium ion not only controls the rate of biosynthesis and secretion of PTH, but also other metabolic and intracellular degradative processes within chief cells.[24] An increase of calcium ions in extracellular fluids rapidly inhibits the uptake of amino acids by chief cells, synthesis of proPTH and conversion to PTH, and secretion of stored PTH. A shift in the percentage of flow of proPTH from the degradative pathway to the secretory route represents a key adaptive response of the parathyroid gland to a low calcium diet. Parathyroid glands from rats fed a low calcium (0.02%) diet convert approximately 40% of proPTH to PTH compared to a 20% conversion in rats fed a control diet (normal calcium).[24] During periods of long-term calcium restriction the enhanced synthesis and secretion of PTH would be accomplished by an increased capacity of the entire pathway in individual hypertrophied chief cells and through hyperplasia of active chief cells. Degradation of "mature PTH" by lysosomal enzymes increases after prolonged exposure to a high calcium environment.

Recently synthesized and processed active PTH may be released directly after passing through the Golgi complex, most likely in small vesicles, in response to increased demand, and bypass the storage pool of mature secretory granules in the cytoplasm of chief cells. Bypass secretion of PTH can be stimulated only by a low circulating concentration of calcium ion whereas β-agonists as well as low calcium can mobilize PTH stored in secretory granules (Fig. 1.3).

Parathyroid chief cells have several adaptive responses to hypocalcemia, which otherwise would be life-threatening. The first is bypass secretion of PTH in response to a low calcium ion signal. The second is to increase the efficiency of conversion of inactive proPTH into active PTH and its subsequent release from chief cells. This process under normal conditions is quite inefficient and, therefore, provides a point of regulation in response to increased demand for hormone. Longer term adaptive responses to hypocalcemia result in hypertrophy and hyperplasia of parathyroid chief cells.

Chief cells synthesize and secrete another major protein termed "parathyroid

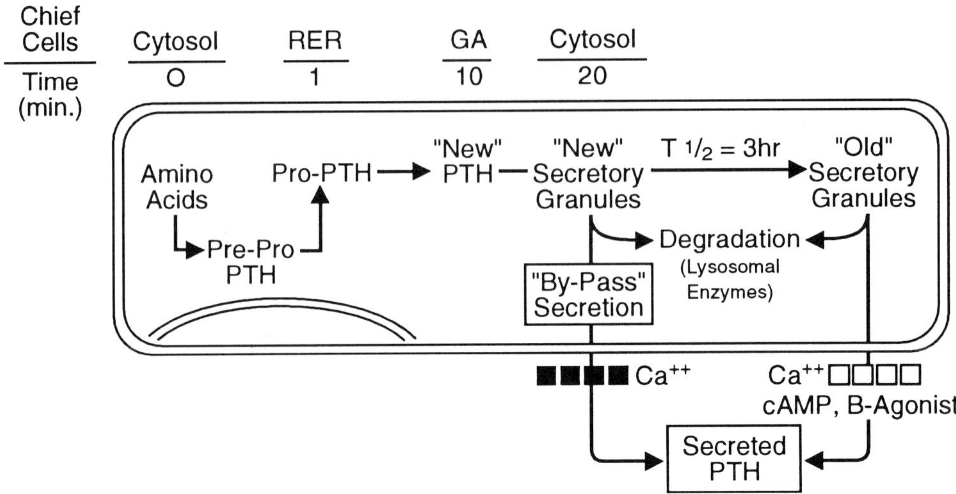

FIG. 1.3. Bypass secretion of parathyroid hormone in response to increased demand signaled by decreased blood calcium ion concentration. Recently synthesized and progressed active PTH(1–84) may be released directly and not enter the storage pool of mature ("old") secretory granules in the cytoplasm of chief cells. PTH from the storage pool can be mobilized by cyclic adenosine monophosphate (*cAMP*) and β (*B*)-agonists (such as epinephrine, norepinephrine, and isoproterenol) as well as by lowered blood calcium ion, whereas secretion from the pool of recently synthesized PTH can be stimulated only by a decreased calcium ion concentration. *RER*, rough endoplasmic reticulum; *GA*, Golgi apparatus. (Redrawn from Cohn, D. V., and MacGregor, R. R. The biosynthesis, intracellular processing, and secretion of parathormone. *Endocr. Rev. 2*:1–20, 1981.)

secretory protein (I)" or chromogranin A. It is a higher molecular weight molecule (70 kD) composed of from 430 to 448 amino acids that is co-stored and secreted with PTH. A similar molecule has been found in secretory granules of a wide variety of hormone peptide-secreting cells and in neurotransmitter secretory vesicles. An internal region of the parathyroid secretory protein or chromogranin A molecule is identical in sequence to pancreastatin, a COOH-terminal amidated peptide that inhibits glucose-stimulated insulin secretion. This proteolytic cleavage product of parathyroid secretory protein has been reported to inhibit low calcium-stimulated secretion of parathyroid hormone and chromogranin A from parathyroid cells. These findings suggest that chromogranin A-derived peptides may act locally in an autocrine manner to inhibit the secretion of active hormone by endocrine cells, such as those of the parathyroid gland.[9,45]

BIOLOGIC ACTIONS

Parathyroid hormone is the principal hormone involved in the minute-to-minute fine regulation of blood calcium in mammals. It exerts its biologic actions by directly influencing the function of target cells primarily in bone and kidney and indirectly in the intestine to maintain plasma calcium at a level sufficient to ensure the optimal functioning of a wide variety of body cells. The action of PTH on bone is to mobilize calcium from skeletal reserves into extracellular fluids.[143] The administration of PTH causes an initial decline followed by a sustained increase in circulating levels of calcium. This transitory decrease in blood calcium is considered to be the result of a sequestration of calcium-phosphate in bone and soft tissues. The subsequent increase in blood calcium results from an interaction of PTH with osteoblasts and osteoclasts in bone and increased tubular reabsorption of calcium in the kidney.[67,185]

BONE

Osteoclasts appear to be primarily responsible for the catabolic action of PTH on bone by increasing bone resorption.[21,22,203] Parathyroid hormone has been known for some time to stimulate an increased activity of preformed osteoclasts. This is interesting in light of recent findings which have failed to demonstrate specific receptors for PTH on osteoclasts; however, receptors were present on osteoblasts.[140,173] Isolated osteoclasts do not respond to PTH without the concurrent presence of osteoblasts.[116]

The mechanisms by which binding of PTH to osteoblasts results in stimulation of osteoblastic secretory products, which are capable of stimulating osteoclastic bone resorption, is not known but may include direct effects on the osteoblast and/or stimulation of osteoblastic secretory products, which are capable of stimulating osteoclastic bone resorption (Fig. 1.4).[194] If the increase in PTH is sustained, the size of the active osteoblast pool in bone is increased by activation of osteoclast-progenitor cells.

The initial binding of PTH to osteoblasts lining bone surfaces appears to cause the cells to contract, thereby exposing the underlying mineral to osteoclasts (Fig. 1.4).[153] The change in shape of osteoblasts associated with PTH may be critical to mediation of osteoclastic bone resorption stimulated by the hormone. Osteoblastic contraction is associated with microfilament disaggregation.[203] The alter-

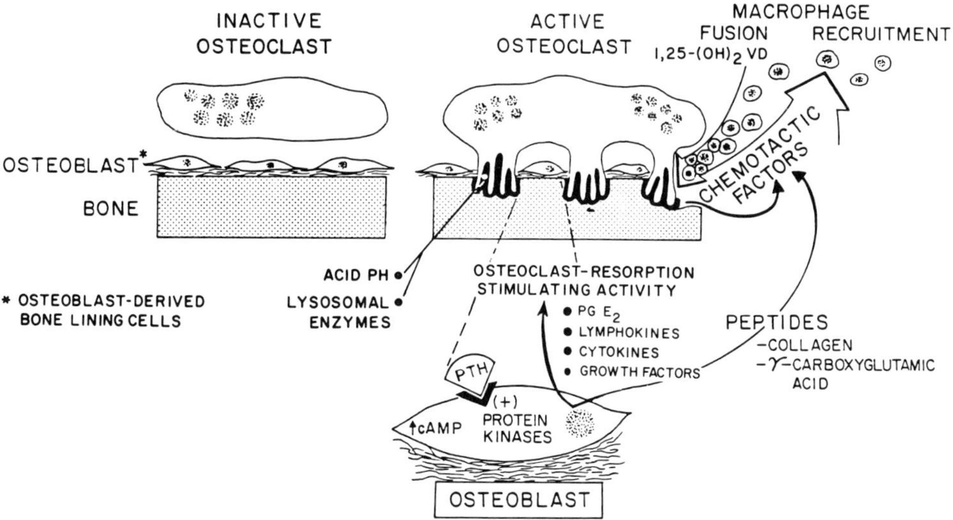

FIG. 1.4. Paracrine control of bone resorption. Specific receptors for parathyroid hormone are present on osteoblasts but not on osteoclasts.

ation in osteoblast shape exposes osteoid-covered bone matrix to osteoclasts; however, osteoclasts attach preferentially to mineralized bone matrix.

Osteoblasts secrete a latent collagenase and neutral proteases (such as plasminogen activator that can activate latent collagenase), which result in degradation of the osteoid matrix and which expose the underlying calcified matrix for osteoclastic bone resorption.[41] Bone-resorbing hormones such as PTH, prostaglandin E_2, and 1,25-dihydroxyvitamin D stimulate plasminogen activator activity in osteoblasts. A collagenase inhibitor (Cl-1, an analogue of collagen α chain sequence) can inhibit PTH-induced bone resorption.[33] Bone resorption products, particularly osteocalcin, can attract osteoclast precursors and enhance the resorption process.

Osteoblasts also may elaborate unidentified paracrine chemical mediators of osteoclastic bone resorption. None of the known bone-resorbing factors (PTH, prostaglandin E_2, lymphokines, growth factors) have been shown to directly stimulate osteoclasts without the presence of osteoblasts.[30] The only substance that was found to stimulate bone resorption by isolated chicken osteoclasts in one investigation was murine splenic conditioned medium.[30] Bone resorption by isolated osteoclasts is inhibited by calcitonin and prostaglandin E_2,which induce 3′,5′-cyclic adenosine monophosphate (cAMP) production in osteoclasts.

Parathyroid hormone stimulation of osteoblasts results in induction of bone resorption due to osteoclast activation and increased osteoclast numbers. The plasma membrane of osteoclasts in intimate contact with the resorbing surfaces is modified to form a series of membranous projections referred to as the brush ("ruffled") border. The brush border of activated osteoclasts is isolated from the extracellular fluids by adjacent transitional ("sealing") zones, thereby localizing the lysosomal enzymes and acidic environment to the immediate area undergoing dissolution. Parathyroid hormone and other bone-resorbing agents increase proteolytic, lysosomal, and acid-producing enzymes in osteoclasts, which include acid phosphatase, β-glucuronidase, and carbonic anhydrase.[203] Carbonic anhydrase is localized to the brush border and induces acidification of the brush border area.

Binding of PTH to specific receptors on bone cells results in the activation of adenylate cyclase in the plasma membrane (Fig. 1.4). The adenylate cyclase catalyzes the conversion of ATP to cAMP in target cells. The accumulation of cAMP in target cells functions as an intracellular messenger of PTH action in osteoblasts. Parathyroid hormone also induces an increase in cytoplasmic calcium and stimulates phosphatidylinositol turnover in osteoblasts; however, it has not been determined which intracellular messenger is required for induction of bone resorption by PTH stimulation of osteoblasts.[37,44,66] The increase in cytosolic calcium is partially dependent on cAMP accumulation. Calcium concentration in the osteoblast also may be increased by the activation of protein kinase C, resulting in the production of inositol triphosphate and subsequent release of calcium from the endoplasmic reticulum.[206]

KIDNEY

Parathyroid hormone has a rapid (within 5–10 min) and direct effect on renal tubular function, leading to decreased reabsorption of phosphate and phosphaturia.[93] The site of PTH on blocking tubular reabsorption of phosphate has been localized by micropuncture methods to the proximal tubule of the nephron. Parathyroidectomy decreases renal phosphate excretion. Parathyroid hormone binds to a receptor on the basolateral aspect of renal epithelial cells. The hormone stimulates adenylate cyclase, increases intracellular cAMP, and inhibits phosphate reabsorption across the brush border through the actions of protein kinases. Parathyroid hormone also increases the transport of calcium across the basolateral renal cell membrane and increases intracellular calcium, which inhibits the formation of cAMP, thus decreasing the phosphaturic effects of PTH.[10,93] Parathyroid hormone is capable of stimulating inositol triphosphate and diacylglycerol production in renal tubular cells.[73] Therefore, regulation of phosphate transport by PTH may be mediated by two classes of receptors and transmembrane-signaling systems, one which activates adenylate cyclase and one which activates protein kinase C and increases intracellular calcium.[26]

Although the effects of PTH on the tubular reabsorption of phosphate have been considered to be of major importance, evidence has accumulated indicating that the ability of PTH to enhance the reabsorption of calcium plays a considerable role in the maintenance of calcium homeostasis. This effect of PTH upon tubular reabsorption of calcium appears to be due to a direct action on the distal convoluted tubule.[185] The biochemical mechanism by which PTH enhances calcium reabsorption is unknown, but it is coupled to increases in intracellular cAMP.[58] There are two calcium-active transport systems in the basolateral membrane of renal cells: a high-affinity calcium ATPase and a Na^+-Ca^{2+} exchanger.

The other important effect of PTH on the kidney is on the regulation of the conversion of 25-hydroxycholecalciferol to 1,25-dihydroxycholecalciferol and other metabolites of vitamin D. Parathyroid hormone has been shown to promote the absorption of calcium from the gastrointestinal tract in animals under a variety of experimental conditions.[132] This effect is not as rapid as the action on the kidney and is not observed in vitamin D-deficient animals. The increase in intestinal calcium transport appears to be an indirect effect of PTH on absorptive cells by its action on stimulating synthesis of the biologically active metabolite of vitamin D by mitochondria in renal tubular epithelial cells.[30] The effects of PTH on the metabolism of 25-hydroxycholecalciferol appear to be mediated by cAMP and not dependent on calcium ion concentration.[65] The active metabolites of vitamin D make bone cells more sensitive to the direct effects of PTH ("permissive effect") as well as greatly enhancing the gastrointestinal absorption of calcium, thereby, amplifying the effect of PTH upon plasma calcium concentration.

The kidney also is a major organ for the degradation of PTH. Biologically active PTH from the peritubular capillaries is degraded by specific proteases on the surface of renal tubular cells. In addition, both biologically active (NH_2 1–34) and inactive (34–84 COOH) fragments are degraded intracellularly by lysosomal enzymes within renal tubular cells.[72]

The parathyroid hormone receptor has been recently cloned and sequenced from cDNA isolated from kidney cells.[87] It belongs to a class of receptors that has seven potential transmembrane domains and is linked to a specific G protein in the target cells (Fig. 1.5). The expressed receptor binds PTH and parathyroid hormone-related protein (PTHrP) with equal affinity, resulting in the activation of adenylate cyclase and phospholipase C. The PTH/PTHrP receptor has a striking degree of sequence homology (approximately 56%) with the calcitonin receptor but lacks similarity with other G protein-linked receptors other than secretin.[101] The receptors for these calcium-regulating hormones appear to belong to a new family of G protein-linked receptors with seven transmembrane spanning domains that activate adenylate cyclase and phospholipase C.

PARATHYROID HORMONE-RELATED PROTEIN

RELATIONSHIP TO PARATHYROID HORMONE

The presence of parathyroid hormone-like activity in tumors associated with humoral hypercalcemia of malignancy (HHM)[156–158,178,200] and the similarities of HHM to primary hyperparathyroidism led to the isolation and discovery of parathyroid hormone-related protein (PTHrP).[104,176] PTHrP was initially purified from human tumors associated with HHM.[17,124,177,183] Subsequently, the cDNA and gene for PTHrP were isolated, sequenced, and characterized.[109,112,187] The PTHrP gene is complicated and contains at least 6 exons, two 5'-untrans-

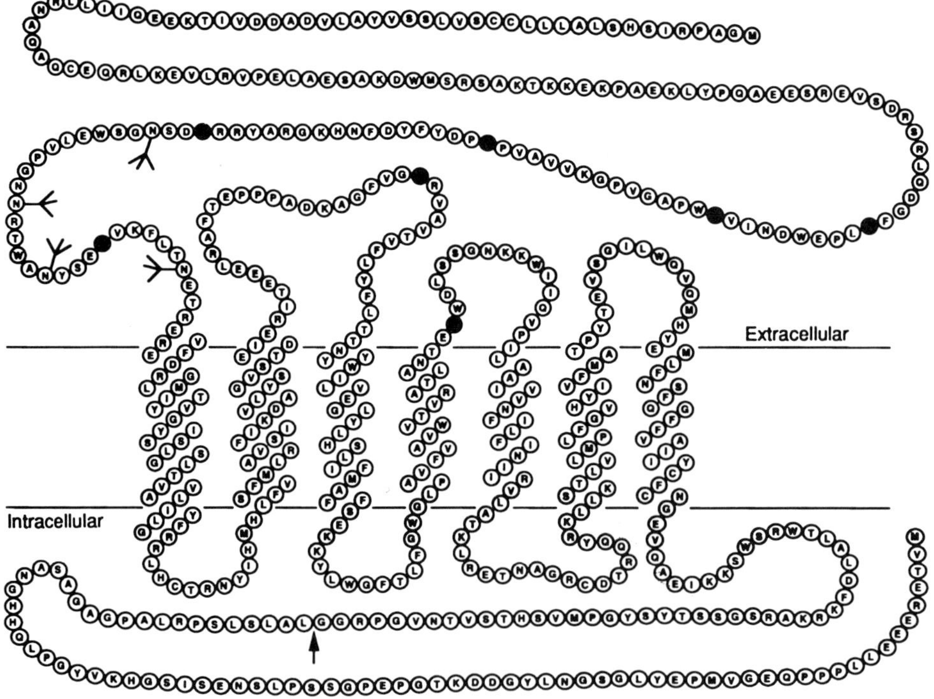

FIG. 1.5. PTH-PTHrP receptor (NH₂ terminus at top) cloned and sequenced from cDNA isolated from kidney cells. Y, potential *N*-glycosylation sites; ●, cysteine residues conserved in the calcitonin receptor. (Reprinted by permission from Jüppner, H., Abou-Samra, A.-B., Freeman, M., *et al.* AG protein-linked receptor for parathyroid hormone and parathyroid hormone-related peptide. *Science* 254:1024–1026, 1991.)

lated regions each with its own promoter, a preprohormone coding region, a main coding region, and 2 additional 3′ regions that have coding and noncoding regions.[55,106,107,186] There is alternate splicing of PTHrP mRNA so that 3 mature peptides can be formed, composed of 139, 141, and 173 amino acid residues.[108,192] The PTHrP gene is located on the short arm of chromosome 12 and is thought to have evolved from the PTH gene on the short arm of chromosome 11 through chromosome duplication.[189,209] The PTH gene is simpler and has only 3 exons (5′-untranslated region, preprohormone coding region, and main coding region with a 3′-noncoding region) and encodes for a mature protein of 84 amino acids.

The rat, mouse, and chicken cDNA or genes for PTHrP also have been isolated and sequenced.[88,105,168] There is extensive primary amino acid sequence homology between the species. The first 111 NH$_2$-terminal amino acids have only two divergent amino acids in the human, rat, and mouse forms of PTHrP. Nonhuman species have only the 139 or 141 amino acid forms of PTHrP and also have a simpler genomic organization with fewer exons. The canine form of PTHrP and its mRNA are similar to human PTHrP as demonstrated by NH$_2$-terminal sequence analysis, immunologic cross-reactivity, and Northern blot analysis.[78,159,199]

Parathyroid hormone-related protein binds to PTH receptors in bone and kidney with similar affinity as PTH (Fig. 1.6).[20,136] The first 34 NH$_2$-terminal

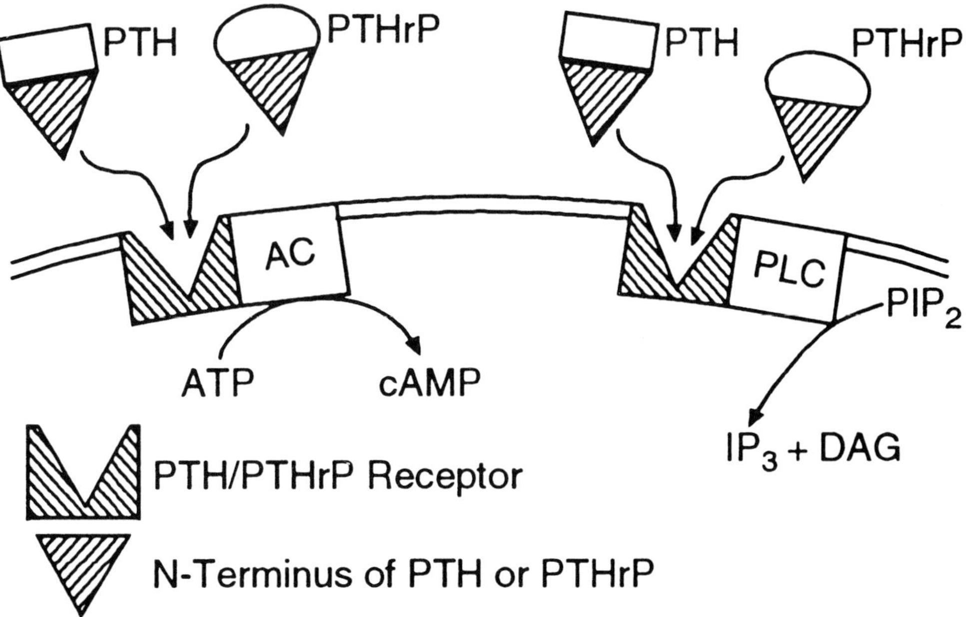

FIG. 1.6. Parathyroid hormone (*PTH*) and parathyroid hormone-related protein (*PTHrP*) have a high degree of homology in the primary or tertiary structures of the NH$_2$-terminal regions. This permits binding and activation of PTH receptors resulting in the stimulation of adenylate cyclase (*AC*) and phospholipase C (*PLC*) in target cells in bone and kidney with the formation of cAMP and conversion of phosphatidylinositol diphosphate (*PIP$_2$*) to inositol triphosphate (*IP$_3$*) and diacylglycerol (*DAG*). (Reprinted by permission from Rosol, T. J., and Capen, C. C. Mechanism of cancer-induced hypercalcemia. *Lab. Invest.* 67:680–702, 1992.)

amino acids of PTHrP contain the PTH-like biologic activity. This is similar to PTH in which the first 34 NH_2-terminal amino acids contain most of the biologic activities. There is 70% sequence homology of the first 13 NH_2-terminal amino acids of PTHrP compared to PTH, but little homology after amino acid 13. The N terminus is important in the activation of the PTH receptor.[142] Sequence homology in this region is important for the ability of PTHrP to stimulate PTH receptors. By comparison, amino acids 20–34 are important for the binding of PTH to its receptor. There is little sequence homology in this region between PTH and PTHrP; however, PTHrP binds to the PTH receptor with this region of its sequence.[1] These findings suggest that two different primary amino acid sequences permit high-affinity binding to the same receptor.

The PTH/PTHrP receptor has recently been cloned and sequenced from cDNA isolated from opossum kidney cells and rat osteoblasts.[2,87] There is 78% homology between the rat and opossum receptors, indicating conservation across mammalian species. The PTH/PTHrP receptor belongs to a newly recognized class of receptors that contains seven transmembrane domains and includes the calcitonin and secretin receptors.[100] Therefore, evidence to date indicates that PTHrP binds to PTH receptors in bone and kidney and that distinct PTHrP receptors do not exist in these organs. It is unknown at present whether PTHrP binds to PTH receptors or whether distinct PTHrP receptors are present in the multitude of other tissues in which PTHrP is produced and functions as an autocrine or paracrine factor.

BIOLOGIC ACTIONS OF PTHrP

The biologic actions of PTHrP in bone and kidney are similar to those of PTH. Both PTHrP and PTH induce their cellular actions in osteoblasts and renal cells by stimulating adenylate cyclase and protein kinase A, phospholipase C and protein kinase C, and pathways leading to increased intracellular calcium concentration (Fig. 1.6).[25,38,39,46,154] The activation of protein kinases A and C by PTH can be dissociated since activation of protein kinase A requires NH_2-terminal amino acids 1 and 2, whereas protein kinase C activation is not dependent on the presence of these amino acids.[86] The efficiency of signal transduction by PTHrP in different cells or membranes may be affected by differences in species specificity for PTHrP.[135] NH_2-terminal PTHrP stimulates osteoclastic bone resorption *in vivo* and *in vitro* with potency similar to that of PTH.[5,47,71,101,161] A COOH-terminal pentapeptide of PTHrP [107–111] and the COOH-terminal region of PTHrP have been reported to inhibit bone resorption. This represents a novel role of PTHrP, but its function *in vivo* and in patients with HHM is unknown. Both PTH and PTHrP have an anabolic effect on bone when administered intermittently, but this effect is less pronounced with PTHrP (1–34) than PTH (1–34).[68]

NH_2-terminal PTHrP mimics most of the effects of PTH in the kidney including increased tubular reabsorption of calcium and increased excretion of inorganic phosphate and cAMP.[40,167,212] There does appear to be a discrepancy in the regulation of acid-base balance and $1,25(OH)_2D$ concentrations in human patients with HHM and primary hyperparathyroidism. Patients with HHM have alkalosis whereas those with primary hyperparathyroidism usually have acidosis.[8] This may be due to the ability of the COOH-terminal region of PTHrP to inhibit bicarbonate excretion by the kidney.[42] Patients with HHM have lower blood concentrations of 1,25(OH)₂D than those with primary hyperparathyroidism; however, the cause for this is unknown.[145] PTHrP stimulates rodent renal 25-hydroxyvitamin D-1α-hydroxylase with equal potency to PTH[196]; however, factors other than PTHrP in patients with HHM may inhibit renal production of 1,25(OH)₂D.[50]

PHYSIOLOGIC SIGNIFICANCE OF PTHrP

In contrast to parathyroid hormone, which is produced only by the parathyroid gland, PTHrP is produced by many normal tissues including stratified squamous epithelium, endocrine glands (adrenal cortex and medulla, fetal and adult parathyroid glands, adenohypophysis, thyroid), skeletal and smooth muscle, kidney, bone, lactating mammary gland, brain, pancreas, ovary, testicle, myometrium, avian oviduct, and placenta.[7,80,94,169,191,198] Present evidence suggests that PTHrP acts as an autocrine or paracrine regulator in most tissues, but its exact function in normal adult tissues is unknown (Fig. 1.7).[55] PTHrP can function as an autocrine growth factor in human renal cell carcinoma.[18]

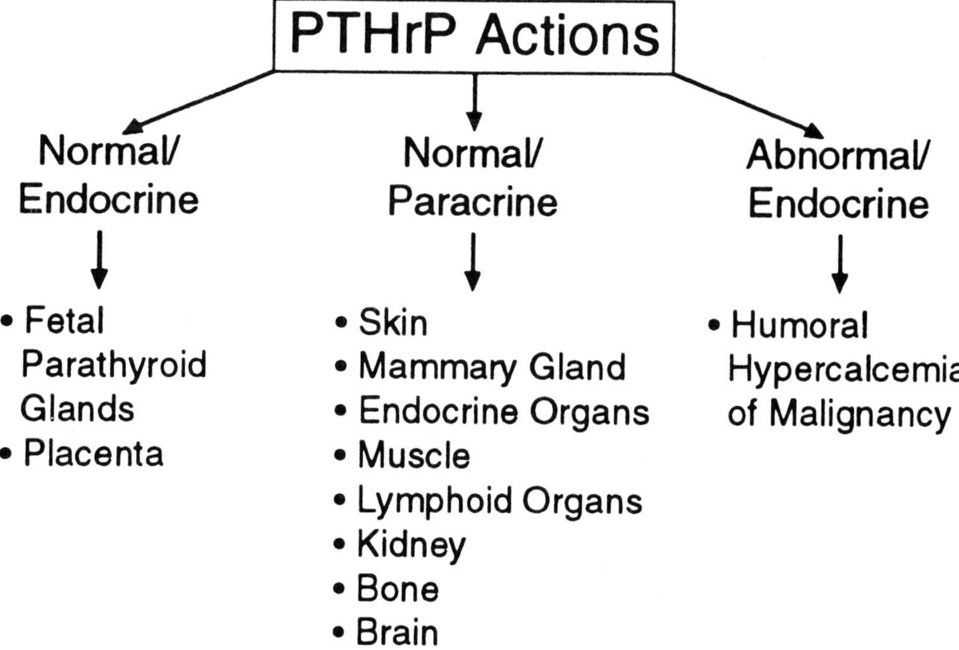

FIG. 1.7.   Sites of parathyroid hormone-related protein (*PTHrP*) production and action. PTHrP can function either in an endocrine or paracrine manner in normal tissues depending on whether it acts locally or is secreted into the circulation or in an abnormal endocrine manner when it is produced by cancer cells. (Reprinted by permission from Rosol, T. J., and Capen, C. C. Mechanism of cancer-induced hypercalcemia. *Lab. Invest.* 67:680–702, 1992.)

Parathyroid hormone-related protein is produced by the fetal parathyroid glands and placenta and appears to function in an endocrine manner to control the serum calcium concentration and calcium and magnesium transport across the placenta.[103,172] In contrast to the PTH-like effects of PTHrP which are associated with the N terminus of PTHrP, the midmolecule region of PTHrP is important in stimulating calcium transport by the placenta. Rat and human fetuses have a wide distribution of PTHrP immunoreactivity which suggests that PTHrP plays a role in cell growth and differentiation.[123] PTHrP is produced by the lactating mammary gland, expression is stimulated by suckling and prolactin,[208] and there are high concentrations of PTHrP in milk.[15,193] PTHrP may have a systemic role in the lactating woman and neonate since suckling increases urinary cAMP and phosphate excretion in lactating rats,[207] nursing calves have increased circulating levels of immunoreactive and bioactive PTHrP,[53] and lactating goats have increased plasma PTHrP levels.[150] However, neutralization of PTHrP by passive immunization did not alter calcium homeostasis in lactating or neonatal mice.[97]

The expression of the PTHrP gene in a variety of normal tissues may explain why so many different types of neoplasms can induce HHM. It is surprising that PTHrP can be produced by many normal tissues of the body and not be associated with significant concentrations in the circulation. PTHrP in most normal tissues appears to act locally and is probably readily metabolized and degraded by the tissues in which it is produced. For example, immunohistochemical studies have demonstrated that epidermal keratinocytes contain abundant PTHrP.[28,60] Total production of PTHrP by the skin and other organs should be much greater than the production of PTH by the parathyroid glands, yet little of the PTHrP produced appears to enter the systemic circulation since circulating concentrations of PTHrP are very low.

PTHrP has been localized to normal, hyperplastic, and adenomatous parathyroid glands by immunohistochemistry[29] and parathyroid adenomas have an increased expression of PTHrP mRNA.[75] PTHrP is secreted in low levels (<1% of the amount of PTH secreted) by normal bovine parathyroid chief cells *in vitro* and is not suppressible by increased extracellular calcium concentration as is PTH.[27] In addition, a rat parathyroid cell line and its subclones have been demonstrated to synthesize and secrete PTHrP but not PTH.[165] PTHrP was inhibited by increased extracellular calcium and secretin concentrations in these cells. Despite the evidence of PTHrP production by normal and abnormal parathyroid tissue, the contribution of PTHrP to the pathogenesis of hyperparathyroidism is probably insignificant compared to the overproduction of PTH.[36]

Parathyroid hormone-related protein may have a role in the regulation of the normal immune system, since it is produced by neoplastic lymphocytes, such as adult T-cell lymphoma/leukemia cells. In addition, PTHrP is produced by activated lymphocytes,[4] lymphocytes have receptors for PTH/PTHrP,[115,139] PTH/PTHrP is a growth inhibitor or stimulator of lymphocytes,[4,92,171] and PTH stimulates lymphocytes to produce bone resorbing activity.[138]

Parathyroid hormone-related protein is secreted by both normal and neoplastic cells *in vitro* under routine culture conditions, which suggests that secretion can occur in a constitutive manner.[31,35] Some investigations have demonstrated that PTHrP production can be regulated *in vitro* or *in vivo*. PTHrP production by neuroendocrine or other carcinomas has been associated with coexpression of calcitonin gene products and chromogranin A, which may influence its secretion.[110] PTHrP secretion and production have been reported to be increased by epidermal growth factor, cholera toxin, $1,25\text{-}(OH)_2D$, hydrocortisone, ionomycin, and calcitonin in squamous carcinoma cells,[32,117] phorbol esters and epidermal growth factor in osteoblasts,[155] high extracellular calcium in rat Leydig tumor cells,[152] and ionomycin and phorbol esters in neuroendocrine carcinoma cells[13] and decreased by chromogranin A in squamous carcinoma cells,[32] monensin in neoplastic keratinocytes,[102,117] and somatostatin in human patients with HHM.[59,205]

Parathyroid hormone-related protein is secreted by normal and neoplastic keratinocytes *in vitro*. Induction of differentiation by hydrocortisone, calcium, or $1,25(OH)_2D$ has been demonstrated to increase or decrease PTHrP production, so the role of epidermal differentiation in relation to PTHrP synthesis and secretion is not clear.[95,202] It appears that PTHrP is produced preferentially by less differentiated keratinocytes since *in vitro* cultures produce PTHrP prior to confluence and then stop producing PTHrP after confluence.[202] There are some human squamous carcinoma cell lines that produce PTHrP spontaneously and others that require the presence of fibroblast feeder layers.[69] Therefore, it appears that stromal cells may regulate PTHrP production by some carcinomas and this interaction may be an important determinant for the production and/or secretion of PTHrP by malignant cells.[90]

Dermal fibroblasts contain PTH/PTHrP receptors which may interact with PTHrP produced by keratinocytes.[141] In addition, immortalized human keratinocytes have been demonstrated to have receptors for PTHrP linked to the stimulation of adenylate cyclase.[63] However, normal human keratinocytes and squamous cell carcinomas do not increase cAMP in response to PTHrP, but do increase intracellular calcium.[134] This indicates that PTHrP receptors on keratinocytes are not classical PTH receptors that are linked to the stimulation of adenylate cyclase. Therefore, keratinocyte-produced PTHrP may have an autocrine and paracrine role in skin. Keratinocytes secrete PTHrP *in vitro* in a glycosylated form, and PTHrP contains many sites of potential proteolytic digestion which indicates that posttranslational modification of PTHrP also may be important in the regulation of PTHrP secretion.[180,204]

Parathyroid hormone-related protein mRNA expression is regulated by growth factors, serum, glucocorticoids, and the degree of cellular differentiation. Transforming growth factor-β may act as an autocrine stimulator of PTHrP production since it is produced by many tumors associated with HHM and it increases PTHrP mRNA expression and secretion.[19,117,134,202] Glucocorticoids have been demonstrated to inhibit PTHrP mRNA expression in a human C-cell line, squamous carcinoma cells, a carcinoid cell line, and normal keratinocytes.[77,134] Fetal bovine serum, epidermal growth factor, or bovine pituitary extract stimulate PTHrP expression in normal and malignant keratinocytes and smooth muscle cells.[95,117,134] $1,25(OH)_2D$ decreased PTHrP expression in a human C-cell line and normal keratinocytes.[77] Cycloheximide (inhibitor of protein synthesis) increased both the rate of PTHrP gene transcription and stabilization of PTHrP mRNA.[76,181] These results led to the hypothesis that control of PTHrP transcription involves a labile repressor protein that regulates a promoter of the PTHrP gene. Stimulation of differentiation of a rat islet cell line or embryonal carcinoma cells increased PTHrP expression, which indicates that PTHrP is involved in the regulation of cell growth and differentiation.[23] The biology and mechanisms that control transcription, translation, post-translational processing, and secretion of PTHrP are important areas for future research.

RELATIONSHIP OF PTHrP TO HYPERCALCEMIA OF MALIGNANCY

Cancer-associated hypercalcemia (CAH) is one of the most frequently occurring paraneoplastic syndromes.[128,130] The hypercalcemia may be subclinical and detected on routine serum analysis or may induce clinical disease including central nervous system depression, muscular weakness, cardiac abnormalities, gastrointestinal disturbances, or renal failure depending on its severity and speed of onset.[147] Cancer-associated hypercalcemia is a syndrome consisting of multiple pathogenic mechanisms and a variety of inciting neoplasms.[56,182] Certain neoplasms are consistently associated with CAH, and there are sporadic reports of a variety of neoplasms that are associated with hypercalcemia. There are two primary mechanisms by which tumors can induce hypercalcemia: 1) release of humoral factors that act systemically to increase osteoclastic bone resorption, increase calcium reabsorption from the kidney, or increase calcium absorption from the intestinal tract; and 2) stimulation of local bone resorption associated with neoplasms metastatic to bone (Fig. 1.8).[126] Some neoplasms that induce

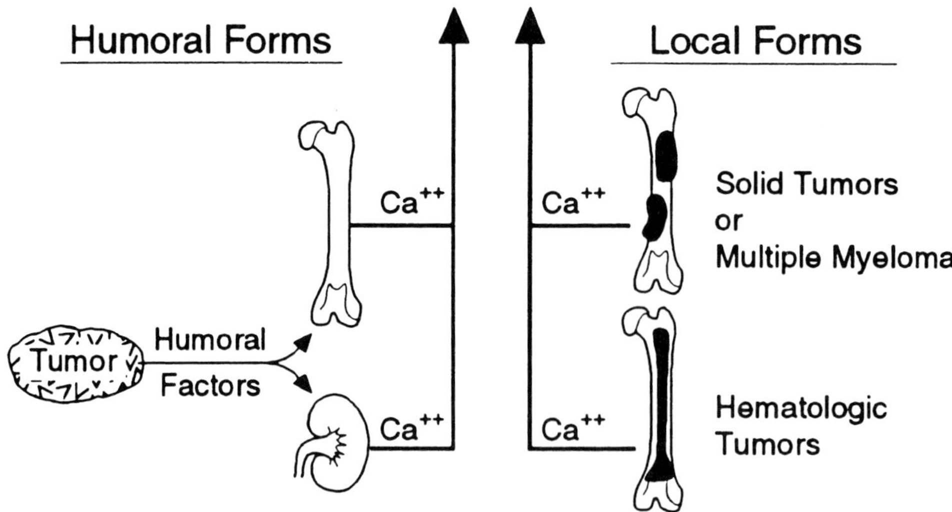

FIG. 1.8.   Humoral and local forms of cancer-associated hypercalcemia increase circulating concentrations of calcium by stimulating osteoclastic bone resorption or increased tubular reabsorption of calcium. (Reprinted by permission from Rosol, T. J., and Capen, C. C. Mechanism of cancer-induced hypercalcemia. *Lab. Invest.* 67:680–702, 1992.)

CAH may stimulate hypercalcemia by both mechanisms simultaneously. The complete syndrome of CAH appears not to be induced by a single factor in individual patients, but rather by the cooperative or synergistic action of multiple factors produced either by neoplastic cells or by host cells.

HHM is a form of cancer-associated hypercalcemia that is induced by the secretion of humoral factors which have effects distant to the site of the neoplasms (Fig. 1.9).[14,111,144] Some neoplasms that cause HHM may metastasize to bone, but the primary mechanism of hypercalcemia is distant effects of humoral factors and not localized bone resorption. This form of CAH has been the focus of intense investigation during the past decade. There are multiple humoral factors that have been associated with HHM, including parathyroid hormone, parathyroid hormone-like protein, cytokines, steroids such as 1,25-dihydroxy-vitamin D, and prostaglandins.[82,127,129,178] It is of interest that many of the humoral factors produced by tumor cells that alter calcium metabolism and bone resorption also can be produced by osteogenic cells, such as osteoblasts.

The clinical syndrome of HHM in human patients and animals mimics primary hyperparathyroidism and a term used previously to describe HHM was pseudo-hyperparathyroidism; however, it has become apparent that HHM does not mimic hyperparathyroidism in all aspects. There are distinct differences in bone remodeling and vitamin D metabolism between patients with HHM and primary hyperparathyroidism.

Humoral Factors and HHM

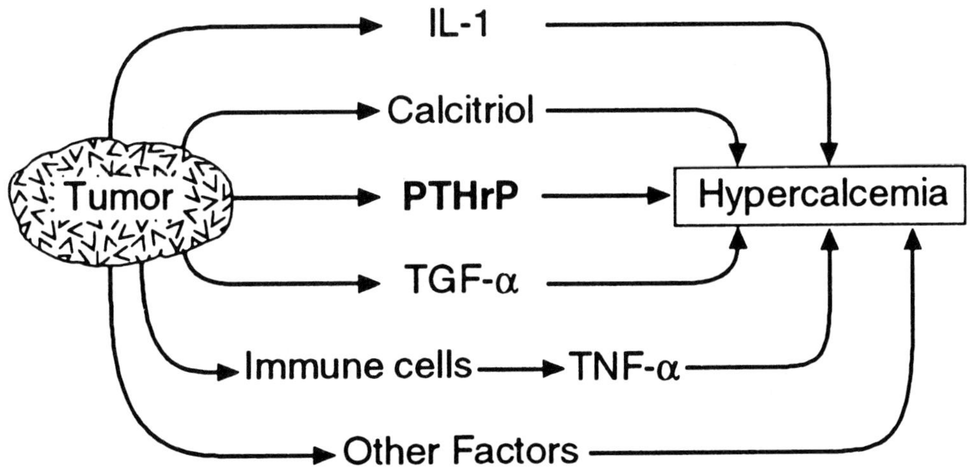

FIG. 1.9. Humoral factors such as parathyroid hormone-related protein (*PTHrP*), interleukin-1 (*IL-1*), tumor necrosis factors (*TNF*), or transforming growth factors (*TGF*) produced by tumors induce humoral hypercalcemia of malignancy (*HHM*) by acting as systemic hormones and stimulating osteoclastic bone resorption or increasing tubular reabsorption of calcium. (Reprinted by permission from Rosol, T. J., and Capen, C. C. Mechanism of cancer-induced hypercalcemia. *Lab. Invest.* 67:680–702, 1992.)

The most consistent feature of HHM in human beings and animals is increased osteoclastic bone resorption distant to the site of the neoplasm. Other features include hypercalciuria, increased renal reabsorption of calcium in spite of increased filtered calcium, increased nephrogenous cAMP, hypophosphatemia, and hyperphosphaturia.[177] The similarities of these clinicopathologic alterations to hyperparathyroidism led to the hypothesis that the neoplasms secrete parathyroid hormone (PTH) or PTH-like substances; however, native PTH is not produced by the vast majority of neoplasms associated with HHM. Immunoreactive PTH is normal or low in patients with HHM, and the tumors do not contain PTH mRNA.[164,174] There have been well-validated reports of ectopic production of PTH by some tumors, but these occurrences are rare.[133,211] Most tumors from patients with HHM do have PTH-like biologic activity even though the tumors do not contain native (1–84) PTH.

Purification of the PTH-like biologic activity from neoplasms associated with HHM has resulted in the discovery of a new hormone currently named parathyroid hormone-related protein [PTHrP, parathyroid hormone-like peptide (PLP), or hypercalcemia of malignancy factor].[112] It is likely that PTHrP plays a central role in the pathogenesis of HHM since it is a consistent feature of HHM and shares most or all of the biologic activities of PTH. Parathyroid hormone-related peptide either acts alone in some forms of HHM or may act synergistically or additively with other humoral factors in the pathogenesis of hypercalcemia (Fig. 1.10). It is also likely that some examples of HHM are not associated with PTHrP production by the inciting neoplasms, but rather are due to recognized or unrecognized humoral factors, cytokines, or hormones that are capable of stimulating osteoclastic bone resorption and result in hypercalcemia.

Tumors of human patients associated with HHM include squamous cell carcinoma (especially of the head, neck, or lungs), renal cell carcinoma, breast carcinoma, ovarian carcinoma, and many examples of neoplasms that induce HHM sporadically.[6,43,170] Humoral hypercalcemia of malignancy also occurs as a spontaneous disease in domestic and laboratory animals. The dog is the species most frequently affected with spontaneous HHM. It occurs in approximately 25% of dogs with lymphoma (usually thymic or multicentric forms) and the majority of dogs with unique adenocarcinomas derived from apocrine glands of the anal sac.[62,118–120,151,201] Lymphoma is a relatively common tumor in older, large-breed dogs, whereas the apocrine adenocarcinoma is less common and occurs most often in older, female dogs. HHM also occurs in dogs as a sporadic form usually due to miscellaneous carcinomas.[131] Spontaneous HHM occurs less commonly in other domestic animals but has been reported in cats and horses.[91,121]

Well characterized animal models of HHM in rodents include two transplantable rat tumors, Leydig cell tumor[83] and Walker mammary carcinosarcoma,[166] a transplantable mammary carcinoma (VX$_2$) in rabbits,[195] dimethylbenzanthracene-induced cutaneous squamous cell carcinomas in mice,[52] among others.[188,190] The rat Leydig cell tumor and Walker mammary carcinosarcoma have been the best characterized and are good models of HHM since they have been shown to produce PTHrP and other cytokines, including transforming growth factors.[74,84]

Humoral Factors and HHM

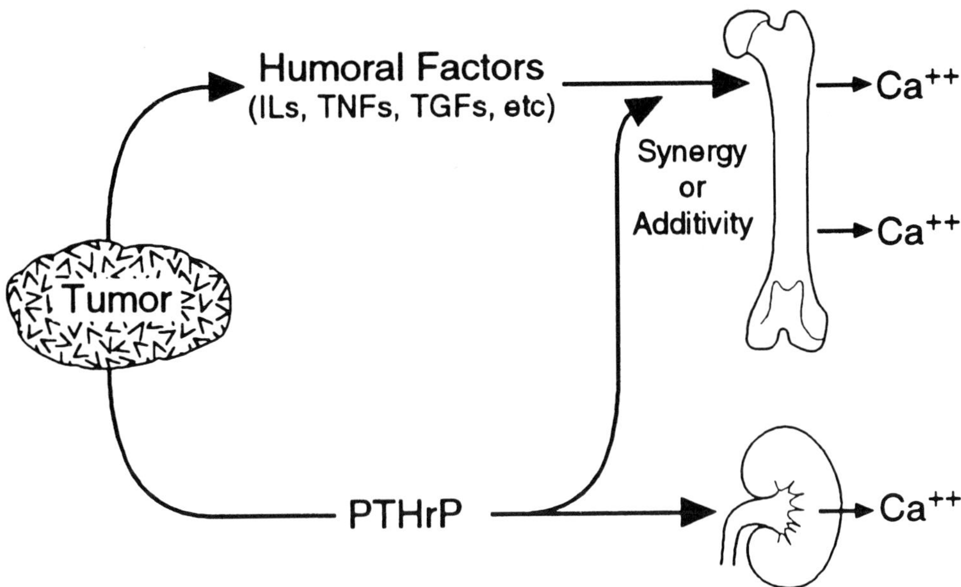

FIG. 1.10. Multiple humoral factors can act additively or synergistically to induce hypercalcemia associated with humoral hypercalcemia of malignancy (*HHM*). (Reprinted by permission from Rosol, T. J., and Capen, C. C. Mechanism of cancer-induced hypercalcemia. *Lab. Invest. 67*:680–702, 1992.)

The rodent and rabbit models of HHM represent a useful exploitation of sporadic occurrences of HHM in these species, but do not represent common spontaneous diseases. Both human and animal tumors associated with HHM have been transplanted to nude mice and rats in order to develop tumor lines that have also been valuable in investigations on the pathogenesis and treatment of HHM *in vivo*.[3,79,113,160,184]

Parathyroid hormone-related protein plays a central role in the pathogenesis of HHM.[156,176] It is produced by most tumors associated with hypercalcemia[12,61,70,210] and is present in the circulation at increased concentrations in human patients and animals with HHM.[64,149,162] The administration of anti-PTHrP antibodies to animal models of HHM has been reported to decrease serum calcium levels and bone resorption.[98,99] Assays for PTHrP include NH_2- and COOH-terminal radioimmunoassays and two-site immunoradiometric assays, which detect PTHrP 1–74 or 1–86.[137,148] An NH_2-terminal PTHrP radioimmunoassay (Incstar Corp., Stillwater, MN) and a two-site two-site immunoradiometric assay (Nichols Institute, Los Angeles, CA) are available commercially. The circulating concentration in normal humans is very low (<0.1–1.0 pM, depending on the assay utilized) and is elevated up to 100 pM in patients with HHM. In general, the two-site immunoradiometric assays are more sensitive and may be more specific for PTHrP but require intact PTHrP.

Parathyroid hormone-related protein contains many potential sites of proteolytic cleavage[14] and may be degraded if samples are not collected appropriately with protease inhibitors.[137] The circulating forms of PTHrP in patients with HHM are not known; however, the speed by which intact PTHrP is degraded in blood suggests that PTHrP is rapidly metabolized into fragments *in vivo*. This is similar to PTH, which is metabolized into an NH_2-terminal fragment (1–34) and COOH-terminal forms *in vivo* by hepatic proteases.[34] Increased concentrations of NH_2-terminal PTHrP or intact PTHrP are relatively specific for HHM, but as with PTH the COOH-terminal region of PTHrP is increased in patients with renal failure.[16] COOH-terminal fragments of PTHrP are excreted into the urine in human patients and animals with HHM.[81] Not all patients with detectable circulating levels of NH_2-terminal or intact PTHrP are hypercalcemic,[11,162] indicating that PTHrP does not always serve as a marker for HHM.

Increased circulating concentrations of PTHrP also have been detected in experimental animal models of HHM and in dogs with spontaneous HHM.[51,162] Dogs with adenocarcinomas derived from apocrine glands of the anal sac have markedly elevated concentrations of PTHrP (10–100 pM), which suggest that PTHrP plays a primary role in the pathogenesis of hypercalcemia with these tumors. In contrast, dogs with HHM and lymphoma have PTHrP concentrations which range from undetectable to 17 pM. PTHrP appears not to be the sole humoral factor responsible for the induction of hypercalcemia in dogs with lymphoma, but may interact cooperatively with other humoral factors.[162]

It is clear that many tumors associated with HHM produce PTHrP, which is important in the pathogenesis of hypercalcemia. However, PTHrP has been shown to be produced by some tumors and not be associated with HHM.[12] Squamous cell carcinomas, benign skin tumors with squamous differentiation, neuroendocrine carcinomas, breast carcinomas, and mesotheliomas, among other neoplasms, stain positive immunohistochemically for PTHrP even though they are not associated with hypercalcemia.[28,89,94] Therefore, production of PTHrP by a tumor does not necessarily confer the ability to induce HHM.[146] Immunohistochemical studies of tumors must be interpreted with caution and correlated with circulating concentrations of PTHrP. The controlling factors which determine whether or not a tumor that produces PTHrP induces HHM are unknown. Possible criteria include: 1) total amount of PTHrP produced by the tumor in relation to the size of the person or animal, 2) biologic activity of the PTHrP produced, 3) ability to secrete the PTHrP in an intact form, 4) degradation of the PTHrP by the tumor, and 5) regulation of PTHrP synthesis and secretion by other factors and cytokines produced by the neoplasm.

There is a high incidence of hypercalcemia in human patients with adult T-cell lymphoma/leukemia (ATLL) induced by human T-lymphotropic virus-1 (HTLV-1).[48] Lymphocytes infected with HTLV-1 and neoplastic cells from lymphoma patients synthesize and secrete PTHrP and express surface receptors for PTHrP.[49,115,122,125] The production of PTHrP by tumor cells is probably important in the pathogenesis of HHM in patients ATLL; however, other hypercalcemia-inducing cytokines also may be produced by the neoplastic cells. The expression of PTHrP is increased by TAX protein, a transactivating regulator produced by expression of the HTLV-1 genome.[197] TAX also stimulates the expression of other genes, including interleukin 2 and the interleukin 2 receptor.[175] Other humoral factors or cytokines may be involved in the pathogenesis of hypercalcemia in ATLL patients since tumor necrosis factor β was increased in hypercalcemic, but not normocalcemic, patients[85] and ATLL cells have been reported to produce interleukin 1.

In summary, cancer-associated hypercalcemia is due to the 1) elaboration of systemically acting humoral factors by neoplasms which alter calcium metabolism in bone, kidney, and intestine or 2) stimulation of bone resorption at sites of tumor metastasis to bone. It is likely that both mechanisms occur in the same patient with certain neoplasms. There are many humoral factors that can be produced by tumors, be secreted into the circulation, and have distant effects which induce hypercalcemia. The stimulation of increased osteoclastic bone resorption by PTHrP is a principal feature of the pathogenesis of humoral hypercalcemia of malignancy, but the kidney also plays an important role. In addition, intestinal absorption of calcium may be a factor in the pathogenesis of hypercalcemia associated with certain neoplasms. Although parathyroid hormone-related protein plays a dominant role in the pathogenesis of HHM, other humoral factors, such as cytokines, can interact with PTHrP to contribute to the development of hypercalcemia.

REFERENCES

1. Abou-Samra, A.-B., Jüppner, H., Force, T., Freeman, M. W., Kong, X.-F., Schipani, E., Urena, P., Richards, J., Bonventre, J. V., Potts, J. T. Jr., Kronenberg, H. M., and Segre, G. V. Expression cloning of a common receptor for parathyroid hormone and parathyroid hormone-related peptide from rat osteoblast-like cells: A single receptor stimulates intracellular accumulation of both cAMP and inositol triphosphates and increases intracellular calcium. *Proc. Natl. Acad. Sci. USA 89*:2732–2736, 1992.

2. Abou-Samra, A., Uneno, S., Jueppner, H., Keutmann, H., Potts, J. T., Jr., Segre, G. V., and Nussbaum, S. R. Non-homologous sequences of parathyroid hormone and the parathyroid hormone-related peptide bind to a common receptor on ROS 17/2.8 cells. *Endocrinology 125*:2215–2217, 1989.

3. Abramson, E. C., Kukla, L. J., Shevrin, D. H., Lad, T. E., McGuire, W. P., and Kukreja, S. C. A model for malignancy-associated humoral hypercalcemia. *Calcif. Tissue Int. 36*:563–567, 1984.

4. Adachi, N., Yamaguchi, K., Miyake, Y., Honda, S., Nagasaki, K., Akiyama, Y., Adachi, I., and Abe, K. Parathyroid hormone-related protein is a possible autocrine growth inhibitor for lymphocytes. *Biochem. Biophys. Res. Commun. 166*:1088–1094, 1990.

5. Akatsu, T., Takahashi, N., Udagawa, N., Sato, K., Nagata, N., Moseley, J. M., Martin, T. J., and Suda, T. Parathyroid hormone (PTH)-related protein is a potent stimulator of osteoclast-like multinucleated cell formation to the same extent as PTH in mouse marrow cultures. *Endocrinology 125*:20–27, 1989.

6. Anstey, A., Gowers, L., Vass, A., and Robson, A. O. Ovarian dysgerminoma presenting with hypercalcaemia. Case report and review of the literature. *Br. J. Obstet. Gynaecol. 97*:641–644, 1990.

7. Asa, S. L., Henderson, J., Goltzman, D., and Drucker, D. J. Parathyroid hormone-like peptide in normal and neoplastic human endocrine tissues. *J. Clin. Endocrinol. Metab. 71*:1112–1118, 1990.

8. Bajorunas, D. R. Clinical manifestations of cancer-related hypercalcemia. *Semin. Oncol. 17*:16–25, 1990.

9. Barbosa, J. A., Gill, B. M., Takiyyuddin, M. A., and O'Connor, D. T. Chromogranin A:

Posttranslational modifications in secretory granules. *Endocrinology 128*:174–190, 1991.

10. Beck N., Singh, H., Reed, S. W., and Davis, B. B. Direct inhibitory effect of hypercalcemia on renal actions of parathyroid hormone. *J. Clin. Invest. 53*:717–725, 1974.

11. Bilezikian, J. P. Clinical utility of assays for parathyroid hormone-related protein. *Clin. Chem. 38*:179–181, 1992.

12. Brandt, D. W., Burton, D. W., Gazdar, A. F., Oie, H. E., and Deftos, L. J. All major lung cancer cell types produce parathyroid hormone-like protein: Heterogeneity assessed by high performance liquid chromatography. *Endocrinology 129*:2466–2470, 1991.

13. Brandt, D. W., Pandol, S. J., and Deftos, L. J. Calcium-stimulated parathyroid hormone-like protein secretion: Potentiation through a protein kinase-C pathway. *Endocrinology 128*:2999–3004, 1991.

14. Broadus, A. E., Mangin, M., Insogna, K. L., Weir, E. C., Burtis, W. J., and Stewart, A. F. Humoral hypercalcemia of malignancy. Identification of a novel parathyroid hormone-like peptide. *N. Engl. J. Med. 319*:556–563, 1988.

15. Budayr, A. A., Halloran, B. P., King, J. C., Diep, D., Nissenson, R. A., and Strewler, G. J. High levels of a parathyroid hormone-like protein in milk. *Proc. Natl. Acad. Sci. USA 86*:7183–7185, 1989.

16. Burtis, W. J., Brady, T. G., Orloff, J. J., Ersbak, J. B., Warrell, R. P. Jr., Olson, B. R., Wu, T. L., Mitnick, M. E., Broadus, A. E., and Stewart, A. F. Immunochemical characterization of circulating parathyroid hormone-related protein in patients with humoral hypercalcemia of malignancy. *N. Engl. J. Med. 322*:1106–1112, 1990.

17. Burtis, W. J., Wu, T., Bunch, C., Wysolmerski, J. J., Insogna, K. L., Weir, E. C., Broadus, A. E., and Stewart, A. F. Identification of a novel 17,000-dalton parathyroid hormone-like adenylate cyclase-stimulating protein from a tumor associated with humoral hypercalcemia of malignancy. *J. Biol. Chem. 262*:7151–7156, 1987.

18. Burton, P. B. J., Moniz, C., and Knight, D. E. Parathyroid hormone related-peptide can function as an autocrine growth factor in human renal cell carcinoma. *Biochem. Biophys. Res. Commun. 167*:1134–1138, 1990.

19. Casey, M. L., Mibe, M., Erk, A., and MacDonald, P. C. Transforming growth factor-β1 stimulation of parathyroid hormone-related protein expression in human uterine cells in culture: mRNA levels and protein secretion. *J. Clin. Endocrinol. Metab. 74*:950–952, 1992.

20. Caulfield, M. P., McKee, R. L., Goldman, M. E., Thiede, M. A., Thompson, D. D., Fisher, J. E., Levy, J. J., Seedor, J. G., Horiuchi, N., Clemens, T. L., Rodan, G. A., and Rosenblatt, M. Parathyroid hormone-related protein (PTHrP): Studies with synthetic peptides indicate that parathyroid hormone and PTHrP interact with the same receptor. *Nucl. Med. Biol. 17*:633–637, 1990.

21. Chambers, T. J. The cellular basis of bone resorption. *Clin. Orthop. Relat. Res. 151*:283–293, 1980.

22. Chambers, T. J., Revell, P. A., Fuller, K., and Athanasou, N. A. Resorption of bone by isolated rabbit osteoclasts. *J. Cell Sci. 66*:383–399, 1984.

23. Chan, S. D. H., Strewler, G. J., King, K. L., and Nissenson, R. A. Expression of a parathyroid hormone-like protein and its receptor during differentiation of embryonal carcinoma cells. *Mol. Endocrinol. 4*:638–646, 1990.

24. Chu, L. L. H., MacGregor, R. R., Anast, C. S., Hamilton, J. W., and Cohn, D. V. Studies on the biosynthesis of rat parathyroid hormone and proparathyroid hormone: Adaptation of the parathyroid gland to dietary restriction of calcium. *Endocrinology 93*:915–924, 1973.

25. Civitelli, R., Martin, T. J., Fausto, A., Gunsten, S. L., Hruska, K. A., and Avioli, L. V. Parathyroid hormone-related peptide transiently increases cytosolic calcium in osteoblastic-like cells: Comparison with parathyroid hormone. *Endocrinology 125*:1204–1210, 1989.

26. Cole, J. A., Eber, S. L., Poelling, R. E., Thorne, P. K., and Forte, L. R. A dual mechanism for regulation of kidney phosphate transport by parathyroid hormone. *Am. J. Physiol. 253*:E221-E227, 1987.

27. Conner, C. S., Drees, B. M., Thurston, A., Forte, L., Hermreck, A. S., and Hamilton, J. W. Bovine parathyroid tissue: A model to compare the biosynthesis and secretion of parathyroid

hormone and parathyroid hormone-related peptide. *Surgery 106*:1057–1062, 1989.
28. Danks, J., Ebeling, P., Hayman, J., Chou, S., Moseley, J., Dunlop, J., Kemp, B., and Martin, T. Parathyroid hormone-related protein: Immunohistochemical localization in cancers and in normal skin. *J. Bone Miner. Res. 4*:273–278, 1989.
29. Danks, J. A., Ebeling, P. R., Hayman, J. A., Diefenbach-Jagger, H., Collier, F. M., Grill, V., Southby, J., Moseley, J. M., Chou, S. T., and Martin, T. J. Immunohistochemical localization of parathyroid hormone-related protein in parathyroid adenoma and hyperplasia. *J. Pathol. 161*:27–33, 1990.
30. de Vernejoul, M.-C., Horowitz, M., Demignon, J., Neff, L., and Baron, R. Bone resorption by isolated chick osteoclasts in culture is stimulated by murine spleen cell supernatant fluids (osteoclast-activating factor) and inhibited by calcitonin and prostaglandin E2. *J. Bone Miner. Res. 3*:69–80, 1988.
31. Deftos, L., Gazdar, A., Ikeda, K., and Broadus, A. The parathyroid hormone-related protein associated with malignancy is secreted by neuroendocrine tumors. *Mol. Endocrinol. 3*:503–508, 1989.
32. Deftos, L. J., Hogue-Angeletti, R., Chalberg, C., and Tu, S. PTHrP secretion is stimulated by CT and inhibited by CgA peptides. *Endocrinology 125*:563–565, 1989.
33. Delaisse, J-M., Eeckhout, Y., Sear, C., Galloway, A., McCullagh, K., and Vaes, G. A new synthetic inhibitor of mammalian tissue collagenase inhibits bone resorption in culture. *Biochem. Biophys. Res. Commun. 133*:483–490, 1985.
34. Diment, S., Martin, K. J., and Stahl, P. D. Cleavage of parathyroid hormone in macrophage endosomes illustrates a novel pathway for intracellular processing of proteins. *J. Biol. Chem. 264*:13403–13406, 1989.
35. Docherty, H. M., Dixon-Lewis, M. J., Milton, P. G., Blight, A., and Heath, D. A. Parathyroid hormone-related proteins in cultured epithelial cells. *J. Endocrinol. 123*:487–493, 1989.
36. Docherty, H. M., Ratcliffe, W. A., Heath, D. A., and Docherty, K. Expression of parathyroid hormone-related protein in abnormal human parathyroids. *J. Endocrinol. 129*:431–438, 1991.
37. Donahue, H. J., Fryer, M. J., Eriksen, E. F., and Heath, H.,III. Differential effects of parathyroid hormone and its analogues on cytosolic calcium ion and cAMP levels in cultured rat osteoblast-like cells. *J. Biol. Chem. 263*:13522–13527, 1988.
38. Donahue, H. J., Fryer, M. J., and Heath, H., III. Structure-function relationships for full-length recombinant parathyroid hormone-related peptide and its amino-terminal fragments: Effects on cytosolic calcium ion mobilization and adenylate cyclase activation in rat osteoblast-like cells. *Endocrinology 126*:1471–1477, 1990.
39. Dunlay, R., and Hruska, K. PTH receptor coupling to phospholipase C is an alternate pathway of signal transduction in bone and kidney. *Am. J. Physiol. 258*:F223-F231, 1990.
40. Ebeling, P. R., Adam, W. R., Moseley, J. M., and Martin, T. J. Actions of synthetic parathyroid hormone-related protein (1–34) on the isolated rat kidney. *J. Endocrinol. 120*:45–50, 1989.
41. Eeckhout, Y., Delaisse, J-M, Ladent, P., and Vaes, G. The proteinases of bone resorption. In: *The Control of Tissue Damage,* edited by A. M. Glauert. Amsterdam, Elsevier Science Publishers, 1988, pp. 297–313.
42. Ellis, A. G., Adam, W. R., and Martin, T. J. Comparison of the effects of parathyroid hormone (PTH) and recombinant PTH-related protein on bicarbonate excretion by the isolated perfused rat kidney. *J. Endocrinol. 126*:403–408, 1990.
43. Fahn, H.-J., Lee, Y.-H., Chen, M.-T., Huang, J.-K., Chen, K.-K., and Chang, L. S. The incidence and prognostic significance of humoral hypercalcemia in renal cell carcinoma. *J. Urol. 145*:248–250, 1991.
44. Farndale, R. W., Sandy, J. R., Atkinson, S. J., Pennington, S. R., Meghi, S., and Meikle, M. C. Parathyroid hormone and prostaglandin E2 stimulate both inositol phosphates and cyclic AMP accumulation in mouse osteoblast cultures. *Biochem. J. 252*:262–268, 1988.
45. Fasciotto, B. H., Gorr, S.-U., Bourdeau, A. M., and Cohn, D. V. Autocrine regulation of parathyroid secretion: Inhibition of secretion by chromogranin-A (secretory protein-I) and potentiation of secretion by chromogranin-A and pancreastatin antibodies. *Endocrinology 127*:1329–1335, 1990.

46. Fujimori, A., Cheng, S.-L., Avioli, L. V., and Civitelli, R. Structure-function relationship of parathyroid hormone: Activation of phospholipase-C, protein kinase-A, and -C in osteosarcoma cells. *Endocrinology* 130:29–36, 1992.

47. Fukayama, S., Bosma, T. J., Goad, D. L., Voelkel, E. F., and Tashjian, A. H., Jr. Human parathyroid hormone (PTH)-related protein and human PTH: Comparative biological activities on human bone cells and bone resorption. *Endocrinology* 123:2841–2848, 1988.

48. Fukumoto, S., Matsumoto, T., Ikeda, K., Yamashita, T., Watanabe, T., Yamaguchi, K., Kiyokawa, T., Takatsuki, K., Shibuya, N., and Ogata, E. Clinical evaluation of calcium metabolism in adult T-cell leukemia/lymphoma. *Arch. Intern. Med.* 148:921–925, 1988.

49. Fukumoto, S., Matsumoto, T., Watanabe, T., Takahashi, H., Miyoshi, I., and Ogata, E. Secretion of parathyroid hormone-like activity from human T-cell lymphotropic virus type I-infected lymphocytes. *Cancer Res.* 49:3849–3852, 1989.

50. Fukumoto, S., Matsumoto, T., Yamoto, H., Kawashima, H., Ueyama, Y., Tamaoki, N., and Ogata, E. Suppression of serum 1,25-dihydroxyvitamin D in humoral hypercalcemia of malignancy is caused by elaboration of a factor that inhibits renal 1,25-dihydroxyvitamin D production. *Endocrinology* 124:2057–2062, 1989.

51. Gaich, G., and Burtis, W. J. Measurement of circulating parathyroid hormone-related protein in rats with humoral hypercalcemia of malignancy using a two-site immunoradiometric assay. *Endocrinology* 127:1444–1449, 1990.

52. Gkonos, P. J., Hayes, T., Burtis, W., Jacoby, R., McGuire, J., Baron, R., and Stewart, A. F. Squamous carcinoma model of humoral hypercalcemia of malignancy. *Endocrinology* 115:2384–2390, 1984.

53. Goff, J. P., Reinhardt, T. A., Lee, S., and Hollis, B. W. Parathyroid hormone-related peptide content of bovine milk and calf blood assessed by radioimmunoassay and bioassay. *Endocrinology* 129:2815–2819, 1991.

54. Goltzman, D., Bennett, H. P. J., Koutsilieris, M., Mitchell, J., Rabbani, S. A., and Rouleau, M. F. Studies of the multiple molecular forms of bioactive parathyroid hormone and parathyroid hormone-like substances. *Recent Prog. Horm. Res.* 42:665–703, 1986.

55. Goltzman, D., Hendy, G. N., and Banville, D. Parathyroid hormone-like peptide: Molecular characterization and biological properties. *Trends Endocrinol. Metab.* 1:39–44, 1989.

56. Gutierrez, G. E., Poser, J. W., Katz, M. S., Yates, A. J. P., Henry, H. L., and Mundy, G. R. Mechanisms of hypercalcaemia of malignancy. *Baillière's Clin. Endocrinol. Metab.* 4:119–138, 1990.

57. Habener, J. F. Recent advances in parathyroid hormone research. *Clin. Biochem.* 14:223–229, 1981.

58. Hanai, H., Ishida, M., Liang, C. T., and Sacktor, B. Parathyroid hormone increases sodium/calcium exchange activity in renal cells and the blunting of the response in aging. *J. Biol. Chem.* 261:5419–5425, 1986.

59. Harrison, M., James, N., Broadley, K., Bloom, S. R., Armour, R., Wimalawansa, S., Heath, D., and Waxman, J. Somatostatin analogue treatment for malignant hypercalcaemia. *Br. Med. J. [Clin. Res.]* 300:1313–1314, 1990.

60. Hayman, J. A., Danks, J. A., Ebeling, P. R., Moseley, J. M., Kemp, B. E., and Martin, T. J. Expression of parathyroid hormone related protein in normal skin and in tumors of skin and skin appendages. *J. Pathol.* 158:293–296, 1989.

61. Heath, D. A., Senior, P. V., Varley, J. M., and Beck, F. Parathyroid-hormone-related protein in tumours associated with hypercalcaemia. *Lancet* 335:66–69, 1990.

62. Heath, H., Weller, R. E., and Mundy, G. R. Canine lymphosarcoma: A model for study of the hypercalcemia of cancer. *Calcif. Tissue Int.* 30:127–133, 1980.

63. Henderson, J. E., Kremer, R., Rhim, J. S., and Goltzman, D. Identification and functional characterization of adenylate cyclase-linked receptors for parathyroid hormone-like peptides on immortalized human keratinocytes. *Endocrinology* 130:449–457, 1992.

64. Henderson, J. E., Shustik, C., Kremer, R., Rabbani, S. A., Hendy, G. N., and Goltzman, D. Circulating concentrations of parathyroid hormone-like peptide in malignancy and in hyperparathyroidism. *J. Bone Miner. Res.* 5:105–113, 1990.

65. Henry, H. L. Parathyroid hormone modulation of 25-hydroxyvitamin D3 metabolism by cultured chick kidney cells is mimicked and enhanced by forskolin. *Endocrinology 116:*503–510, 1985.
66. Herrmann-Erlee, M. P. M., van deer Meer, J. M., Lowik, C. W. G. M., van Leeuwen, J. P. T. M., and Boonekamp, P. M. Different roles for calcium and cyclic AMP in the action of PTH: Studies in bone explants and isolated bone cells. *Bone 9:*93–100, 1988.
67. High, W. B., Black, H. E., and Capen, C. C. Histomorphometric evaluation of the effects of low dose parathyroid hormone administration on cortical bone remodeling in adult dogs. *Lab. Invest. 44:*449–454, 1981.
68. Hock, J. M., Fonseca, J., Gunness-Hey, M., Kemp, B. E., Martin, and T. J. Comparison of the anabolic effects of synthetic parathyroid hormone-related protein (PTHrP) 1–34 and PTH 1–34 on bone in rats. *Endocrinology 125:*2022–2027, 1989.
69. Hoekman, K., Löwik, C. W. G. M., v.d. Ruit, M., Kempenaar, J., Bijvoet, O. L. M., and Ponec, M. Modulation of the production of a parathyroid hormone-like protein in human squamous carcinoma cell lines by interaction with fibroblasts. *Cancer Res. 50:*3589–3594, 1990.
70. Honda, S., Yamaguchi, K., Suzuki, M., Sato, Y., Adachi, I., Kimura, S., and Abe, K. Expression of parathyroid hormone-related protein mRNA in tumors obtained from patients with humoral hypercalcemia of malignancy. *Jpn. J. Cancer Res. 79:*677–681, 1988.
71. Horiuchi, N., Caulfield, M. P., Fisher, J. E., Goldman, M. E., McKee, R. L., Reagan, J. E., Levy, J. J., Nutt, R. F., Rodan, S. B., Schofield, T. L., Clemens, T. L., and Rosenblatt, M. Similarity of synthetic peptide from human tumor to parathyroid hormone *in vivo* and *in vitro. Science 238:*1566–1568, 1987.
72. Hruska, K. A., Martin, K., Mennes, P., Greenwalt, A., Anderson, C., Klahr, S., and Slatopolsky, E. Degradation of parathyroid hormone and fragment production by the isolated perfused dog kidney. The effect of glomerular filtration rate and perfusate Ca++ concentrations. *J. Clin. Invest. 60:*501–510, 1977.
73. Hruska, K. A., Moskowitz, D., Esbrit, P., Civitelli, R., Westbrook, S., and Huskey, M. Stimulation of inositol trisphosphate and diacylglycerol production in renal tubular cells by parathyroid hormone. *J. Clin. Invest. 79:*230–239, 1987.
74. Ibbotson, K. J., D'Souza, S. M., Ng, K. W., Osborne, C. K., Niall, M., Martin, T. J., and Mundy, G. R. Tumor-derived growth factor increases bone resorption in a tumor associated with humoral hypercalcemia of malignancy. *Science 221:*1292–1294, 1983.
75. Ikeda, K., Arnolds, A., Mangin, M., Kinder, B., Vydelingum, N. A., Brennan, M. F., and Broadus, A. E. Expression of transcripts encoding a parathyroid hormone-related peptide in abnormal human parathyroid tissues. *J. Clin. Endocrinol. Metab. 69:*1240–1248, 1989.
76. Ikeda, K., Lu, C., Weir, E. C., Mangin, M., and Broadus, A. E. Regulation of parathyroid hormone-related peptide gene expression by cycloheximide. *J. Biol. Chem. 265:*5398–5402, 1990.
77. Ikeda, K., Lu, C., Weir, E. C., Mangin, M., and Broadus, A. E. Transcriptional regulation of the parathyroid hormone-related peptide gene by glucocorticoids and vitamin D in a human C-cell line. *J. Biol. Chem. 264:*15743–15746, 1989.
78. Ikeda, K., Mangin, M., Dreyer, B. E., Webb, A. C., Posillico, J. T., Stewart, A. F., Bander, N. H., Weir, E. C., Insogna, K. L., and Broadus, A. E. Identification of transcripts encoding a parathyroid hormone-like peptide in messenger RNAs from a variety of human and animal tumors associated with humoral hypercalcemia of malignancy. *J. Clin. Invest. 81:*2010–2014, 1988.
79. Ikeda, K., Matsumoto, T., Fukumoto, S., Kurokawa, K., Ueyama, Y., Fujishige, K., Tamaoki, N., Saito, T., Ohtake, K., and Ogata, E. A hypercalcemic nude rat model that completely mimics human syndrome of humoral hypercalcemia of malignancy. *Calcif. Tissue Int. 43:*97–102, 1988.
80. Ikeda, K., Weir, E., Mangin, M., Dannies, P., Kinder, B., Deftos, L., Brown, E., and Broadus, A. Expression of messenger ribonucleic acids encoding a parathyroid hormone-like peptide in normal human and animal tissues with abnormal expression in human parathyroid adenomas. *Mol. Endocrinol. 2:*1230–1236, 1988.
81. Imamura, H., Sato, K., Shizume, K., Satoh, T., Kasono, K., Ozawa, M., Ohmura, E., Tsushima,

T., and Demura, H. Urinary excretion of parathyroid hormone-related protein fragments in patients with humoral hypercalcemia of malignancy and hypercalcemia tumor-bearing nude mice. *J. Bone Miner. Res. 6:*77–84, 1991.

82. Insogna, K. L. Humoral hypercalcemia of malignancy: The role of parathyroid hormone-related protein. *Endocrinol. Metab. Clin. North Am. 18:*779–794, 1989.

83. Insogna, K. L., Stewart, A. F., Vignery, A. M.-C., Weir, E. C., Namnum, P. A., Baron, R. E., Kirkwood, J. M., Deftos, L. M., and Broadus, A. E. Biochemical and histomorphometric characterization of a rat model for humoral hypercalcemia of malignancy. *Endocrinology 114:*888–896, 1984.

84. Insogna, K. L., Weir, E. C., Wu, T. L., Stewart, A. F., Broadus, A. E., Burtis, W. J., and Centrella, M. Co-purification of transforming growth factor β-like activity with PTH-like and bone-resorbing activities from a tumor associated with humoral hypercalcemia of malignancy. *Endocrinology 120:*2183–2185, 1987.

85. Ishibashi, K., Ishitsuka, K., Chuman, Y., Otsuka, M., Kuwazuru, Y., Iwahashi, M., Utsunomiya, A., Hanada, S., Sakarami, T., and Arima, T. Tumor necrosis factor-β in the serum of adult T-cell leukemia with hypercalcemia. *Blood 77:*2451–2455, 1991.

86. Jouishomme, H., Whitfield, J. F., Chakravarthy, B., Durkin, J. P., Gagnon, L., Isaacs, R. J., MacLean, S., Neugebauer, W., Willick, G., and Rixon, R. H. The protein kinase-C activation domain of the parathyroid hormone. *Endocrinology 130:*53–60, 1992.

87. Jüppner, H., Abou-Samra, A.-B., Freeman, M., Kong, X. F., Schipani, E., Richards, J., Kolakowski, L. F., Jr., Hock, J., Potts, J. T., Jr., Kronenberg, H. M., and Segre, G. V. A G protein-linked receptor for parathyroid hormone and parathyroid hormone-related protein. *Science 254:*1024–1026, 1991.

88. Karaplis, A. C., Yasuda, T., Hendy, G. N., Goltzman, D., and Banville, D. Gene-encoding parathyroid hormone-like peptide: Nucleotide sequence of the rat gene and comparison with the human homologue. *Mol. Endocrinol. 4:*441–446, 1990.

89. Kitazawa, S., Fukase, M., Kitazawa, R., Takenaka, A., Gotoh, A., Fujita, T., and Maeda, S. Immunohistologic evaluation of parathyroid hormone-related protein in human lung cancer and normal tissue with newly developed monoclonal antibody. *Cancer 67:*984–989, 1991.

90. Kitazawa, S., Kitazawa, R., Fukase, M., Fujimori, T., and Maeda, S. Immunohistochemical evaluation of parathyroid hormone-related protein (PTHrP) in the uterine cervix. *Int. J. Cancer 50:*731–735, 1992.

91. Klausner, J. S., Bell, F. W., Hayden, D. W., Hegstad, R. L., and Johnston, S. D. Hypercalcemia in two cats with squamous cell carcinomas. *J. Am. Vet. Med. Assoc. 196:*103–105, 1990.

92. Klinger, M., Alexiewicz, J. M., Linker-Israeli, M., Pitts, T. O., Gaciong, Z., Fadda, G. Z., and Massry, S. G. Effect of parathyroid hormone on human T cell activation. *Kidney Int. 37:*1543–1551, 1990.

93. Knox, F. G., and Haramati, A. Renal regulation of phosphate excretion. In: *The Kidney: Physiology and Pathophysiology,* edited by D. W. Seldin, and G. Giebisch. New York, Raven Press, 1985.

94. Kramer, S., Reynolds, F. H., Castillo, M., Valenzuela, D. M., Thorikay, M., and Sorvillo, J. M. Immunological identification and distribution of parathyroid hormone-like protein polypeptides in normal and malignant tissues. *Endocrinology 128:*1927–1937, 1991.

95. Kremer, R., Karaplis, A. C., Henderson, J., Gulliver, W., Banville, D., Hendy, G. N., and Goltzman, D. Regulation in parathyroid hormone-like peptide in cultured normal human keratinocytes. *J. Clin. Invest. 87:*884–893, 1991.

96. Kronenberg, H. M., Igarashi, T., Freeman, M. W., Okazaki, T., Brand, S. J., Wiren, K. M., and Potts, J. T., Jr. Structure and expression of the human parathyroid hormone gene. *Recent Prog. Horm. Res. 42:*641–663, 1986.

97. Kukreja, S. C., D'Anza, J. J., Melton, M. E., Wimbicus, S. A., Grill, V., and Martin, T. J. Lack of effects of neutralization of parathyroid hormone-related protein on calcium homeostasis in neonatal mice. *J. Bone Miner. Res. 6:*1197–1201, 1991.

98. Kukreja, S. C., Rosol, T. J., Wimbicus, S. A., Shevrin, D. H., Grill, V., Barengolts, E. I., and Martin, T. J. Tumor resection and antibodies to parathyroid hormone-related protein cause

similar changes on bone histomorphometry in hypercalcemia of cancer. *Endocrinology* *127*:305–310, 1990.

99. Kukreja, S. C., Shevrin, D. H., Wimbicus, S. A., Ebeling, P. R., Danks, J. A., Rodda, C. P., Wood, W. I., and Martin, T. J. Antibodies to parathyroid hormone-related protein lower serum calcium in athymic mouse models of malignancy-associated hypercalcemia due to human tumors. *J. Clin. Invest. 82*:1798–1802, 1988.

100. Lin, H. Y., Harris, T. L., Flannery, M. S., Aruffo, A., Kaji, E. H., Gorn, A., Kolakowski, L. F., Jr., Lodish, H. F., and Goldring, S. R. Expression cloning of an adenylate cyclase-coupled calcitonin receptor. *Science 254*:1022–1024, 1991.

101. Loveridge, N., Dean, V., Goltzman, D., and Hendy, G. N. Bioactivity of parathyroid hormone and parathyroid hormone-related peptide: Agonist and antagonist activities of amino-terminal fragments as assessed by the cytochemical bioassay and *in situ* hybridization. *Endocrinology 128*:1938–1946, 1991.

102. Löwik, C. W. G. M., Hoekman, K., Offringa, R., Groot, C. G., Hendy, G. N., Papapoulos, S. E., and Ponec, M. Regulation of parathyroid hormone-like protein production in cultured normal and malignant keratinocytes. *J. Invest. Dermatol. 98*:198–203, 1992.

103. MacIsaac, R. J., Heath, J. A., Rodda, C. P., Moseley, J. M., Care, A. D., Martin, T. J., and Caple, I. W. Role of the fetal parathyroid glands and parathyroid hormone-related protein in the regulation of placental transport of calcium, magnesium, and inorganic phosphate. *Reprod. Fertil. Dev. 3*:447–457, 1991.

104. Mallette, L. E. The parathyroid polyhormones: New concepts in the spectrum of peptide hormone action. *Endocr. Rev. 12*:110–117, 1991.

105. Mangin, M., Ikeda, K., and Broadus, A. E. Structure of the mouse gene encoding parathyroid hormone-related protein. *Gene 95*:195–202, 1990.

106. Mangin, M., Ikeda, K., Dreyer, B. E., and Broadus, A. E. Identification of an up-stream promoter of the human parathyroid hormone-related peptide gene. *Mol. Endocrinol. 4*:851–858, 1990.

107. Mangin, M., Ikeda, K., Dreyer, B., and Broadus, A. Isolation and characterization of the human parathyroid hormone-like peptide gene. *Proc. Natl. Acad. Sci. USA 86*:2408–2412, 1989.

108. Mangin, M., Ikeda, K., Dreyer, B. E., Milstone, L., and Broadus, A. E. Two distinct tumor-derived, parathyroid hormone-like peptides result from alternative ribonucleic acid splicing. *Mol. Endocrinol. 2*:1049–1055, 1988.

109. Mangin, M., Webb, A. C., Dreyer, B. E., Posillico, J. T., Ikeda, K., Weir, E. C., Stewart, A. F., Bander, N. H., Milstone, L., Barton, D. E., Francke, U., and Broadus, A. E. Identification of a cDNA encoding a parathyroid hormone-like peptide from a human tumor associated with humoral hypercalcemia of malignancy. *Proc. Natl. Acad. Sci. USA 85*:597–601, 1988.

110. Martin, E. M. E., Gould, V. E., Hoog, A., Rosen, S. T., Radosevich, J. A., and Deftos, L. J. Parathyroid hormone-related protein, chromogranin A, and calcitonin gene products in the neuroendocrine skin carcinoma cell lines MKL1 and MKL2. *Bone Miner. 14*:113–120, 1991.

111. Martin, T. J. Humoral hypercalcemia of malignancy. *Horm. Res. 32*:84–88, 1989.

112. Martin, T. J., Allan, E. H., Caple, I. W., Care, A. D., Danks, J. A., Diefenbach-Jagger, H., Ebeling, P. R., Gillespie, M. T., Hammonds, G., Heath, J. A., Hudson, P. J., Kemp, B. E., Kubota, M., Kukreja, S. C., Moseley, J. M., Ng, K. W., Suva, L. J., Wettenhall, R. E. H., and Wood, W. I. Parathyroid hormone-related protein: Isolation, molecular cloning, and mechanism of action. *Recent Prog. Horm. Res. 45*:467–506, 1989.

113. Matthews, P. N., Nisbet, J., Grant, A. G., and Hermon-Taylor, J. Tumor cachexia and hypercalcemia in nude rats and mice bearing human renal carcinomas. *J. Urol. 135*:1308–1311, 1986.

114. Mayer, G. P., and Hurst, J. G. Comparison of the effects of calcium and magnesium on parathyroid hormone secretion rate in calves. *Endocrinology 102*:1803–1807, 1978.

115. McCauley, L. K., Rosol, T. J., Merryman, J. I., and Capen, C. C. Parathyroid hormone-related protein binding to human T cell lymphotrophic virus type 1-infected lymphocytes. *Endocrinology 130*:300–306, 1992.

116. McSheehy, P. M., and Chambers, T. J. Osteoblastic cells mediate osteoclastic responsiveness to parathyroid hormone. *Endocrinology 118*:824–828, 1986.

117. Merryman, J. I., Rosol, T. J., McCauley, L. K., Werkmeister, J. R., and Capen, C. C. Production of parathyroid hormone-related protein by two squamous cell carcinoma cell lines in vitro. *J. Bone Min. Res. 6(Suppl. 1):*232, 1991 (abstract).
118. Meuten, D. J., Cooper, B. J., Capen, C. C., Chew, D. J., and Kociba, G. J. Hypercalcemia associated with an adenocarcinoma derived from the apocrine glands of the anal sac. *Vet. Pathol. 18:*454–471, 1981.
119. Meuten, D. J., Kociba, G. J., Capen, C. C., Chew, D. J., Segre, G. V., Levine, L., Tashjian, A. H., Jr., Voelkel, E. F., and Nagode, L. A. Hypercalcemia in dogs with lymphosarcoma: Biochemical, ultrastructural, and histomorphometric investigations. *Lab. Invest. 49:*553–562, 1983.
120. Meuten, D. J., Segre, G. V., Capen, C. C., Kociba, G. J., Voelkel, E. F., Levine, L., Tashjian, A. H., Chew, D. J., and Nagode, L. A. Hypercalcemia in dogs with adenocarcinoma derived from apocrine glands of the anal sac: Biochemical and histomorphometric investigations. *Lab. Invest. 48:*428–435, 1983.
121. Meuten, D. J., Price, S. M., Seiler, R. M., and Krook, L. Gastric carcinoma with pseudohyperparathyroidism in a horse. *Cornell Vet. 68:*179–195, 1978.
122. Moseley, J. M., Danks, J. A., Grill, V., Lister, T. A., and Horton, M. A. Immunocytochemical demonstration of PTHrP protein in neoplastic tissue of HTLV-1 positive human adult T cell leukaemia/lymphoma: Implications for the mechanism of hypercalcemia. *Br. J. Cancer 64:*745–748, 1991.
123. Moseley, J. M., Hayman, J. A., Danks, J. A., Alcorn, D., Grill, V., Southby, J., and Horton, M. A. Immunohistochemical detection of parathyroid hormone-related protein in human fetal epithelia. *J. Clin. Endocrinol. Metab. 73:*478–484, 1991.
124. Moseley, J. M., Kubota, M., Diefenbach-Jagger, H., Wettenhall, R. E. H., Kemp, B. E., Suva, L. J., Rodda, C. P., Ebeling, P. R., Hudson, P. J., Zajac, J. D., and Martin, T. J. Parathyroid hormone-related protein purified from a human lung cancer cell line. *Proc. Natl. Acad. Sci. USA 84:*5048–5052, 1987.
125. Motokura, T., Fukumoto, S., Matsumoto, T., Takahashi, S., Fujita, A., Yamashita, T., Igarashi, T., and Ogata, E. Parathyroid hormone-related protein in adult T-cell leukemia-lymphoma. *Ann. Intern. Med. 111:*484–488, 1989.
126. Mundy, G. R. Pathophysiology of cancer-associated hypercalcemia. *Semin. Oncol. 17:*10–15, 1990.
127. Mundy, G. R. Hypercalcemic factors other than parathyroid hormone-related protein. *Endocrinol. Metab. Clin. North Am. 18:*795–806, 1989.
128. Mundy, G. R. Hypercalcemia of malignancy revisited. *J. Clin. Invest. 82:*1–6, 1988.
129. Mundy, G. R., Ibbotson, K. J., and D'Souza, S. M. Tumor products and the hypercalcemia of malignancy. *J. Clin. Invest. 394:*391–394, 1985.
130. Mundy, G. R., Ibbotson, K. J., D'Souza, S. M., Simpson, E. L., Jacobs, J. W., and Martin, T. J. The hypercalcemia of cancer. Clinical implications and pathogenic mechanisms. *N. Engl. J. Med. 310:*1718–1727, 1984.
131. Nafe, L. A., Patnaik, A. K., and Lyman, R. Hypercalcemia associated with epidermoid carcinoma in a dog. *J. Am. Vet. Med. Assoc. 176:*1253–1254, 1980.
132. Nemere, I., and Norman, A. W. Parathyroid hormone stimulates calcium transport in perfused duodena from normal chicks. Comparison with the rapid (transcaltachic) effect of 1,25-dihydroxyvitamin D3. *Endocrinology 119:*1406–1408, 1986.
133. Nussbaum, S. R., Gaz, R. D., and Arnold, A. Hypercalcemia and ectopic secretion of parathyroid hormone by an ovarian carcinoma with rearrangement of the gene for parathyroid hormone. *N. Engl. J. Med. 323:*1324–1328, 1990.
134. Orloff, J. J., Ganz, M. B., Ribaudo, A. E., Burtis, W. J., Reiss, M., Milstone, L. M., and Stewart, A. F. Analysis of PTHRP binding and signal transduction mechanisms in benign and malignant squamous cells. *Am. J. Physiol. 262:*E599-E607, 1992.
135. Orloff, J. J., Goumas, D., Wu, T. L., and Stewart, A. F. Interspecies comparison of renal cortical receptors for parathyroid hormone and parathyroid hormone-related protein. *J. Bone Miner. Res. 6:*279–287, 1991.

136. Orloff, J. J., Wu, T. L., and Stewart, A. F. Parathyroid hormone-like proteins: Biochemical responses and receptor interactions. *Endocr. Rev. 10:*476–494, 1989.

137. Pandian, M. R., Morgan, C. H., Carlton, E., and Segre, G. V. Modified immunoradiometric assay of parathyroid hormone-related protein: Clinical application in the differential diagnosis of hypercalcemia. *Clin. Chem. 38:*282–288, 1992.

138. Perry, H. M., III. Parathyroid hormone-lymphocyte interactions modulate bone resorption. *Endocrinology 119:*2333–2339, 1986.

139. Perry, H. M., III, Chappel, J. C., Bellorin-Font, E., Tamao, J., and Martin, K. J. Parathyroid hormone receptors in circulating human mononuclear leukocytes. *J. Biol. Chem. 259:*5531–5535, 1984.

140. Pliam, N. B., Nyiredy, K. O., and Arnaud, C. D. Parathyroid hormone receptors in avian bone cells. *Proc. Natl. Acad. Sci. USA 79:*2061–2063, 1982.

141. Pun, K. K., Arnaud, C. D., and Nissenson, R. A. Parathyroid hormone receptors in human dermal fibroblasts: Structural and functional characterization. *J. Bone Miner. Res. 3:*453–460, 1988.

142. Rabbani, S. A., Mitchell, J., Roy, D. R., Hendy, G. N., and Goltzman, D. Influence of the amino-terminus on *in vitro* and *in vivo* biological activity of synthetic parathyroid hormone-like peptides of malignancy. *Endocrinology 123:*2709–2716, 1988.

143. Raisz, L. G., and Kream, B. E. Regulation of bone formation. *N. Engl. J. Med. 309:*83–89, 1983.

144. Ralston, S. H. The pathogenesis of humoral hypercalcaemia of malignancy. *Lancet 8573:*1443–1446, 1987.

145. Ralston, S. H., Cowan, R. A., Robertson, A. G., Gardner, M. D., and Boyle, I. T. Circulating vitamin D metabolites and hypercalcaemia of malignancy. *Acta Endocrinol. (Copenh.) 106:*556–563, 1984.

146. Ralston, S. H., Danks, J., Hayman, J., Fraser, W. D., Stewart, C. S., and Martin, T. J. Parathyroid hormone-related protein of malignancy: Immunohistochemical and biochemical studies in normocalcemic and hypercalcemic patients with cancer. *J. Clin. Pathol. 44:*472–476, 1991.

147. Ralston, S. H., Gallacher, S. J., Patel, U., Campbell, J., and Boyle, I. T. Cancer-associated hypercalcemia: Morbidity and mortality clinical experience in 126 treated patients. *Ann. Intern. Med. 112:*499–504, 1990.

148. Ratcliffe, W. A., Norbury, S., Heath, D. A., and Ratcliffe, J. G. Development and validation of an immunoradiometric assay of parathyrin-related protein in unextracted plasma. *Clin. Chem. 37:*678–685, 1991.

149. Ratcliffe, W. A., Norbury, S., Stott, R. A., Heath, D. A., and Ratcliffe, J. G. Immunoreactivity of plasma parathyrin-related peptide: Three region-specific radioimmunoassays and a two-site immunoradiometric assay compared. *Clin. Chem. 37:*1781–1787, 1991.

150. Ratcliffe, W. A., Thompson, G. E., Care, A. D., and Peaker, M. Production of parathyroid hormone-related protein by the mammary gland of the goat. *J. Endocrinol. 133:*87–93, 1992.

151. Rijnberk, A., Elsinghorst, A. M., Koeman, J. P., Hackeng, W. H. L., and Lequin, R. M. Pseudohyperparathyroidism associated with perirectal adenocarcinomas in elderly female dogs. *Tijdschr. Diergeneeskd. 103:*1069–1075, 1978.

152. Rizzoli, R., Bonjour, J.-P. High extracellular calcium increases the production of a parathyroid hormone-like activity by cultured Leydig tumor cells associated with humoral hypercalcemia. *J. Bone Miner. Res. 4:*839–844, 1989.

153. Rodan, G. A., and Martin, T. J. Role of osteoblasts in hormonal control of bone resorption - a hypothesis. *Calcif. Tissue Int. 33:*349–351, 1981.

154. Rodan, S. B., Noda, M., Wesolowski, G., Rosenblatt, M., and Rodan, G. A. Comparison of postreceptor effects of 1–34 human hypercalcemia factor and 1–34 human parathyroid hormone in rat osteosarcoma cells. *J. Clin. Invest. 81:*924–927, 1988.

155. Rodan, S. B., Wesolowski, G., Ianacone, J., Thiede, M. A., and Rodan, G. A. Production of parathyroid hormone-like peptide in a human osteosarcoma cell line: Stimulation by phorbol esters and epidermal growth factor. *J. Endocrinol. 122:*219–227, 1989.

156. Rosol, T. J., and Capen, C. C. Biology of disease. Mechanisms of cancer-induced hypercalcemia. *Lab. Invest. 67:*680–702, 1992.

157. Rosol, T. J., and Capen, C. C. Inhibition of *in vitro* bone resorption by a parathyroid hormone receptor antagonist in the canine adenocarcinoma model of humoral hypercalcemia of malignancy. *Endocrinology 122*:2098–2102, 1988.

158. Rosol, T. J., Capen, C. C., and Brooks, C. L. Bone and kidney adenylate cyclase-stimulating activity produced by a hypercalcemic canine adenocarcinoma line (CAC-8) maintained in nude mice. *Cancer Res. 47*:690–695, 1987.

159. Rosol, T. J., Capen, C. C., Danks, J. A., Suva, L. J., Steinmeyer, C. L., Hayman, J., Ebeling, P. R., and Martin, T. J. Identification of parathyroid hormone-related protein in canine apocrine adenocarcinoma of the anal sac. *Vet. Pathol. 27*:89–95, 1990.

160. Rosol, T. J., Capen, C. C., Weisbrode, S. E., and Horst, R. L. Humoral hypercalcemia of malignancy in nude mouse model of a canine adenocarcinoma derived from apocrine glands of the anal sac. *Lab. Invest. 54*:679–688, 1986.

161. Rosol, T. J., Merryman, J. I., Nohutcu, R. M., McCauley, L. K., and Capen, C. C. Effects of transforming growth factor-α on parathyroid hormone- and parathyroid hormone-related protein-mediated bone resorption and adenylate cyclase stimulation *in vitro*. *Domest. Anim. Endocrinol. 8*:501–508, 1991.

162. Rosol, T. J., Nagode, L. A., Couto, C. G., Hammer, A. S., Chew, D. J., Peterson, J. L., Ayl, R. D., Steinmeyer, C. L., and Capen, C. C. Parathyroid hormone (PTH)-related protein, PTH, and 1,25-dihydroxyvitamin D in dogs with cancer-associated hypercalcemia. *Endocrinology 131*:1157–1164, 1992.

163. Roth, S. I., and Raisz, L. G. Effect of calcium concentration on the ultrastructure of rat parathyroid in organ culture. *Lab. Invest. 13*:331–345, 1964.

164. Rousseau-Merck, M. F., de Keyzer, Y., Bourdeau, A., Cournot, G., Mercier, F., and Nezelof, C. PTH mRNA transcription analysis in infantile tumors associated with hypercalcemia. *Cancer 62*:303–308, 1988.

165. Sakaguchi, K., Ikeda, K., Curcio, F., Aurbach, G. D., and Brandi, M. L. Subclones of a rat parathyroid cell line (PT-r): Regulation of growth and production of parathyroid hormone-related peptide (PTHrP). *J. Bone Miner. Res. 5*:863–869, 1990.

166. Scharla, S. H., Minne, H. W., Lempert, U. G., Krieg, P., Rappel, S., Maurer, E., Grohe, U., and Ziegler, R. Osteolytic activity of Walker carcinosarcoma 256 is due to parathyroid hormone-related protein (PTHrP). *Horm. Metab. Res. 23*:66–69, 1991.

167. Scheinman, S. J., Mitnick, M. E., and Stewart, A. F. Quantitative evaluation of anticalciuric effects of synthetic parathyroid hormone-like peptides. *J. Bone Miner. Res. 6*:653–658, 1990.

168. Schermer, D. T., Chan, S. D. H., Bruce, R., Nissenson, R. A., Wood, W. I., and Strewler, G. J. Chicken parathyroid hormone-related protein and its expression during embryologic development. *J. Bone Miner. Res. 6*:149–155, 1991.

169. Selvanayagam, P., Graves, K., Cooper, C., and Rajaraman, S. Expression of the parathyroid hormone-related peptide gene in rat tissues. *Lab. Invest. 64*:713–717, 1991.

170. Shanberg, A. M., Baghdassarian, R., Tansey, L. A., Bacon, D., Greenberg, P., and Perley, M. Pheochromocytoma with hypercalcemia: Case report and review of literature. *J. Urol. 133*:258–259, 1985.

171. Shasha, S. M., Kristal, B., Barzilai, M., Makov, U. E., and Shkolnik, M. T. *In vitro* effect of PTH on normal T cell functions. *Nephron. 50*:212–216, 1988.

172. Shaw, A. J., Mughal, M. Z., Maresh, M. J. A., and Sibley, C. P. Effects of two synthetic parathyroid hormone-related protein fragments on maternofetal transfer of calcium and magnesium and release of cyclic AMP by the in-situ perfused rat placenta. *J. Endocrinol. 129*:399–404, 1991.

173. Silve, C. M., Hradek, G. T., Jones, A. L., and Arnaud, C. D. Parathyroid hormone receptor in intact embryonic chicken bone: Characterization and cellular localization. *J. Cell Biol. 94*:379–386, 1982.

174. Simpson, E. L., Mundy, G. R., D'Souza, S. M., Ibbotson, K. J., Bockman, R., and Jacobs, J. W. Absence of parathyroid hormone messenger RNA in nonparathyroid tumors associated with hypercalcemia. *N. Engl. J. Med. 309*:325–330, 1983.

175. Smith, M. R., and Greene, W. C. Molecular biology of the type I human T-cell leukemia virus

(HTLV-I) and adult T-cell leukemia. *J. Clin. Invest. 87:*761–766, 1991.

176. Stewart, A. F., and Broadus, A. E. Clinical review 16: Parathyroid hormone-related proteins: Coming of age in the 1990s. *J. Clin. Endocrinol. Metab. 71:*1410–1414, 1990.

177. Stewart, A. F., Horst, R., Deftos, L. J., Cadman, E. C., and Lang, R., Broadus, A. E. Biochemical evaluation of patients with cancer-associated hypercalcemia evidence for humoral and non-humoral groups. *N. Engl. J. Med. 303:*1377–1383, 1980.

178. Stewart, A. F., Insogna, K. L., Burtis, W. J., Aminiafshar, A., Wu, T., Weir, E. C., and Broadus, A. E. Frequency and partial characterization of adenylate cyclase-stimulating activity in tumors associated with humoral hypercalcemia of malignancy. *J. Bone Miner. Res. 1:*267–276, 1986.

179. Stewart, A. F., Wu, T., Goumas, D., Burtis, W. J., and Broadus, A. E. N-terminal amino acid sequence of two novel tumor-derived adenylate cyclase-stimulated proteins: Identification of parathyroid hormone-like and parathyroid hormone-unlike domains. *Biochem. Biophys. Res. Commun. 146:*672–678, 1987.

180. Stewart, A. F., Wu, T. L., Insogna, K. L., Milstone, L. M., and Burtis, W. J. Immunoaffinity purification of parathyroid hormone-related protein from bovine milk and human keratino-cyte-conditioned medium. *J. Bone Miner. Res. 6:*305–311, 1991.

181. Streutker, C., and Drucker, D. J. Rapid induction of parathyroid hormone-like gene expression by sodium butyrate in a rat islet cell line. *Mol. Endocrinol. 5:*703–708, 1991.

182. Strewler, G. J., and Nissenson, R. A. Nonparathyroid hypercalcemia. *Adv. Intern. Med. 32:*235–258, 1987.

183. Strewler, G. J., Stern, P. H., Jacobs, J. W., Eveloff, J., Klein, R. F., Leung, S. C., Rosenblatt, M., and Nissenson, R. A. Parathyroid hormone-like protein from human renal carcinoma cells. Structural and functional homology with parathyroid hormone. *J. Clin. Invest. 80:*1803–1807, 1987.

184. Strewler, G. J., Wronski, T. J., Halloran, B. P., Miller, S. C., Leung, S. C., Williams, R. D., and Nissenson, R. A. Pathogenesis of hypercalcemia in nude mice bearing a human renal carcinoma. *Endocrinology 119:*303–310, 1986.

185. Sutton, R. A. L., and Dirks, J. H. Renal handling of calcium. *Fed. Proc. 37:*2112–2119, 1978.

186. Suva, L. J., Mather, K. A., Gillespie, M. T., Webb, G. C., Ng, K. W., Winslow, G. A., Wood, W. I., Martin, T. J., and Hudson, P. J. Structure of the 5′ flanking region of the gene encoding human parathyroid-hormone-related protein (PTHrP). *Gene 77:*95–105, 1989.

187. Suva, L. J., Winslow, G. A., Wettenhall, R. E. H., Hammonds, R. G., Moseley, J. M., Diefenbach-Jagger, H., Rodda, C. P., Kemp, B. E., Rodriquez, H., Chen, E. Y., Hudson, P. J., Martin, T. J., and Wood, W. I. A parathyroid hormone-related protein implicated in malignant hyper-calcemia: Cloning and expression. *Science 237:*893–896, 1987.

188. Suzuki, K., and Yamada, S. Ascites sarcoma 180, an animal model of humoral hypercalcemia of malignancy, produces a factor(s) exhibiting potent bone-resorbing activity without any para-thyroid hormone-like activity. *Bone Miner. 14:*1–13, 1991.

189. Szpirer, C., Riviere, M., Szpirer, J., Hanson, C., Levan, G., and Hendy, G. N. Assignment of the rat parathyroid hormone-related peptide gene (PTHLH) to chromosome 4: Evidence for conserved synteny between human chromosome 12, mouse chromosome 6, and rat chromo-some 4. *Cytogenet. Cell Genet. 56:*193–195, 1991.

190. Tashjian, A. H., Voelkel, E. F., Levine, L., and Goldhaber, P. Evidence that the bone resorption-stimulating factor produced by mouse fibrosarcoma cells is prostaglandin E_2: A new model for the hypercalcemia of cancer. *J. Exp. Med. 136:*1329–1343, 1972.

191. Thiede, M. A., Daifotis, A. G., Weir, E. C., Brines, M. L., Burtis, W. J., Ikeda, K., Dreyer, B. E., Garfield, R. E., and Broadus, A. E. Intrauterine occupancy controls expression of the parthyroid hormone-related peptide gene in preterm rat myometrium. *Proc. Natl. Acad. Sci. USA 87:*6969–6973, 1990.

192. Thiede, M. A., Strewler, G. J., Nissenson, R. A., Rosenblatt, M., and Rodan, G. A. Human renal carcinoma expresses two messages encoding a parathyroid hormone-like peptide: Evidence for the alternative splicing of a single copy gene. *Proc. Natl. Acad. Sci. USA 85:*4605–4609, 1988.

193. Thurston, A. W., Cole, J. A., Hillman, L. S., Im, J. H., Thorne, P. K., Krause, W. J., Jones, J. R., Eber, S. L., and Forte, L. R. Purification and properties of parathyroid hormone-related peptide isolated from milk. *Endocrinology 126*:1183–1190, 1990.
194. Vaes, G. Cellular biology and biochemical mechanism of bone resorption. A review of recent developments on the formation, activation, and mode of action of osteoclasts. *Clin. Orthop. Relat. Res. 231*:239–271, 1988.
195. Voelkel, E. F., Tashjian, A. H., Franklin, R., Wasserman, E., and Levine, L. Hypercalcemia and tumor-prostaglandins: The VX2 carcinoma model in the rabbit. *Metabolism 24*:973–986, 1975.
196. Walker, A. T., Stewart, A. F., Korn, E. A., Shiratori, T., Mitnick, M. A., and Carpenter, T. O. Effect of parathyroid hormone-like peptides on 25-hydroxyvitamin D-1α-hydroxylase activity in rodents. *Am. J. Physiol. 258*:E297-E303, 1990.
197. Watanabe, T., Yamaguchi, K., Takatsuki, K., Osame, M., and Yoshida, M. Constitutive expression of parathyroid hormone-related protein gene in human T cell leukemia virus type I (HTLV-1) carriers and adult T cell leukemia patients that can be transactivated by HTLV-1 tax gene. *J. Exp. Med. 172*:759–765, 1990.
198. Weir, E. C., Brines, M. L., Ikeda, K., Burtis, W. J., Broadus, A. E., and Robbins, R. J. Parathyroid hormone-related peptide gene is expressed in the mammalian central nervous system. *Proc. Natl. Acad. Sci. USA 87*:108–112, 1990.
199. Weir, E. C., Burtis, W. J., Morris, C. A., Brady, T. G., and Insogna, K. L. Isolation of 16,000-dalton parathyroid hormone-like proteins from two animal tumors causing humoral hypercalcemia of malignancy. *Endocrinology 123*:2744–2751, 1988.
200. Weir, E. C., Insogna, K. L., Brownstein, D. G., Bander, N. H., and Broadus, A. E. *In vitro* adenylate cyclase-stimulating activity predicts the occurrence of humoral hypercalcemia of malignancy in nude mice. *J. Clin. Invest. 81*:818–821, 1988.
201. Weir, E. C., Norrdin, R. W., Matus, R. E., Brooks, M. B., Broadus, A. E., Mitnick, M., Johnston, S. D., and Insogna, K. L. Humoral hypercalcemia of malignancy in canine lymphosarcoma. *Endocrinology 122*:602–608, 1988.
202. Werkmeister, J. R., Rosol, T. J., Merryman, J. I., McCauley, L. K., Horton, J. E., and Capen, C. C. Regulation of parathyroid hormone-related protein in normal human keratinocytes. *J. Bone Min. Res. 6(Suppl. 1)*:230, 1991 (abstract).
203. Wong GL. Skeletal effects of parathyroid hormone. In: *Bone and Mineral Research*, 4th ed., edited by W. A. Peck. Amsterdam, Elsevier Science Publishers, 1986, pp. 103–129.
204. Wu, T. L., Soifer, N. E., Burtis, W. J., Milstone, L. M., and Stewart, A. F. Glycosylation of parathyroid hormone-related peptide secreted by human keratinocytes. *J. Clin. Endocrinol. Metab. 73*:1002–1007, 1991.
205. Wynick, D., Ratcliffe, W. A., Heath, D. A., Ball, S., Barnard, M., and Bloom, S. R. Treatment of a malignant pancreatic endocrine tumour secreting parathyroid hormone related protein. *Br. Med. J. [Clin. Res.] 300*:1314–1315, 1990.
206. Yamaguchi, D. T., Kleeman, C. R., and Muallem, S. Protein kinase C-activated calcium channel in the osteoblast-like clonal osteosarcoma cell line UMR-106. *J. Biol. Chem. 262*:14967–14973, 1987.
207. Yamamoto, M., Duong, L. T., Fisher, J. E., Thiede, M. A., Caulfield, M. P., and Rosenblatt, M. Suckling-mediated increases in urinary phosphate and 3',5'-cyclic adenosine monophosphate excretion in lactating rats: Possible systemic effects in parathyroid hormone-related protein. *Endocrinology 129*:2614–2622, 1991.
208. Yamamoto, M., Fisher, J. E., Thiede, M. A., Caulfield, M. P., Rosenblatt, M., and Duong, L. T. Concentrations of parathyroid hormone-related protein in rat milk change with duration of lactation and interval from previous suckling, but not with milk calcium. *Endocrinology 130*:741–747, 1992.
209. Yasuda, T., Banville, D., Hendy, G. N., and Goltzman, D. Characterization of the human parathyroid hormone-like peptide gene functional and evolutionary aspects. *J. Biol. Chem. 264*:7720–7725, 1989.
210. Yasuda, T., Banville, D., Rabbani, S., Hendy, G., and Goltzman, D. Rat parathyroid hormone-like peptide: Comparison with the human homologue and expression in malignant and normal

tissue. *Mol. Endocrinol. 3:*518–525, 1989.
211. Yoshimoto, K., Yamasaki, R., Sakai, H., Tezuka, U., Takahashi, M., Iizuka, M., Sekiya, T., and Saito, S. Ectopic production of parathryoid hormone by small cell lung cancer in a patient with hypercalcemia. *J. Clin. Endocrinol. Metab. 68:*976–981, 1989.
212. Zhou, H., Leaver, D. D., Moseley, J. M., Kemp, B., Ebeling, P. R., and Martin, T. J. Actions of parathyroid hormone-related protein on the rat kidney *in vivo. J. Endocrinol. 122:*229–235, 1989.

Chapter 2

Pathology of Hyperparathyroidism: A Practical Approach

J. AIDAN CARNEY

Hyperparathyroidism was discovered almost simultaneously in Europe and the United States just over 60 years ago. The disorder is the result of inappropriately increased secretion of parathyroid hormone (PTH) by one or more of the parathyroid glands. The increased secretion is caused by a defect in the parathyroid gland(s) or by an extraparathyroid condition, such as chronic renal failure or intestinal malabsorption, that tends to lower serum calcium, thereby producing secondary parathyroid hyperfunction (secondary hyperparathyroidism).

Primary hyperparathyroidism is a relatively common disease that is two to three times more common in women than in men. After the introduction of routine measurement of serum calcium, the annual age-adjusted incidence in Rochester, Minnesota, was 27.7 ± 5.8 per 100,00 population.[31] In most cases, the cause of the disorder is unknown. Recently, Prinz and associates[44] reported that two-thirds of patients with parathyroid and thyroid tumors had a history of exposure to radiation. In a minority of cases, primary hyperparathyroidism is a familial disorder (familial hyperparathyroidism) or a component of a multiple endocrine neoplasia syndrome. Nonfamilial primary hyperparathyroidism usually affects older individuals, whereas familial cases commonly are seen in the third and fourth decades of life. Although various nonspecific symptoms are associated with hyperparathyroidism, most patients are asymptomatic, and the disorder is identified by screening for serum calcium.

Primary hyperparathyroidism ordinarily is not a serious condition. It should be relieved by a single surgical procedure, the objective of which is to achieve a lasting cure for hypercalcemia and avoidance of permanent postoperative hypocalcemia. Minor and major complications sometimes arise in the course of treatment and are occasionally caused by excessive operation as a result of pathologic misinterpretation. Rarely, the cause of the disorder is not found at the primary operation, and another operation(s) is necessary. It is interesting to recall that in the first patient operated on in the United States for primary hyperparathyroidism—this was in 1926—seven operations were required before his mediastinal parathyroid tumor was finally found.

In order to achieve permanent cure, the physicians (internist, radiologist, surgeon, and pathologist) involved should be knowledgeable about the pitfalls in the diagnosis and treatment of hyperparathyroidism and be willing to cooperate and interact closely with one another. It is well for all concerned to keep in mind the Hippocratic adage *primum non nocere*, because serious adverse effects—most important, permanent hypoparathyroidism—can result from overly zealous treatment. Thus, the approach to pathologic diagnosis of hyperparathyroidism that is outlined in this chapter is pragmatic and designed to achieve a successful outcome for the patient rather than to obtain absolute pathologic accuracy. The approach suggested certainly is *not intended* to stifle interest in the nosology and pathogenesis of parathyroid hyperfunction, about which there is much to learn.

For the pathologist to analyze parathyroid specimens appropriately, it is helpful to have knowledge of some aspects of calcium homeostasis, and the embryology, anatomy, and histology of normal parathyroid glands. Therefore, these subjects are briefly reviewed below.

NORMAL PARATHYROID GLANDS

CALCIUM HOMEOSTASIS

Adequate amounts of ionized calcium are needed for a wide range of cellular processes, including cell division, muscle contraction, and secretion. The concentration of calcium in the extracellular fluid is normally maintained within narrow limits; deviations in either direction are not well tolerated and, if large, may be life-threatening.

Dietary intake of calcium is usually offset by urinary loss. Maintenance of adequate concentrations of calcium in extracellular fluid requires two hormones, PTH and 1,25-dihydroxycholecalciferol, a derivative of vitamin D. PTH is secreted by the parathyroid chief cells and facilitates the transfer of calcium into the extracellular fluid by promoting mobilization of calcium from bone. It stimulates the formation of 1,25-dihydroxycholecalciferol in the kidney and indirectly causes the intestinal uptake of calcium and phosphate and the reabsorption of these substances by the kidney. PTH secretion is regulated by the serum calcium level through a negative feedback mechanism: low calcium levels stimulate PTH secretion and high calcium levels inhibit it.

The total calcium concentration in the blood is nearly twice that in the interstitial fluid, because calcium is avidly bound to albumin and other circulating proteins. Total calcium in blood plasma is normally about 10 mg/dL, but only the ionized fraction appears to be regulated. When the extracellular concentration of calcium is low (hypocalcemia), the electrical excitability of cell membranes is increased, eventually resulting in involuntary contractions of skeletal muscle (tetany). In the opposite condition, hypercalcemia, calcium salts may precipitate from solution because of their low solubility at physiologic pH. In the kidney, calculi commonly form and cause infection, renal damage, and ultimately renal failure. With prolonged severe hypercalcemia, metastatic calcification occurs, and calcium salts are precipitated in arterial walls, pulmonary alveolar walls, and gastric fundal mucosa.

In primary hyperparathyroidism, one or more parathyroid glands secrete excessive amounts of PTH, which produces hypercalcemia by the mechanisms outlined above. However, the phenomenon of hypercalcemia has many causes besides hyperparathyroidism (Table 2.1). Thus, the diagnosis of hyperparathyroidism is made after exclusion of these other conditions and after finding increased levels of PTH in the blood plasma. In practice, the triad of hypercalcemia, hypophosphatemia, and hypercalciuria suggests primary hyperparathyroidism. The symptomatology resulting from hypercalcemia involves many organs and systems (Table 2.2).

EMBRYOLOGY OF PARATHYROID GLANDS

The parathyroid glands are generally thought to develop from the primitive branchial pouches and, thus, have an endodermal origin.[27] This idea was recently challenged, and it was proposed that the glands have an ectodermal, specifically neuroectodermal, origin.[42] According to the classical description, the upper pair of glands (parathyroid IV) develop from the fourth branchial pouch, as does the lateral thyroid anlage. These structures remain associated during development, hence, the proximity of the upper glands to the thyroid and the likelihood that an intrathyroid parathyroid gland will be an upper gland (that was presumably trapped between the lateral and medial thyroid anlagen as they fused).

The lower pair of parathyroid glands (parathyroid III) and the thymus arise from the third branchial pouch. The two organs descend in the neck and stay associated in about 50% of cases, with the parathyroid gland being located within a cervical thymic extension at the thoracic inlet. The parathyroid may descend into the anterior mediastinum and migrate as far as the pericardium. Rarely, the thymus and the inferior gland (parathymus) remain high in the neck. The supernumerary glands that are often associated with a lobule of the thymus are

TABLE 2.1. CAUSES OF HYPERCALCEMIA

Common	Uncommon
Cancer with or without bone metastasis	Leukemia
Thiazide therapy	Hyperthyroidism
Myeloma	Myxedema
Sarcoidosis	Addisonian crisis
Hypervitaminosis D	Immobilization
Milk-alkali syndrome	Diuretic phase of renal tubular damage
	Idiopathic hypercalcemia of infancy
	Acromegaly

TABLE 2.2. CLINICAL MANIFESTATIONS OF HYPERCALCEMIA

Gastrointestinal:	Anorexia, constipation, nausea, vomiting, peptic ulcer, acute pancreatitis
Genitourinary:	Polyuria, nephrocalcinosis, renal calculi, renal insufficiency, polydypsia
Neurologic:	Fatigue, muscle weakness, depressed tendon reflexes, disorientation, stupor, coma
Psychiatric:	Apathy, depression
Metastatic calcification:	Ocular keratopathy, nephrocalcinosis, vascular calcification, periarticular calcification, chondrocalcinosis

probably the result of subdivision of parathyroid III during its embryologic descent.

ANATOMY AND HISTOLOGY OF PARATHYROID GLANDS

The parathyroid glands, which are usually four in number, are located in the lower neck, posterior to the thyroid gland. In a study of 352 cases, Alveryd[3] found five parathyroid glands in 3.5%, four in 90.8%, three in 5.1%, and two in 0.6%. In only one of the cases with two or three parathyroid glands was the combined weight of the glands sufficient to suggest that none had been overlooked. The conclusion is that four or more parathyroid glands occur in almost every case. The glands are arranged in two pairs, an upper pair and a lower pair. The former are located at the cricothyroid junction posteriorly (approximately 75% of cases) or behind the upper pole of the thyroid gland (approximately 20% of cases). They are rarely behind the pharyngoesophageal junction.[53] They should be found within the zone bounded by the upper border of the larynx and the lower border of the thyroid gland. The position of the lower parathyroid glands is more variable, but they usually lie somewhere between the lower pole of the thyroid gland and the thymus. In approximately 40% of cases, the lower pair is located on the anterior or posterior surface of the lower pole of the thyroid gland, and in another 40%, they are enclosed in a cervical tongue of the thymus gland in the lower neck. However, as indicated above, they may be found as high as the carotid artery bifurcation or considerably lateral to the inferior pole of the thyroid gland or as low as the pericardium.

It is well to remember that enlarged parathyroid glands may be displaced caudally. Upper parathyroid glands are anterior to the thyroid fascia and tend to migrate inferiorly along the tracheoesophageal groove into the posterior mediastinum. Lower parathyroid glands are located posterior to the thyroid fascia and may be displaced into either the anterior or posterior mediastinum.

GROSS APPEARANCE AND CONSISTENCY

The color of normal parathyroid glands varies with the amount of stromal fat, which increases with advancing age. Before puberty, the glands contain little or no fat and are reddish-brown in color; in older individuals, increasing amounts of fatty stroma (as much as 30% or more) produce a characteristic yellowish-brown appearance. By contrast, adjacent structures have a slightly different color—thyroid tissue is redder, lymph nodes are paler and pinker, and the thymus is faintly grayish-yellow.

Parathyroid glands are soft and flabby; hence, they tend to be molded by adjacent structures. This accounts for their various shapes and dimensions. Ordinarily, the glands are oval and have rounded margins, but they may be flattened and have sharp margins if adjacent structures press on them (this occurs when they are located beneath the capsule of the thyroid gland). The consistency of parathyroid glands is useful in distinguishing them from lymph nodes or thyroid nodules, which are firmer and more elastic.

Size and Weight

On average, parathyroid glands measure 5 × 3 × 1 mm and weigh 35–40 mg.[28] The total parathyroid mass (parenchyma and stroma) weighs only 5–9 mg at birth and increases until the third or fourth decade when the weight is about 120 and 130 mg in men and women, respectively; total parenchymal cell weight is about 85 and 90 mg in men and women, respectively.[1,48] Glandular weights are less in patients with chronic illnesses, in men than in women, and in whites than in blacks.[24] Obese patients have more and emaciated patients have fewer fat cells than normal for their age.[1] Usually, the parathyroid glands are approximately equal in size and weight, but one gland is often smaller than the remaining three. In some cases, two glands are distinctly smaller than the others.[24] Total parathyroid mass is directly dependent on the amount of fat tissue in the body as a whole. Thus, it is the amount of stromal fat tissue in the parathyroid glands and not the amount of parenchyma that is positively correlated with the size (mass) of the glands. Nevertheless, parathyroid gland weight is a good simple index of parenchymal cell mass. Clearly, accurate determinations of parenchymal cell weight have greater diagnostic value,[1] but this measurement is not practical for routine diagnosis.

Histology of Parathyroid Glands

The parathyroid parenchyma is enclosed within a very thin fibrous capsule (Fig. 2.1). In children, the gland is composed of uniform sheets and cords of epithelial cells in a vascular stroma that contains few mature fat cells. After puberty, the stromal content of adipose tissue increases progressively (Fig. 2.1).

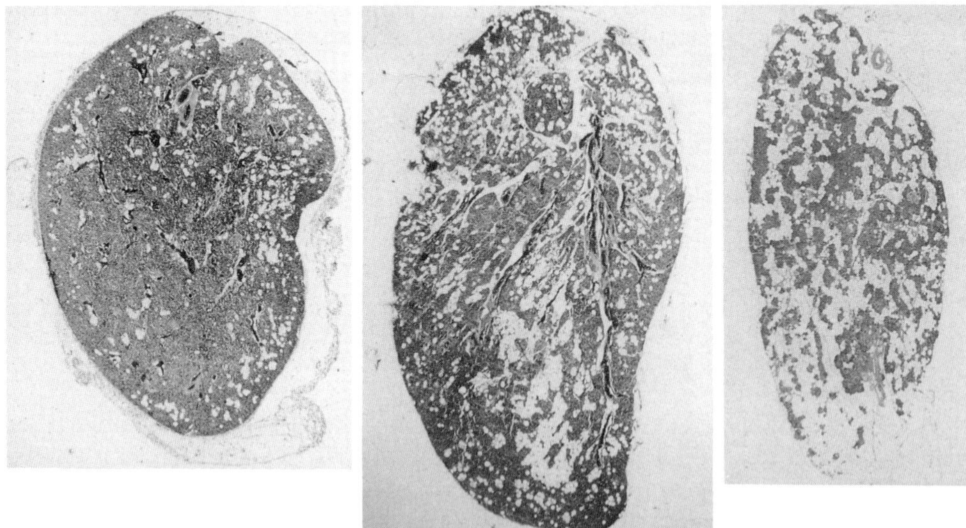

Fig. 2.1.   Low-power appearance of normal parathyroid glands showing variation in the quantity of stromal fat.

In the past, misinterpretation of the classic study of Gilmour and Martin[28] resulted in the belief[15] that there was more stromal fat in the gland than there actually is; until recently, a 50:50 parenchymal/stromal fat ratio in adults was considered normal. Recent studies have shown that three-quarters of adult parathyroid glands have less than 30% fat, and one-half have less than 10%.[20,23] Thus, in the glands of many older, normal people there is relatively little stromal fat—the ratio of parenchymal to stromal fat may be 90:10, a finding that increases the difficulty of diagnosis of minimal parathyroid hyperplasia in glands that are normal size or minimally enlarged.

Two principal types of epithelial cells, chief and oxyphil (with several intermediate forms), occur in the parathyroid gland. Chief cells are round or polygonal, sharply outlined, 6–10 μ in diameter and have central pyknotic nuclei and inconspicuous nucleoli. Slight cytoplasmic eosinophilia permits separating them into a minority of cells with stainable cytoplasm (dark chief cells) and cells with lightly stained or clear, glycogen-containing cytoplasm (light chief cells). The light chief cells are more abundant; however, it is the dark chief cells that synthesize and secrete PTH.

The light chief cells, whose delicate staining reflects a paucity of cytoplasmic organelles, are thought to be inactive; they frequently have a spherical or crescentic juxtanuclear clear zone that is the relic of a lipid organelle dissolved during tissue processing.[49] This body, which is 0.5–1.5 μ in size, is readily visualized in frozen sections stained with Sudan IV (positively stained and an orange color) or with polychrome methylene blue (negatively stained and refractile). The organelle is important because it marks parathyroid cells that are resting or suppressed. Use of alcoholic stains, mounting of sections in fat-solubilizing media, and routine dehydration procedures remove the sudanophilic granules from tissue sections.

Oxyphil cells appear in late childhood and increase in number with age. In the elderly, they form irregular sheets or small nodules or are randomly scattered in the gland (Fig. 2.1). Typically, they are large cells (as much as 20 μ in diameter) with eosinophilic, finely granular cytoplasm and a central nucleus. Transitional forms between the chief and oxyphilic cells (transitional oxyphil cells), intermediate in size and cytoplasmic tinctorial quality, are common. Oxyphil cells are thought to be nonfunctional.

Theoretically, hypercalcemia would be expected to cause atrophy of normal parathyroid glands, that is, a decrease in the weight of the glands accompanied by a decrease in the size and number of the parenchymal cells. However, this atrophy does not occur. Instead, the parathyroid glands maintain their normal size and a variable number of parenchymal cells (as many as 25%) undergo a distinctive histologic change[22]: they increase in size, acquire clear, vacuolated cytoplasm, and become arranged in a trabecular pattern with peripherally palisaded nuclei (Fig. 2.2). These histologic changes should not be misinterpreted as parathyroid hyperplasia. In theory, the alteration should also occur in the compressed rim of "normal" parathyroid at the periphery of at least some parathyroid adenomas, but this has not been described.

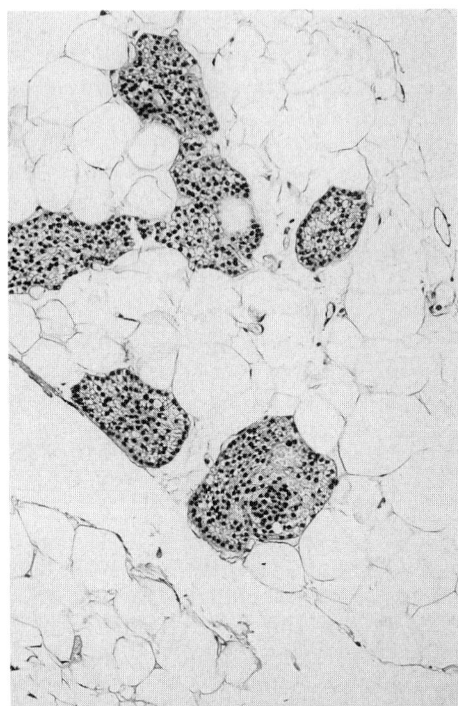

FIG. 2.2. Effect of hypercalcemia on normal parathyroid gland. Uniform population of moderately enlarged chief cells with clear cytoplasm and peripherally palisaded nuclei.

EVOLUTION OF HISTOPATHOLOGY OF HYPERPARATHYROIDISM

The first resection of a parathyroid adenoma for primary hyperparathyroidism was performed by Felix Mandl[37] in Vienna in 1926. Three years later, the first functioning "malignant adenoma" (on review, a parathyroid carcinoma) was excised by Russell Wilder[57] at the Mayo Clinic. In less than a decade after Mandl's report, more than 100 cases of hyperparathyroidism had been reported; most were due to a single functioning adenoma, rarely to two adenomas, and exceptionally, to carcinoma.

In 1934, Fuller Albright and associates[2] at the Massachusetts General Hospital in Boston reported three cases of primary hyperparathyroidism in which all four glands were enlarged. This was a new entity whose microscopic features included uniformity of structure, enormous cells, and extremely clear cytoplasm. This condition became known as "water-clear cell," or "wasserhelle-cell," hyperplasia. The affected glands were easily distinguishable grossly and microscopically from the usual adenoma and from glands associated with secondary hyperplasia, a condition that was well recognized at time time.[16] Subsequently, water-clear cell hyperplasia was observed by others, but for unknown reasons, the condition disappeared about 30 years ago.

In 1958, Cope and colleagues[19] at the Massachusetts General Hospital described a third type of hyperplasia that affected all the glands; they called it "chief-cell hyperplasia." The disorder occurred in 10% of their first 200 patients with primary hyperparathyroidism. It was the most common cause of parathyroid enlargement in patients with multiple endocrine adenopathy (usually referred to currently as "multiple endocrine neoplasia") and in patients with nonfamilial enlargement of multiple parathyroid glands. Grossly and microscopically, an individual gland with chief-cell hyperplasia could not be distinguished from the usual adenoma.

In 1966, Cope[18] wrote: "The only way the surgeon can be sure [of whether he is dealing with a parathyroid adenoma or chief-cell hyperplasia] is to see at least two glands. If one is normal, and the other is enlarged, the enlargement is presumably a neoplasm, either adenoma or carcinoma. If both are enlarged, presumably both are hyperplastic." Subsequently, on the basis of the relatively common occurrence of chief-cell hyperplasia and on Cope's authority, the notion gradually became accepted that if two (or three) parathyroid glands were enlarged, the disorder was parathyroid chief-cell hyperplasia and affected all four glands, with uneven involvement (sometimes microscopically only) of smaller or normal-sized glands.

This approach to diagnosis assumed increased importance in the 1970s when a number of influential groups in the United States concluded that there were many more cases of chief-cell hyperplasia than previously thought—as many as 65% of cases of primary hyperparathyroidism were attributed to it.[25,40,41] The basis for this assertion was that many cases that featured enlargement of one or two glands purportedly showed microscopic evidence of hyperplasia in biopsy specimens from apparently normal-sized glands. Clearly, this interpretation had potential for considerable consequences because cases of chief-cell hyperplasia were treated with subtotal parathyroidectomy (removal of three and one-half glands) or total parathyroidectomy with autotransplantation of parathyroid tissue, major procedures that carried an increased risk of permanent postoperative hypoparathyroidism. In the reports mentioned, diagnosis of chief-cell hyperplasia was often based on the finding of a parenchymal/stromal fat ratio greater than 50:50 (a ratio that at the time was thought to be normal for adults but, as pointed out above, is now known to reflect too low a normal parenchymal content) and a gland weight greater than 40 mg. Thus, the diagnosis of chief-cell hyperplasia in some earlier series is questionable; it is likely that many of the glands so interpreted were normal. But, on the basis of enlargement of one or two parathyroid glands and microscopic evidence of "hyperplasia" in other glands, subtotal parathyroidectomy was advised.[10] The justification for the potentially hazardous operation was that there would be recurrence if most of the parathyroid parenchyma was not removed. The result for patients so treated was an increased incidence of permanent postoperative hypoparathyroidism.[9,14] More recently, the occurrence of adenoma in two and three glands has become accepted as an occasional occurrence.[7,30]

Pathologists should be aware of the consequences of overdiagnosis of microscopic hyperplasia as a result of misinterpretation of parenchymal/stromal fat ratio or small "increases" in weight of an individual parathyroid gland, or both.

Most surgeons are now aware of the serious sequelae of overtreatment of cases in which the hyperplasia is "microscopic" only. Return of serum calcium to normal levels after successful surgical treatment of hyperparathyroidism is gratifying, but development of permanent postoperative hypoparathyroidism after surgical overtreatment (possibly influenced by pathologic misinterpretation) is a tragedy.

PRACTICAL APPROACH TO PATHOLOGIC DIAGNOSIS OF HYPERPARATHYROIDISM

Neoplastic and hyperplastic conditions of the parathyroid glands that cause hyperparathyroidism account for the majority of parathyroid operations. Experience has shown that these conditions generally are *successfully treated by removing enlarged gland(s) and leaving normal-sized glands undisturbed.* Therefore, as far as therapy is concerned, the importance of intraoperative precise pathologic categorization of enlarged parathyroid glands as "adenoma" or "hyperplasia" has diminished. In this practical setting, the traditional role of the pathologist as arbiter of the final diagnosis of "adenoma" or "hyperplasia" has decreased in importance. Nevertheless, the pathologist is still an important member of the team who treat patients with parathyroid overactivity.

The following is a description of the role of the surgical pathologist at the Mayo Clinic as a member of the team responsible for treating patients with hyperparathyroidism. A laboratory devoted to performance of frozen sections is located in the operating room suite, and the pathology team has easy access to preoperative and intraoperative clinical formation. The frozen section technique we use permits sections to be prepared (frozen, cut, stained, and mounted) at the rate of 1/min, which is ideal for examining multiple specimens quickly. The pathology team's involvement commences with preoperative review of the basis of the diagnosis of hyperparathyroidism and results of localization tests. It continues with the intraoperative monitoring, assessment and cataloguing of tissue removed at operation, and consultation with the surgeon by voice intercom system, or if necessary, a visit to the operating room. The pathologist's involvement includes postoperative correlation of the pathologic diagnosis with the patient's level of serum calcium and additional discussion with the surgeon, if indicated.

Preoperative Evaluation

The serum levels of calcium and PTH are of interest, because there is some correlation between the amount of increase in these substances and the mass of abnormal parathyroid tissue likely to be found at operation. Minimal increases in serum levels of calcium are unlikely to be associated with massive parathyroid disease. By contrast, serum calcium levels that exceed 13 mg/mL and substantially increased serum PTH are commonly associated with an amount of abnormal parathyroid tissue that can be measured in grams rather than milligrams or with parathyroid carcinoma. If, however, serum calcium is greatly increased and serum PTH level is only slightly increased, the presence of a nonparathyroid malignant tumor that produces a PTH-like substance or other hypercalcemic substance (ectopic hyperparathyroidism) is a possibility.[43] If a parathyroid tumor was palpated on physical examination, the patient probably has a carcinoma.[52]

The patient's medical records should reveal whether the operation is primary or a reexploration for persistent hyperparathyroidism or recurrent hyperparathyroidism after an apparent cure. A prior operation for an endocrine disorder or a family history of 1) parathyroid disease (familial hyperparathyroidism),[36] 2) pituitary or pancreatic islet cell tumors or both (multiple endocrine neoplasia, type 1),[56] or 3) medullary thyroid carcinoma or pheochromocytoma or both (multiple endocrine neoplasia, type 2)[51] should be apparent. If any of these conditions have occurred in the patient or the patient's family, the pathologic condition probably involves multiple parathyroid glands.

INTRAOPERATIVE TISSUE EXAMINATION

On occasion, small fat lobules (particularly when they have been discolored by hemorrhage), lymph nodes, thymic remnants, and exophytic thyroid nodules may be mistaken for parathyroid tissue, even by experienced surgeons. Therefore, at the Mayo Clinic, all specimens that are removed at parathyroidectomy are examined by frozen section technique for identification purposes.

PARATHYROID GLANDS

The anatomic location of parathyroid specimens submitted for pathologic examination is identified by the surgeon. Specifically, resected parathyroid tissue is identified as right or left and upper or lower gland, and whether it is an entire parathyroid gland or a biopsy specimen. This is particularly important if a parathyroid abnormality is not found at the primary operation and another operation is necessary, perhaps by a different surgeon. Gross examination of specimens that are submitted as parathyroid tissue or as parathyroid tumors is often informative. Parathyroid adenomas usually shell out readily from their fatty beds. They appear as discrete, oval, slightly flattened, tan-colored lesions with a thin glistening capsule. Hyperplastic glands have a similar appearance but frequently are more lobulated or nodular. A tumor with a thick fibrous capsule or poor circumscription or an invasive appearance is suggestive of parathyroid carcinoma.

Each gland is measured and weighed (to the nearest 5 mg) after extraneous tissue, usually fat, has been trimmed from the gland. Excess blood and moisture are removed by placing the specimen on filter paper before weighing it. Parathyroid glands weighing 60 mg or more are considered abnormal, providing that the surgeon has identified three other normal-sized glands.[48] The trimmed tissue is also weighed, because subsequent histologic examination may show that it was parathyroid tissue that had a deceptively high content of adipose tissue. Often, the fatty-appearing tissue is thymus, an observation that is conveyed to the surgeon because it identifies the removed gland as an inferior one and, thus, may influence the search for the other parathyroid gland on that side.

The pathologist's usual task has been to distinguish parathyroid adenoma from parathyroid hyperplasia.[8] Distinction between the two conditions is complicated and often frustrated by overlap of some of their pathologic features. It is made difficult because the gross appearance of the remaining glands, on which the diagnosis largely depends, usually is not known to the pathologist at the time of microscopic examination of the first excised parathyroid gland. Additionally, a rim of parent gland, even if it is present, may not be evident on the slide because it was inadvertently excluded by the plane of sectioning.

In regard to terminology, we have adopted an arbitrary and pragmatic approach: single gland enlargement in association with three normal-sized glands is designated "adenoma," even if on microscopic examination the enlarged gland has some nodularity or contains minimal stromal fat (both features of hyperplasia) (Fig. 2.3). On the other hand, if all glands are enlarged, the disorder is considered hyperplasia, irrespective of the microscopic appearance of the glands, even though one or more of them resemble adenoma (Fig. 2.4). If two or three glands are enlarged, a descriptive diagnosis or a diagnosis of multiple adenomas or of hyperplasia may be made, depending on the findings. There is no danger for misunderstanding and consequent overtreatment to occur if the diagnosis "chief-cell hyperplasia" is made, because the surgeons are aware of the difficulty in separating adenoma from hyperplasia histologically. They rely heavily on the

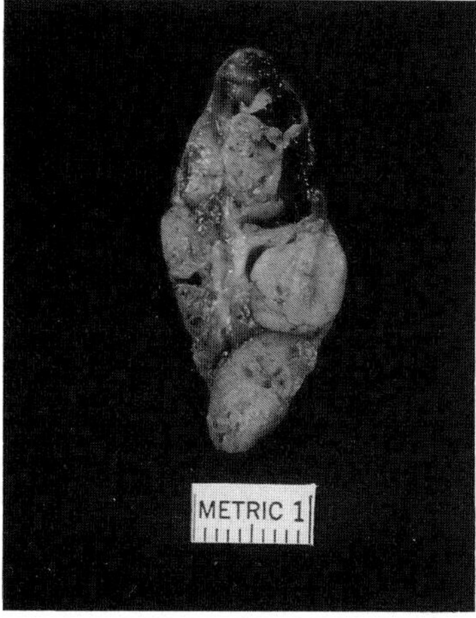
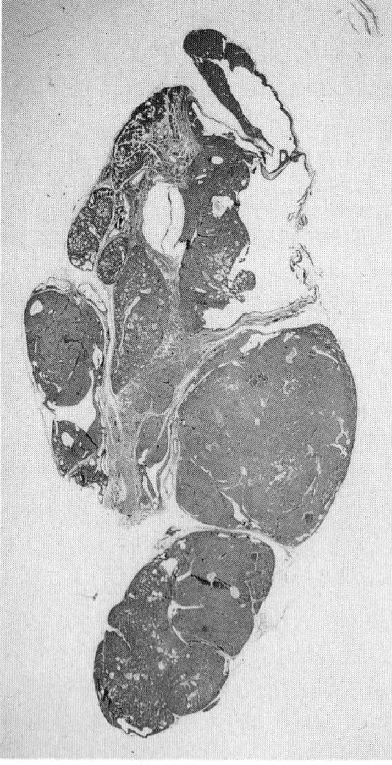

FIG. 2.3.   Parathyroid adenoma simulating chief-cell hyperplasia. Parathyroid gland weighing 2.2 g with gross (*left*) and microscopic (*right*) features suggesting parathyroid chief-cell hyperplasia. The parathyroid enlargement was designated adenoma because the three remaining glands were normal in size and histologic appearance. (Reprinted by permission from Carney, J. A. Parathyroid glands. In: *Practical Surgical Pathology*, edited by Z. A. Karcioglu and A. Someren. New York, Macmillan Publishing Company, 1985.)

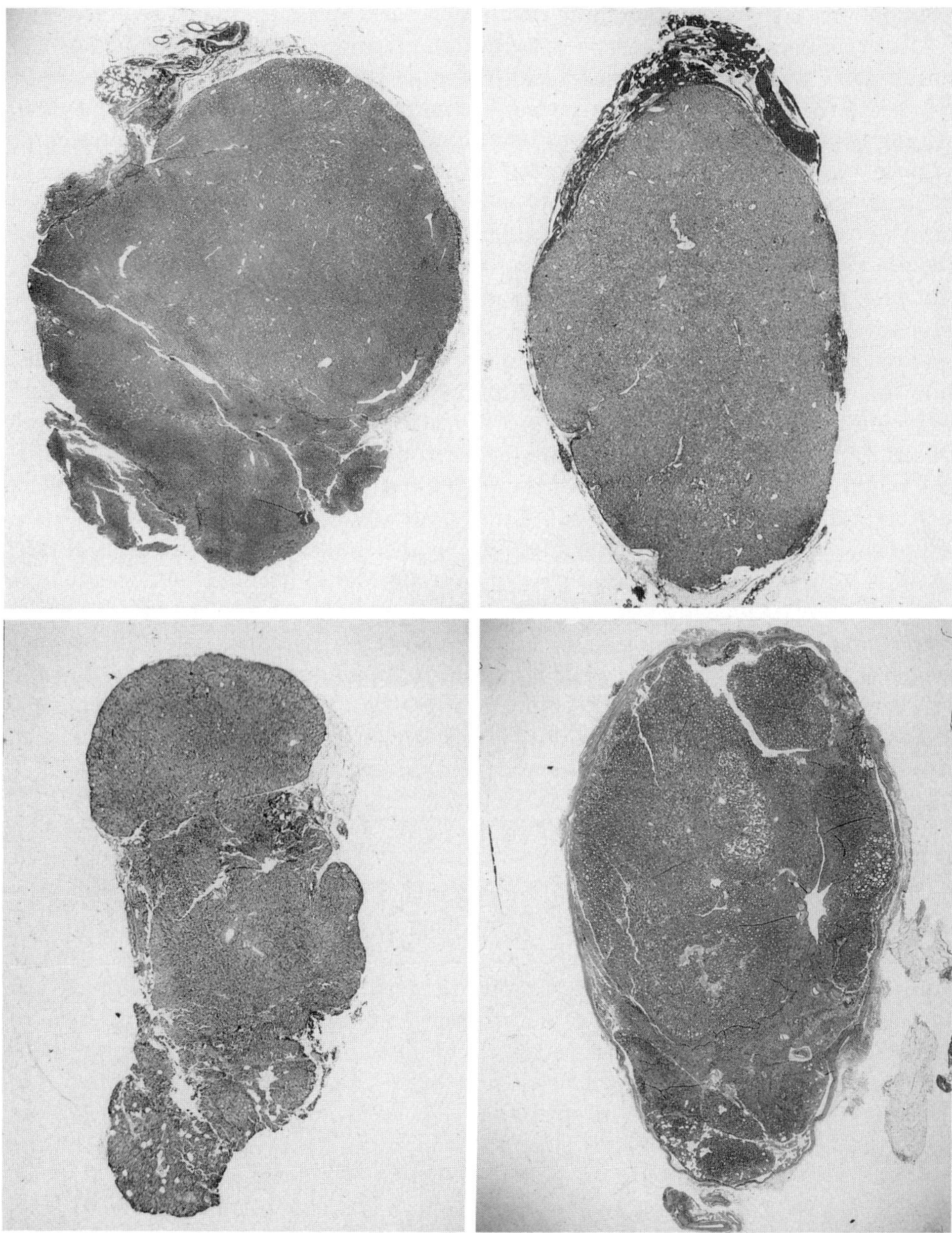

FIG. 2.4. Parathyroid chief-cell hyperplasia simulating parathyroid adenoma. Two glands (*upper right and left*) have appearances consistent with diagnosis of parathyroid adenoma: a single tumorous nodule with a rim of residual parathyroid gland (*above*). The two other glands (*lower right and left*) are slightly nodular and feature some residual fat cells (*below*). (Reprinted by permission from Carney, J. A. Parathyroid glands. In: *Practical Surgical Pathology*, edited by Z. A. Karcioglu and A. Someren. New York, Macmillan Publishing Company, 1985.)

gross operative findings in judging how much parathyroid tissue to resect.

After studying an enlarged parathyroid gland and concluding that it has the morphologic attributes of parathyroid adenoma (to be outlined), we convey our opinion to the surgeon. However, we are prepared to hear (on occasion) that one, two, or the remaining three glands are enlarged. This occurrence is infrequent because approximately 85% of cases of primary hyperparathyroidism are caused by single gland enlargement. The converse situation may occur: an enlarged parathyroid gland may appear lobulated or nodular. This suggests a diagnosis of nodular chief-cell hyperplasia, a diagnosis that becomes untenable if the surgeon indicates that the remaining three glands are normal-sized and biopsies show they are normal.

Microscopic description of an obviously enlarged parathyroid gland includes notation of whether there is a single tumor nodule devoid of mature fat cells and with cells having no cytoplasmic lipid (tentatively, adenoma) or whether there are multiple nodules, several of which may contain some mature fat cells (provisionally, hyperplasia). The condition of the parent gland, if it is present in the section, should be assessed. A semilunar-compressed parent gland with small cells that contain intracytoplasmic lipid bodies (easily seen in fresh frozen sections stained with methylene blue or toluidine blue) with a pseudocapsule or fibrous capsule separating it from the pathologic mass of parathyroid cells is good evidence that the lesion is an adenoma. But, as indicated below, the rim of the parent gland may be normal or hyperplastic in an adenoma, a fibrous capsule between the nodule and parent gland may not be present, and the tumor cells occasionally contain various amounts of intracytoplasmic lipid. If the tumor has extended through its capsule to invade surrounding fat, muscle, or thyroid, it is a carcinoma.

PARATHYROID BIOPSIES

Our assessment of a parathyroid biopsy includes: 1) accurate weighing of the specimen (if the surgeon indicates what proportion of the gland or lesion the biopsy represents, its approximate weight can be estimated), 2) microscopic confirmation that the specimen is parathyroid tissue, 3) estimation of the parenchymal/stromal fat ratio, 4) notation of a nodular parenchymal pattern, 5) search for the hypercalcemia-associated cytologic and histologic findings mentioned above under "Histology of the Parathyroid Glands," and 6) estimation of the approximate percentage of epithelial cells with intracytoplasmic large lipid droplets. The presence of cytoplasmic lipid droplets in the majority of the epithelial cells and a modest quantity of stromal fat suggest that the gland is normal. Conversely, parenchymal cells that have few intracytoplasmic lipid granules and that are arranged in nodules suggest that the gland is abnormal and probably hyperplastic. After a frozen section diagnosis has been made, accurately labeled specimens are immersed in 10% buffered formaldehyde for subsequent processing for permanent sections. Tissue remaining after adequate sampling of large tumors is placed on dry ice and used to produce antibodies to human PTH for radioimmunoassay purposes.

In 1978, Wang and Rieder[54] introduced the so-called "Density Test" for distinguishing between normal and abnormal parathyroid glands as an ancillary intraoperative help in diagnosis. The test is based on the finding of little or no stromal fat or intracellular fat granules in diseased parathyroid glands. Whereas normal parathyroid tissue floats in a mannitol solution with a density between 1.049 and 1.069, abnormal tissue (adenoma and hyperplasia) sinks. We have not used the test nor have we used another technique, cytologic imprints,[50] for intraoperative evaluation of parathyroid disease.

POSTOPERATIVE CORRELATION

The success or failure of surgical treatment of primary hyperparathyroidism may be gauged by measuring the serum calcium level postoperatively. Restoration of increased serum calcium to permanently normal levels (often after transient hypocalcemia, as a result of bone "hunger" for calcium) signals success of the operation. If the final pathologic assessment is parathyroid chief-cell hyperplasia, the diagnosis is discussed with the surgeon in terms of the disease possibly being associated with the multiple endocrine neoplasia syndrome or of its being familial.

In a small number of patients, the hypercalcemia persists. This may be caused by: 1) failure of the surgeon to locate a cervical or ectopically located parathyroid adenoma, 2) failure of the surgeon to remove an adequate amount of parathyroid tissue from a patient with chief-cell hyperplasia and disproportionate involvement of one gland, thus simulating adenoma, or 3) misdiagnosis of primary hyperparathyroidism in a patient with familial benign hypercalcemia, a condition that is not corrected by subtotal parathyroidectomy. Uncommonly, the serum calcium level may decrease postoperatively from a high preoperative value to a lower but still not normal one, to be followed in the ensuing months by a progressive increase to preoperative levels. These findings suggest recurrence of parathyroid carcinoma.

Among 153 patients with persistent hyperparathyroidism,[13] the cause was parathyroid adenoma that was not found at the first operation in 60%, parathyroid hyperplasia in 32%, parathyroid carcinoma in 3%, and nonparathyroid causes in 5%. True recurrent hyperparathyroidism is much less common than persistent hyperparathyroidism. Criteria[38] that have been proposed to identify such cases include: 1) histologic identification by biopsy of all parathyroid glands at the first operation, 2) total removal of the enlarged gland(s), 3) normocalcemia for at least 1 year postoperatively, and 4) finding of tumor at reoperation at the site of a previously normal-sized gland.

Transplanted parathyroid tissue rarely proliferates and hyperfunctions to cause recurrent hyperparathyroidism. In an exceptional case, tissue that in retrospect was identified as parathyroid carcinoma was transplanted to the forearm and subsequently metastasized to an axillary lymph node (C. S. Feind, personal communication).

PATHOLOGY OF HYPERPARATHYROIDISM

PRIMARY HYPERPARATHYROIDISM

PARATHYROID ADENOMA

Parathyroid adenoma is the most common cause of primary hyperparathyroidism and accounts for 80–85% of cases.[17,40] Recent studies using techniques of molecular biology[4,5] have indicated that parathyroid adenomas are true neoplasms; this is in contrast to earlier studies[6] that suggested a polyclonal origin for these lesions. At operation, one parathyroid gland is enlarged and the remaining three glands are normal-sized. Hyperparathyroidism due to single gland enlargement (adenoma) is almost always cured by removal of the enlarged gland. Among 198 patients with primary hyperparathyroidism thus treated at the Mayo Clinic, the serum calcium level was restored to normal in 196.[45] The neoplasm commonly weighs from 200 to 1000 mg, but the range may be from as little as 60 mg to 10 g or more. Grossly, the tumor is discrete, oval or pear-shaped or slightly lobulated and often slightly flattened (Fig. 2.5). The external surface is smooth, glistening, and light tan to brown in color, and there is a thin transparent capsule. It has a soft, flaccid consistency. The cut surface is solid and homogeneous, tan or brown in color, and commonly features cysts (single or multiple) that contain a clear or brownish fluid. Occasionally, there is focal calcification in the tumor or its capsule.

A variable histology is characteristic, both within a single tumor and from case to case. A parathyroid adenoma may show any of the following microscopic appearances: 1) a single compact nodule without stromal and cytoplasmic fat and with or without an atrophic, normal, or hyperplastic rim of parathyroid gland (Fig. 2.6), 2) multiple compact nodules with or without fatty stroma and without residual normal gland, and 3) no nodule but diffuse enlargement with some residual fatty stroma or a fibrous stroma. The tumors vary in cellular composition, ranging from masses of light and dark chief cells, small water-clear cells, small and large oxyphilic cells, or mixtures of these cell types (Fig. 2.7). Occasionally, columnar cells are present and rarely a tumor is composed of water-clear cells. Adenomas featuring spindle cells are rare. The low-power microscopic appearance is one of sheets of small polygonal cells with central pyknotic nuclei and distinct

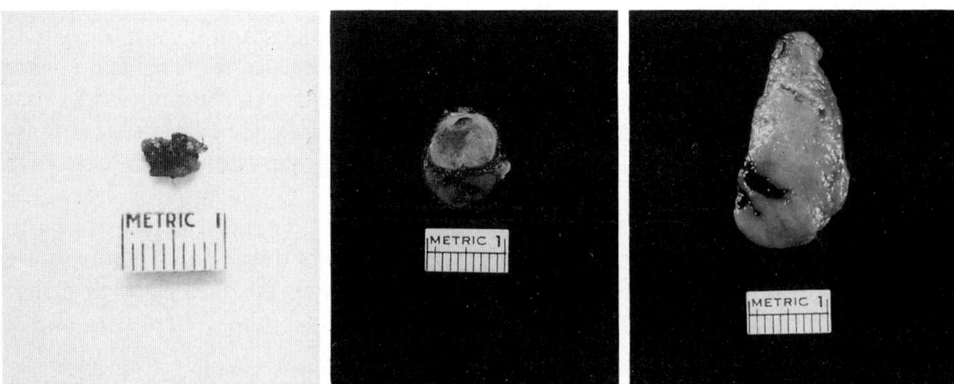

FIG. 2.5.   Variable gross appearance of parathyroid adenoma. *Left,* nondescript parathyroid lesion (54 mg). *Center,* tumor (550 mg) composed of juxtaposed spherical and semilunar masses. *Right,* homogeneous tan-colored tumor (1.54 g) with a zone of hemorrhage (*below*) and fine nodularity (*above*). (Reprinted by permission from Carney, J. A. Parathyroid glands. In: *Practical Surgical Pathology,* edited by Z. A. Karcioglu and S. Someren. New York, Macmillan Publishing Company, 1985.)

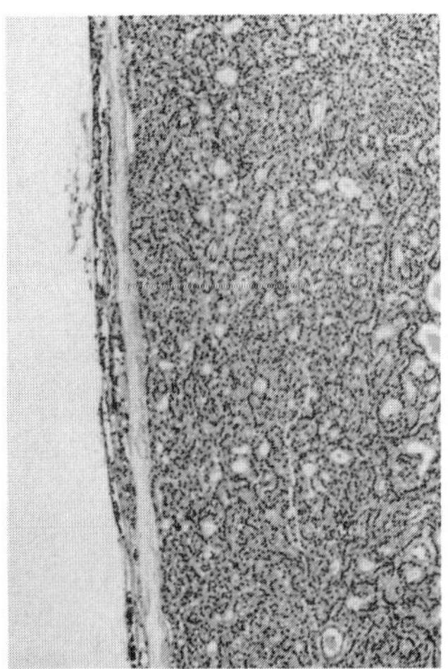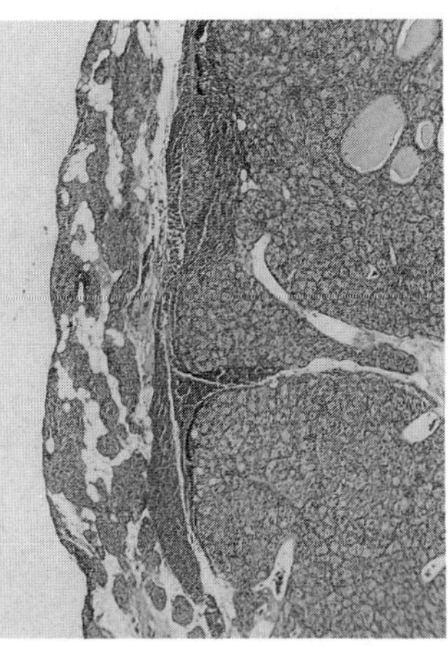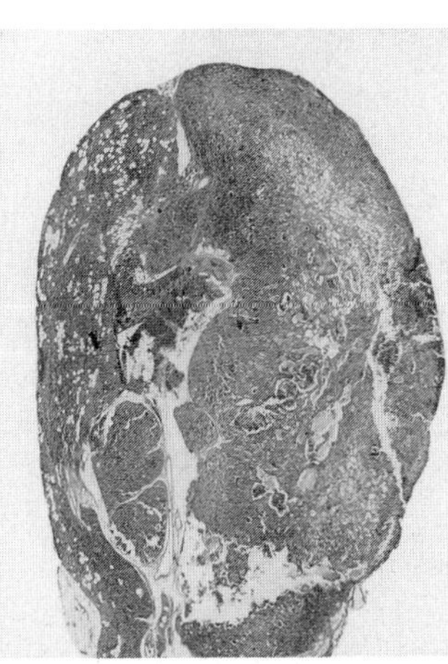

FIG. 2.6.   Range of appearance of rim of parathyroid gland associated with parathyroid adenoma. *Left,* thin compressed rim. *Center,* rim with approximately normal parenchymal/stromal fat ratio. *Right,* rim with cellular appearance. (Reprinted by permission from Carney, J. A. Parathyroid glands. In: *Practical Surgical Pathology,* edited by Z. A. Karcioglu and A. Someren. New York, Macmillan Publishing Company, 1985.)

cell membranes. The intracytoplasmic lipid granules seen in normal chief cells generally are absent from the chief cells in parathyroid adenoma; if present, they are smaller than normal. Mitoses are infrequent and the nucleoli usually are not prominent.

Diffuse, trabecular, perivascular, and acinar patterns may be encountered (Fig. 2.8). Acini may contain colloid-like material and, thus, mimic the appearance of thyroid microfollicular adenoma. It may be difficult to distinguish between the latter and a parathyroid adenoma, particularly in frozen sections. The presence of unequivocal normal thyroid tissue at the periphery of the tumor, central degeneration and edema, calcification, thick-walled blood vessels, thick fibrous capsule, and immunocytochemical demonstration of thyroglobulin are indicative of thyroid neoplasm. A parathyroid origin is suggested by the presence of occasional typical parathyroid intracytoplasmic lipid bodies, cytoplasmic periodic acid-Schiff positivity (glycogen), nuclear pleomorphism, and immunoperoxidase positivity for PTH.

A distinct capsule separating the tumor from the residual gland is not usual but may be present. Large intracytoplasmic lipid droplets seen with fat stains (better morphologic detail is seen in fresh frozen sections stained with methylene blue or toluidine blue) are conspicuous in the rim of residual gland (Fig. 2.9). A few adult fat cells are occasionally present focally in the stroma of the tumor. Rarely, myxoid alteration of the stroma may be prominent. Small lymphocyte accumulations sometimes occur.

Degenerative changes are common. Smudged, giant, and atypical nuclei unaccompanied by appreciable mitotic activity are characteristic of parathyroid adenoma (especially the oxyphilic type) (Fig. 2.10). Cyst formation is frequent.

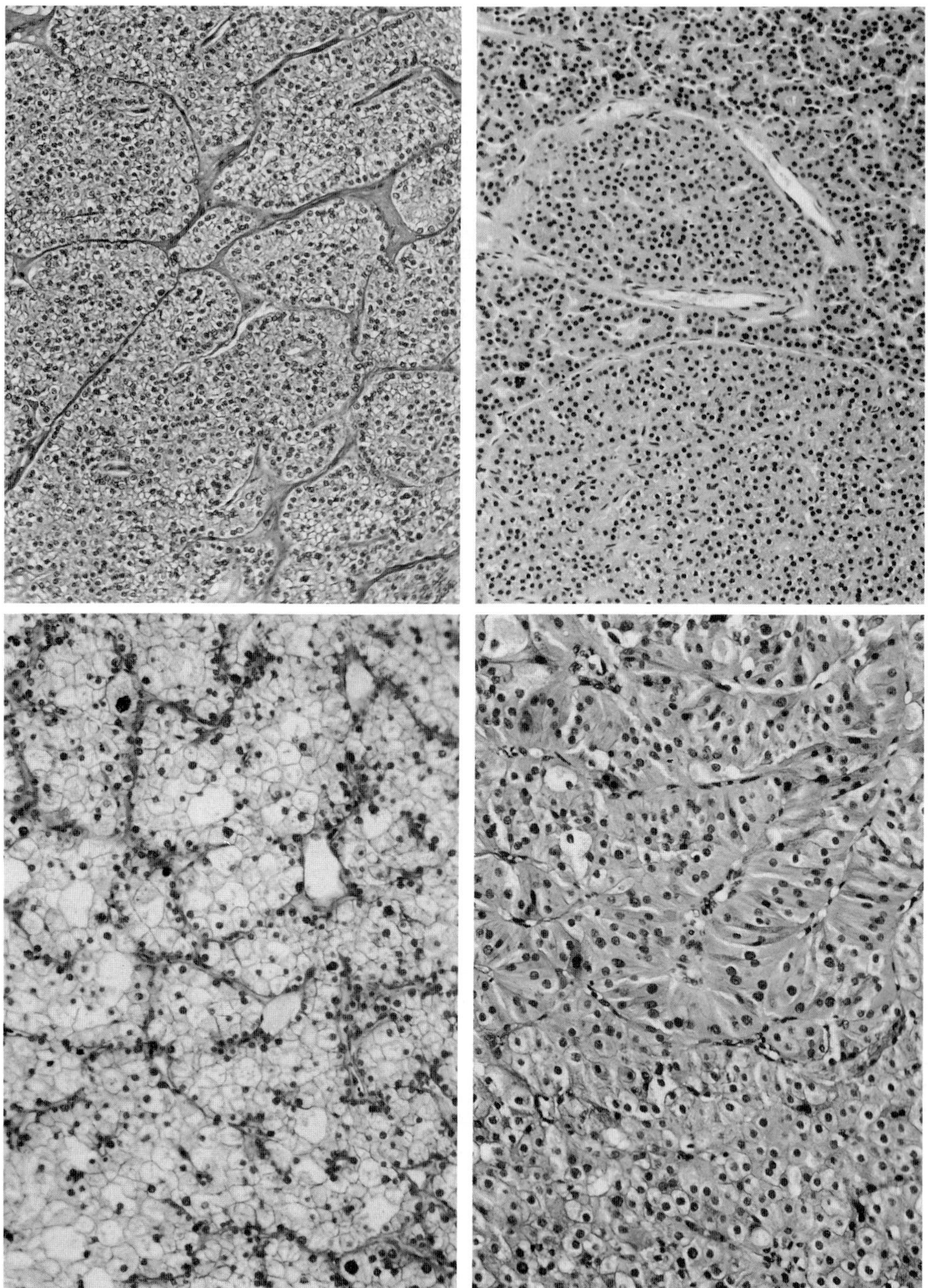

Fig. 2.7. Variable cellular composition of parathyroid adenoma. *Upper left,* light chief cells arranged in irregular masses and clusters supported by a scanty hyalinized fibrous tissue stroma. *Upper right,* zones of transitional oxyphil cells (*left and center*) and small oxyphil cells (*right*). *Lower left,* cells with clear cytoplasm, well-defined cytoplasmic membranes, and nuclei oriented toward the vascular pole of the cells are arranged in clusters supported by a scanty vascularized stroma. *Lower right,* sheet of oxyphilic cells, transitional oxyphils (*left*), and elongated oxyphil cells (*right*). (Reprinted by permission from Carney, J. A. Parathyroid glands. In: *Practical Surgical Pathology,* edited by Z. A. Karcioglu and A. Someren. New York, Macmillan Publishing Company, 1985.)

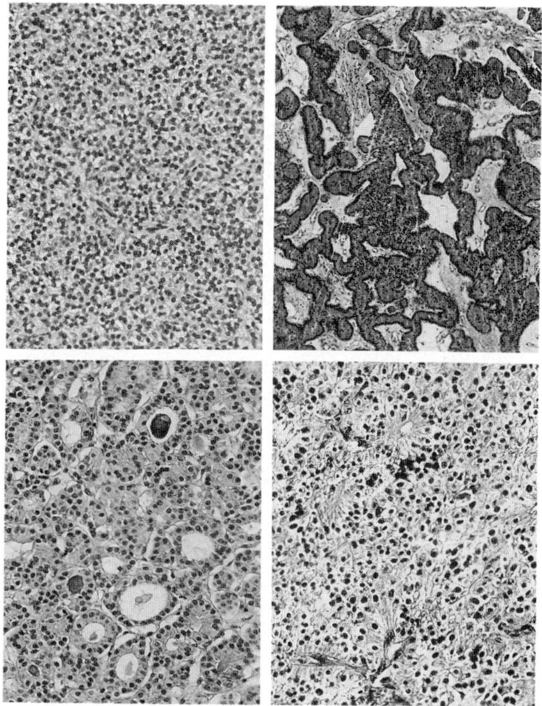

FIG. 2.8.   Different histologic patterns in parathyroid adenoma. *Upper left,* monotonous-appearing sheet of chief cells. *Upper right,* anastomosing trabecular pattern of oxyphil cells with peripherally palisaded nuclei. *Lower left,* cells forming acini (follicles) that contain thick, acidophilic colloid-like material. *Lower right,* tumor cells arranged in rosette-like pattern. (Reprinted by permission from Carney, J. A. Parathyroid glands. In: *Practical Surgical Pathology,* edited by Z. A. Karcioglu and A. Someren. New York, Macmillan Publishing Company, 1985.)

Hemorrhage and subsequent scarring may result in the development of a thick fibrous capsule, sometimes with entrapment of tumor cells. This appearance should not be interpreted as carcinomatous invasion of the capsule. Dystrophic calcification and cholesterol granulomas may be present in the capsule and tumor, respectively.

As a result of the long migration of the parathyroid gland during its development, parathyroid tumors may be found ectopically, most commonly in the anterior mediastinum in association with the thymus. These tumors can usually be retrieved by extraction of the thymus from the mediastinum during cervical exploration. Splitting the sternum for a formal mediastinal exploration is necessary in less than 2% of cases. To qualify for the designation "intrathyroid," the parathyroid tumor should be completely surrounded by thyroid parenchyma and not be just subcapsular, that is, sandwiched between the thyroid capsule and thyroid parenchyma.

Rare cases of multiple parathyroid adenomas have been reported.[7,30] Long-term follow-up of such cases with more than one and less than four enlarged parathyroid glands is necessary to be sure that they are not examples of chief-cell hyperplasia with uneven enlargement of the glands.

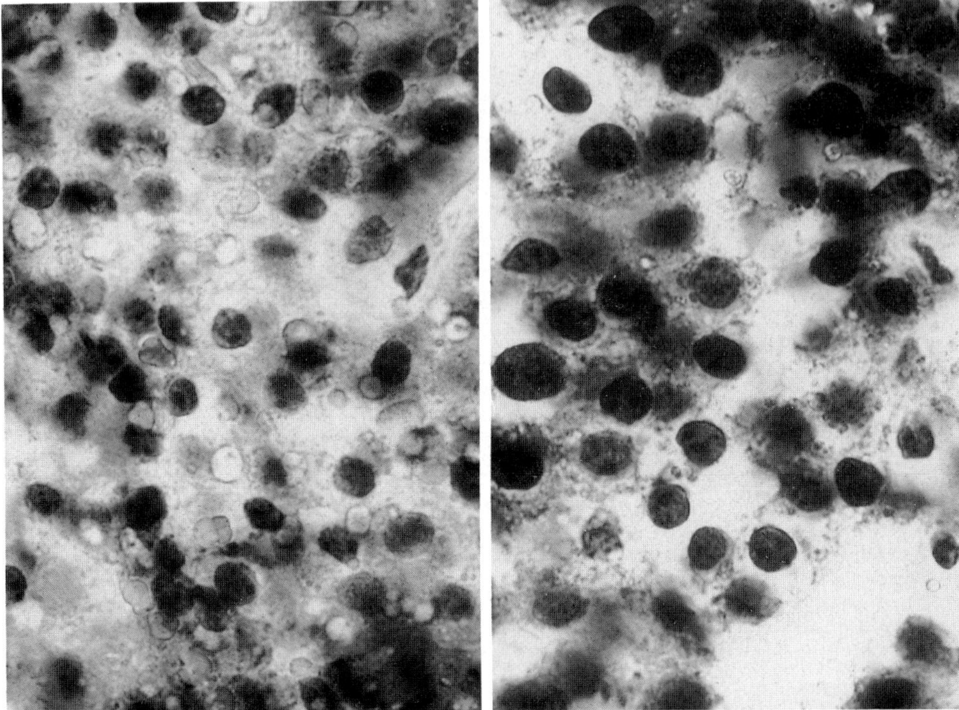

FIG. 2.9.   Intracytoplasmic lipid seen on fresh frozen section examination of parathyroid adenoma. *Left,* large, spherical lipid bodies (nearly as large as the nuclei of parathyroid cells) in the residual gland at the periphery of parathyroid adenoma. *Right,* parathyroid adenoma with a few, small lipid cytoplasmic bodies. (Reprinted by permission from Carney, J. A. Parathyroid glands. In: *Practical Surgical Pathology,* edited by Z. A. Karcioglu and A. Someren. New York, Macmillan Publishing Company, 1985.)

Sporadic (nonfamilial) occurrence of parathyroid adenoma with other endocrine tumors, including papillary carcinoma of the thyroid, intestinal carcinoid, and pheochromocytoma, has been reported. Whether these findings represent true associations (*i.e.,* rare nonfamilial forms of multiple endocrine neoplasia) or random events remains to be determined. The most common association is that of parathyroid adenoma and papillary thyroid carcinoma. This association has been attributed to cervical irradiation in childhood, but the combination could be explained equally well by the finding of two relatively common disorders in anatomically contiguous locations.

Parathyroid Carcinoma

Parathyroid carcinoma is a rare cause of primary hyperparathyroidism (approximately 1% of cases).[17,52] It should be suspected when a tumor in the neck is palpable, serum calcium and PTH levels are high, or hyperparathyroidism recurs several months after initial apparent surgical cure. Parathyroid carcinoma rarely is nonfunctioning.[39]

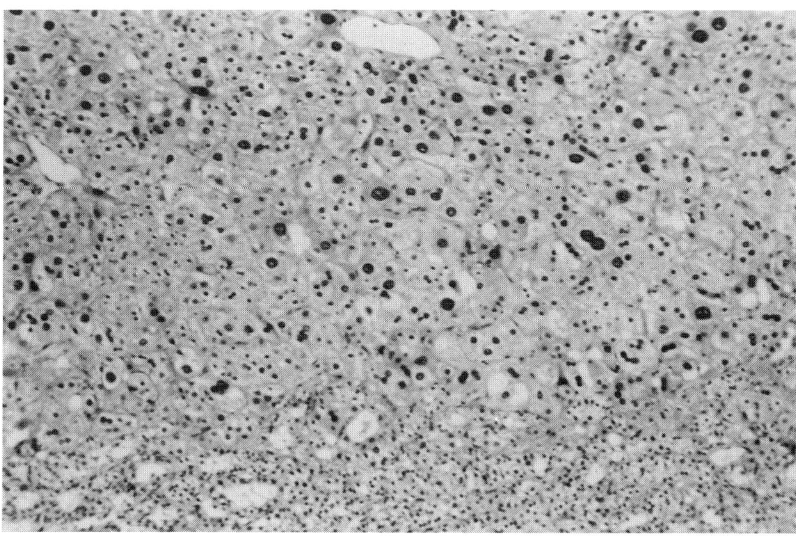

FIG. 2.10.　Parathyroid adenoma with atypical nuclei. Enlarged, hyperchromatic degenerative nuclei in oxyphil cells (*top*) contrast with the small nuclei of chief cells (*bottom*). (Reprinted by permission from Carney, J. A. Parathyroid glands. In: *Practical Surgical Pathology*, edited by Z. A. Karcioglu and A. Someren. New York, Macmillan Publishing Company, 1985.)

Usually, a large hard tumor adherent to surrounding structures is found at operation. Grossly, the ragged external surface suggests an "inflammatory" mass or invasive tumor (Fig. 2.11). A thick fibrous capsule is common, and central necrosis and calcification are sometimes present.

Microscopically, the tumor capsule of hyalinized fibrous tissue and the surrounding structures are invaded by sheets of monotonous-appearing cells that lack pleomorphism but often have prominent nucleoli or, rarely, by masses of mitotically active anaplastic cells. Wide hyalinized fibrous septa that extend from the capsule into the tumor and separate it into cell masses of various sizes are common. Mitotic figures usually are not numerous (Fig. 2.11). Metastasis occurs to lung, liver, bone, and cervical lymph nodes. Five-year survival is approximately 30%. Death usually results from ventricular fibrillation caused by uncontrolled hypercalcemia, not from the burden of tumor metastasis.

Measurement of nuclear DNA content by flow cytometry and cell cycle analysis has been useful in predicting patient survival and the malignant potential of many neoplasms. The technique has been applied to study of parathyroid lesions,[12,29,33] but the results have been inconclusive. Most studies report that normal parathyroid cells are diploid. Among the neoplasms, approximately 70% of carcinomas are aneuploid or tetraploid and the remainder are diploid; approximately 70% of adenomas are diploid and the remainder are aneuploid or tetraploid. About 30% of glands showing primary chief cell and secondary hyperplasia are aneuploid. Thus, DNA aneuploidy or tetraploidy may be present in many parathyroid abnormalities. The results indicate that flow cytometric

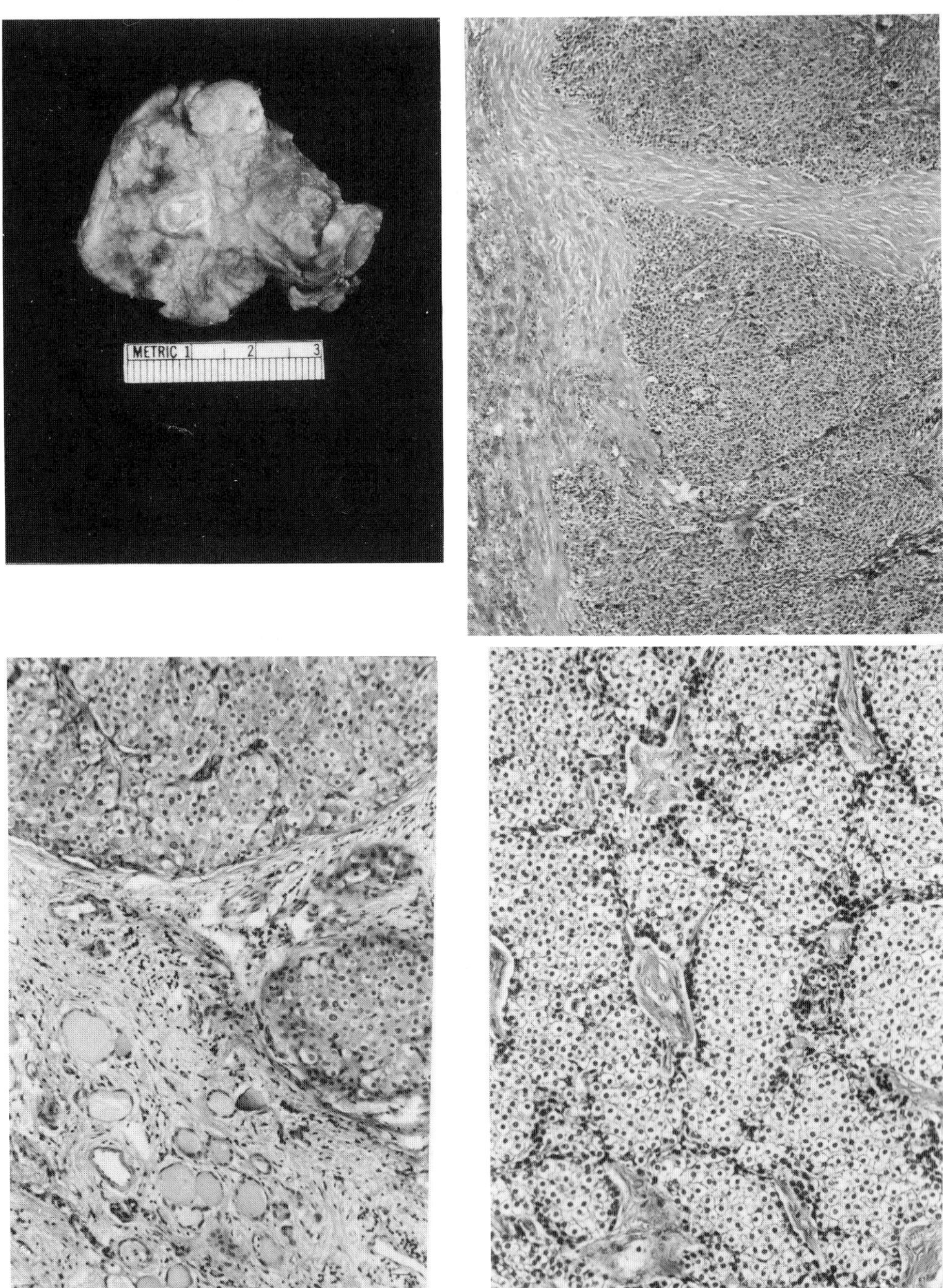

Fig. 2.11. Parathyroid carcinoma. *Upper left,* irregular mass of parathyroid carcinoma with central necrosis. *Upper right,* thick fibrous septa subdivide a sheet of tumor cells. *Lower left,* population of well-differentiated carcinoma cells in organoid and vaguely trabecular patterns. *Lower right,* invasion of thyroid by parathyroid carcinoma. (*Upper left and lower right* from van Heerden, J. A., Weiland, L. H., ReMine, W. H., Walls, J. T., and Purnell, D. C. Cancer of the parathyroid glands. *Arch. Surg. 114:*475–480, 1979. Copyright ©1979, American Medical Association. Used by permission of Mayo Foundation.) (*Upper right and lower left* reprinted by permission from Carney, J. A. Parathyroid glands. In: *Practical Surgical Pathology,* edited by Z. A. Karcioglu and A. Someren. New York, Macmillan Publishing Company, 1985.)

analysis of nuclear DNA in parathyroid lesions is of little diagnostic use in individual cases.

PARATHYROID LIPOADENOMA

Parathyroid lipoadenoma (parathyroid hamartoma) is rarely a cause of hyperparathyroidism.[17,55] The tumor may weigh 1 to 10 g or more. Grossly, it is circumscribed and encapsulated. The cut surface is homogeneous, yellow, and sometimes lobulated (Fig. 2.12). Microscopically, a mixture of parenchymal cells and mature fat cells is apparent, and the latter account for 20–90% of the tumor area (Fig. 2.12). Many areas have an appearance that is indistinguishable from that of normal parathyroid gland. Parenchymal cells are usually the chief cell type, but they vary. The lesion reportedly has occurred outside the neck.

CHIEF-CELL HYPERPLASIA

Chief-cell hyperplasia is the cause of about 10% of the cases of hyperparathyroidism.[17,19] The disorder is treated by subtotal parathyroidectomy (resection of three and one-half glands) or by total parathyroidectomy with autotransplantation of a portion of one gland. All four glands are enlarged, about equally in half the cases (Fig. 2.13). The upper glands are often enlarged to a greater degree

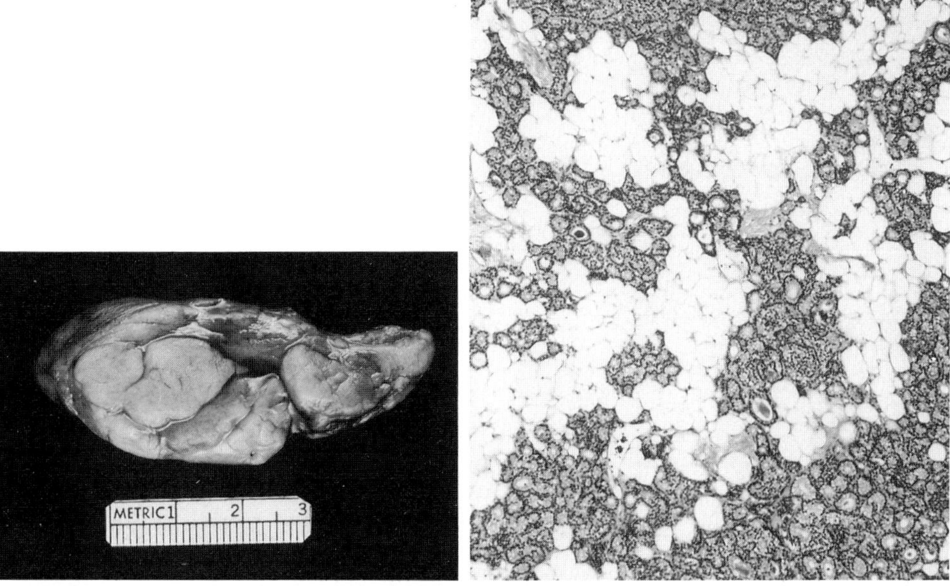

FIG. 2.12. Parathyroid lipoadenoma. *Left,* circumscribed tumor with a smooth external surface and a coarsely lobulated yellow cut surface. *Right,* equal proportions of parenchyma and adipose tissue simulate appearance of normal parathyroid gland. (Reprinted by permission from Weiland, L. H., Garrison, R. C., and ReMine, W. H. Lipoadenoma of the parathyroid gland. *Am. J. Surg. Pathol.* 2:3–7, 1978.)

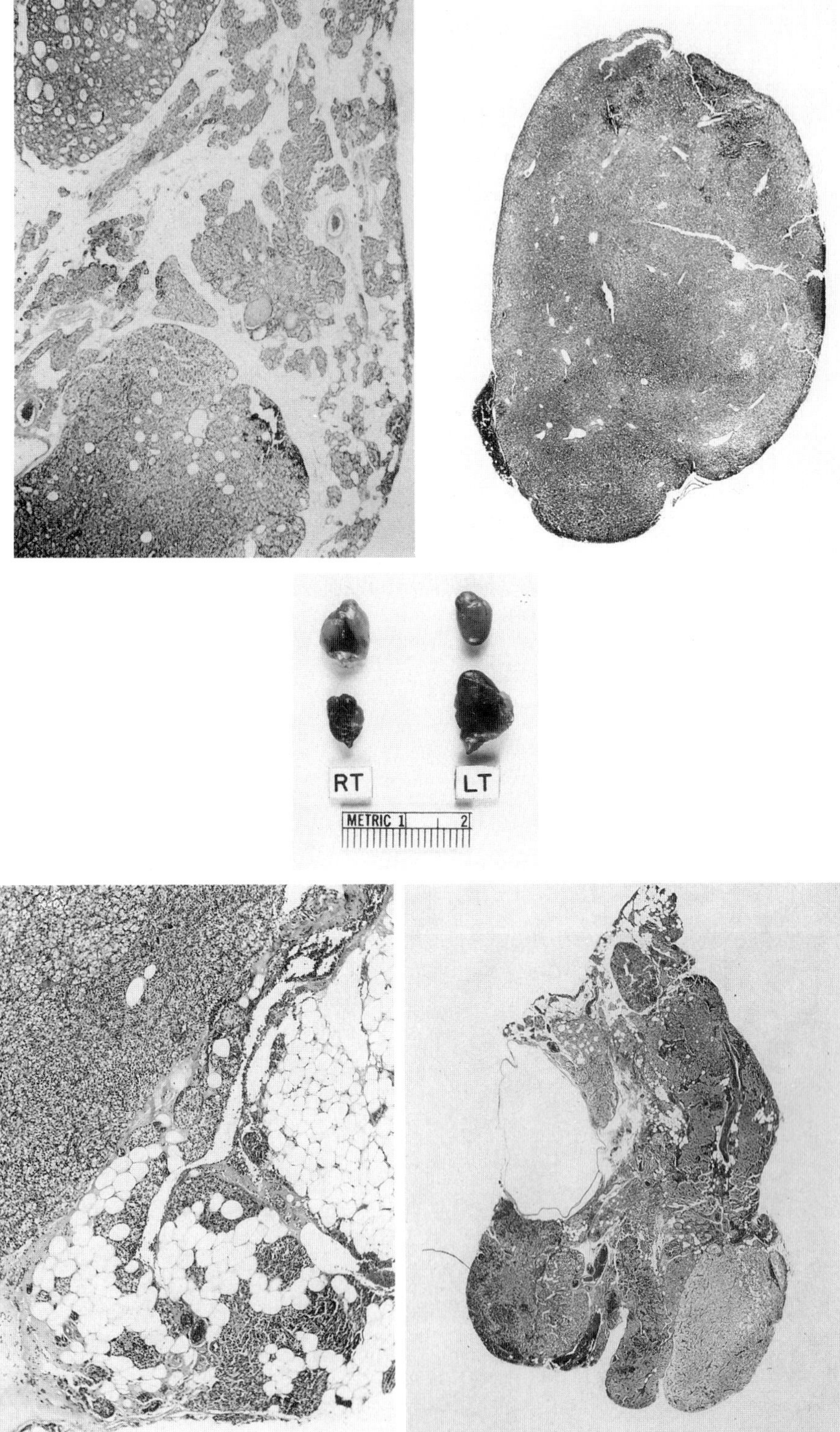

FIG. 2.13. Parathyroid chief-cell hyperplasia. *Center,* gross appearance of enlarged right superior (subtotally resected), right inferior, left superior, and left inferior glands that weighed 220, 100, 130, and 370 mg, respectively. *Upper left,* nodular arrangement of cells with acinar pattern and residual paraparathyroid gland at left. *Upper right,* solid proliferation of cells without nodules. *Lower left,* enlarged parathyroid gland featuring multiple nodules and a cyst. *Lower right,* residual parathyroid gland (*bottom and left*) abutting a nodule of hyperlastic parathyroid cells. (Reprinted by permission from Carney, J. A. Parathyroid glands. In: *Practical Surgical Pathology,* edited by Z. A. Karcioglu and A. Someren. New York, Macmillan Publishing Company, 1985.)

than the lower ones, although the difference is not as prominent as in cases of water-clear cell hyperplasia. The glands appear smooth, shiny, and tan to reddish-brown in color. Commonly, they exhibit nodularity of the external surface or the cut surface or both. However, this appearance cannot be relied on to distinguish a parathyroid gland that is hyperplastic from one that contains an adenoma. Single or multiple fluid-filled cysts are frequently present. The total weight of hyperplastic parathyroid glands is from 150 mg to 10 g or more.

In the full-blown case of chief-cell hyperplasia, sheets, cords, or acinar arrangements of cells almost completely replace the stromal fat cells. The predominant cell is a small (6–8 μ) or large (10 μ) chief cell that is disposed in nodules of various size, suggesting multiple foci of growth rather than a single focus. Large tumorlike masses with some residual fat cells may replace one or several glands. A mixture of cell types—chief, pale oxyphilic, and transitional oxyphilic—is commonly present. The cells usually lack the large intracytoplasmic lipid granule seen in normal chief cells. Fat cells are present in 40% of the glands. It is only when the gland is grossly enlarged (increased in mass) and cytoplasmic lipid in the chief cells is reduced that decreased amounts of stromal fat are additional evidence of hyperplasia.[21]

Early involvement of a gland may be evidenced by small scattered islands or nodules of hyperplastic cells in a gland with an otherwise normal parenchymal stromal fat relationship (nodular hyperplasia) or a diffuse non-nodular increase in parenchymal cells (diffuse hyperplasia). Both patterns may be seen in normal-sized glands or slightly enlarged glands. Because the parenchymal/stromal fat ratio in the parathyroid glands of some older normal patients may be as high as 90:10, it is not justified to make a diagnosis of early hyperplasia on the basis of low stromal fat content in a gland of normal weight. The chronic parathyroiditis that rarely is associated with parathyroid hyperplasia has been interpreted as an autoimmune phenomenon.[11]

Parathyromatosis is a very rare condition that is characterized by the presence of multiple nodules of hyperfunctioning parathyroid tissue scattered throughout the lower neck and upper mediastinum. It usually occurs after rupture and spillage of a parathyroid adenoma[46] or after deliberate transplantation of parathyroid tissue in cases of primary and secondary hyperparathyroidism.[26,40,47] However, it has been found at primary operation to accompany chief-cell hyperplasia.[40] Some have thought that the condition represents spread of low-grade carcinoma.

WATER-CLEAR CELL HYPERPLASIA

Water-clear cell hyperplasia (wasserhelle-cell hyperplasia)[2,17] was seen occasionally until the 1950s but is rarely, if ever, encountered today. It was usual for all four glands to be enlarged. Typically, they were bulky and often symmetrically enlarged on the right and left sides, but upper and lower glands were not enlarged equally (Fig. 2.14). The total mass of tissue resected usually exceeded 3 g. The chocolate-colored glands occasionally exhibited smooth pseudopodium-like extensions. Cystic degeneration was common.

Characteristically, the glands were composed of very large cells (larger than

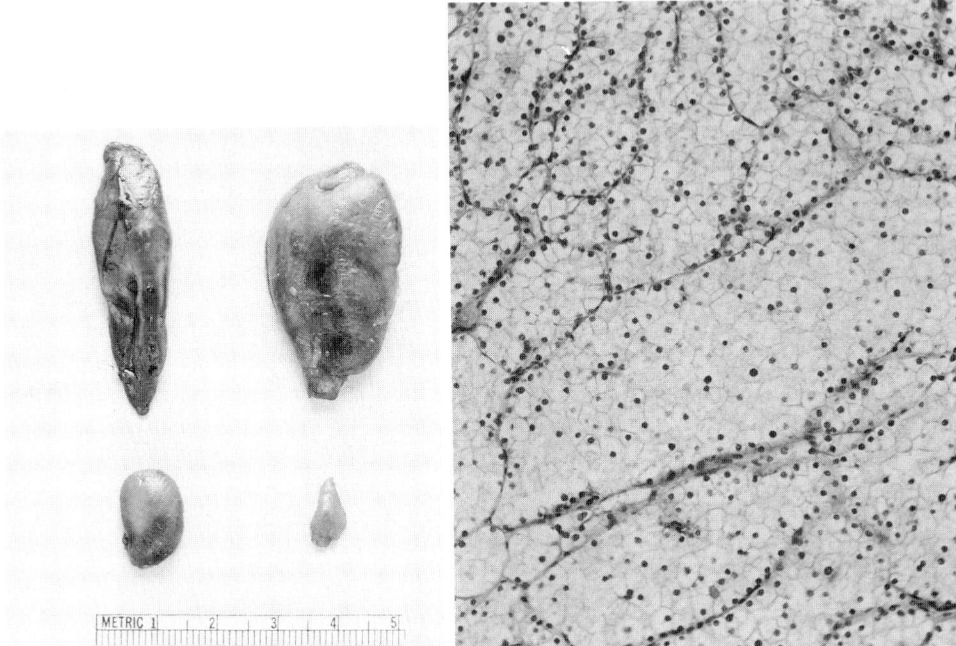

FIG. 2.14.   Clear-cell (wasserhelle-cell) hyperplasia. *Left,* chocolate-colored glands with smooth external surface that weight from 100 mg to 6.5 g. *Right,* large cells with clear cytoplasm and basally oriented nuclei. The cells are arranged in clusters separated by delicate fibrovascular stroma. (Reprinted with permission from Hoehn, J. G., Beahrs, O. H., and Woolner, L. B. Unusual surgical lesions of the parathyroid gland. *Am. J. Surg. 118:*770–779, 1969.)

normal oxyphil cells) with clear cytoplasm. On close examination, the cytoplasm was finely reticular or exhibited fine eosinophilic granularity (Fig. 2.14). In approximately 10% of cases, an admixture of small cells was present. The hyperplastic cells were arranged in sheets or in an alveolar or acinar pattern with basally oriented nuclei. The resemblance of the histologic features to those of clear-cell renal carcinoma was striking. The treatment for water-clear cell hyperplasia was the same as that for chief-cell hyperplasia.

SECONDARY HYPERPARATHYROIDISM

Secondary hyperparathyroidism, a result of secondary parathyroid hyperplasia, occurs as a compensatory response to hypocalcemia (and possibly to other factors) in cases of chronic renal glomerular failure and severe chronic intestinal malabsorption.[16] The differential diagnosis between primary and secondary chief-cell hyperplasia often cannot be made with certainty on histologic grounds, although secondary hyperplasia tends to be more diffuse and to exhibit fewer cell types.

Grossly, secondary parathyroid hyperplasia is similar to primary chief-cell hyperplasia. All four glands are enlarged, although not always equally. Microscopically, there is a significant decrease or absence of stromal fat, with more or less complete replacement of the glands by diffuse sheets of light or partly vacuolated chief cells. The cell pattern may vary and include nodules of oxyphilic or water-clear cells.

Treatment is the same as that for primary chief cell hyperplasia.

TERTIARY HYPERPARATHYROIDISM

Tertiary hyperparathyroidism is a state of apparently autonomous parathyroid hyperfunction that develops in the presence of long-standing secondary hyperparathyroidism.[34] It is usually encountered after successful renal transplantation for chronic renal failure. The gross and microscopic features, as well as the mode of treatment, are similar to those for secondary hyperparathyroidism.

FAMILIAL HYPERPARATHYROIDISM

Familial hyperparathyroidism, transmitted as an autosomal dominant trait, may occur 1) alone, 2) with pituitary or pancreatic islet cell tumors or both (multiple endocrine neoplasia, type 1, formerly known as Wermer's syndrome), or 3) with bilateral medullary thyroid carcinoma or bilateral pheochromocytoma or both (multiple endocrine neoplasia, type 2a, formerly known as Sipple's syndrome) (Fig. 2.15).[51] The gross and microscopic appearance and the treatment for familial hyperparathyroidism are similar to those of primary chief-cell hyper-

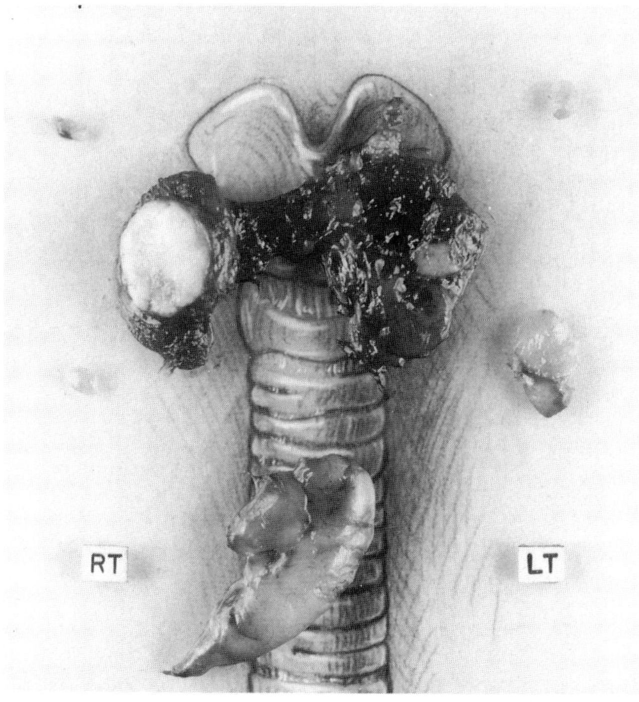

FIG. 2.15.   Multiple endocrine neoplasia, type 2a. Medullary carcinoma in mid-portion of right and left lobes of thyroid. The four parathyroid glands are enlarged, with the largest weighing 570 mg. (Reprinted by permission from Carney, J. A. Parathyroid glands. In: *Practical Surgical Pathology*, edited by Z. A. Karcioglu and A. Someren. New York, Macmillan Publishing Company, 1985.)

plasia. Rarely, familial hyperparathyroidism is caused by a solitary adenoma[32,36] and associated with ossifying fibroma of the jaw bones.

ECTOPIC HYPERPARATHYROIDISM

The clinical syndrome of nonparathyroid tumor associated with hypercalcemia, hypophosphatemia, and detectable serum PTH[43] has been referred to as "ectopic hyperparathyroidism" and "pseudohyperparathyroidism." This disorder is usually caused by malignant nonendocrine tumors, of which the two most common are squamous cell carcinoma of the lung and renal cell carcinoma.

FAMILIAL BENIGN HYPERCALCEMIA

Familial benign hypercalcemia (familial hypocalciuric hypercalcemia), a rare condition, is the cause of persistent hypercalcemia after subtotal parathyroidectomy.[35] It is characterized by an autosomal dominant pattern of inheritance, the onset of hypercalcemia in the first two decades of life, moderate hypercalcemia without hypercalciuria, a relatively greater increase of serum calcium level than PTH level, the uncommon occurrence of complications of hypercalcemia (nephrolithiasis or peptic ulcer disease), and the failure of subtotal parathyroidectomy to abolish the hypercalcemia. The pathogenetic mechanisms may include renal hypersensitivity to PTH. On gross examination, the parathyroid glands are almost invariably of normal size. Microscopically, they appear normal or mildly hyperplastic.

ACKNOWLEDGMENT

The author thanks G. B. Thompson, M.D., for review of the manuscript and his comments.

REFERENCES

1. Åkerström, G., Grimelius, L., Johannson, H., Lundqvist, H., Pertoft, H., and Bergström, R. The parenchymal cell mass in normal human parathyroid glands. *Acta Pathol. Microbiol. Scand.* [A] *89*:367–375, 1981.
2. Albright, F., Bloomberg, E., Castleman, B., and Churchill, E. D. Hyperparathyroidism due to diffuse hyperplasia of all parathyroid glands rather than adenoma of one. Clinical studies on three such cases. *Arch. Intern. Med. 54*:315–329, 1934.
3. Alveryd, A. Parathyroid glands in thyroid surgery. I. Anatomy of parathyroid glands. *Acta. Chir. Scand.* [Suppl.] *389*:1–48, 1968.
4. Arnold, A., and Kim, H. G. Clonal loss of one chromosome II in a parathyroid adenoma. *J. Clin. Endocrinol. Metab. 69*:496–499, 1989.
5. Arnold, A., Kim, H. G., Gaz, R. D., Eddy, R. R., Fukushima, Y., Beyers, M. G., Shows, T. B., and Kronenberg, H. M. Molecular cloning and chromosomal mapping of DNA rearranged with the parathyroid hormone gene in a parathyroid adenoma. *J. Clin. Invest. 83*:2034–2040, 1989.
6. Arnold, A., Staunton, C. E., Kim, H. G., Gaz, R. D., and Kronenberg, H. M. Monoclonality and abnormal parathyroid hormone genes in parathyroid adenomas. *N. Engl. J. Med. 318*:658–662, 1988.
7. Attie, J. N., Bock, G., and Auguste, L.-J. Multiple parathyroid adenomas: Report of thirty-three cases. *Surgery 108*:1014–1020, 1990.
8. Black, W. C., and Utley, J. R. The differential diagnosis of parathyroid adenoma and chief cell hyperplasia. *Am. J. Clin. Pathol. 49*:761–775, 1968.

9. Block, M. A., Frame, B., Jackson, C. E., and Horn, R. C. The extent of operation for primary hyperparathyroidism. *Arch. Surg. 109:*798–801, 1974.

10. Block, M. A., Frame, B., Jackson, C. E., and Horn, R. C. Primary diffuse microscopical hyperplasia of the parathyroid glands. Surgical importance. *Arch. Surg. 111:*348–354, 1976.

11. Bondeson, A.-G., Bondeson, L., and Ljungberg, O. Chronic parathyroiditis associated with parathyroid hyperplasia and hyperparathyroidism. *Am. J. Surg. Pathol. 8:*211–215, 1984.

12. Bowlby, I. S., DeBault, L. E., and Abraham, S. R. Flow cytometric DNA analysis of parathyroid glands. Relationship between nuclear DNA and pathologic classifications. *Am. J. Pathol. 128:*338–344, 1987.

13. Brennan, M. F., and Norton, J. A. Reoperation for persistent and recurrent hyperparathyroidism. *Ann. J. Surg. 201:*40–44, 1985.

14. Bruining, H. A. *Surgical treatment of hyperparathyroidism.* Springfield, IL, Charles C Thomas, 1971.

15. Castleman, B. Tumors of the parathyroid glands. In: *Atlas of Tumor Pathology.* Washington, DC, Armed Forces Institute of Pathology, 1952.

16. Castleman, B., and Mallory, T. B. Parathyroid hyperplasia in chronic renal insufficiency. *Am. J. Pathol. 13:*553–574, 1937.

17. Castleman, B., and Roth, S. I. Tumors of the parathyroid glands. In: *Atlas of Tumor Pathology,* Series 2, Fascicle 14. Washington, DC, Armed Forces Institute of Pathology, 1977.

18. Cope, O. The story of hyperparathyroidism at the Massachusetts General Hospital. *N. Engl. J. Med. 274:*1174–1182, 1966.

19. Cope, O., Keynes, W. M., Roth, S. I., and Castleman, B. Primary chief-cell hyperplasia of the parathyroid glands: A new entity in the surgery of hyperparathyroidism. *Ann. Surg. 148:*375–388, 1958.

20. Dekker, A., Dunsford, H. A., and Geyer, S. J. The normal parathyroid gland at autopsy: The significance of stromal fat in adult patients. *J. Pathol. 128:*127–132, 1979.

21. Dekker, A., Watson, C. G., and Barnes, E. L. The pathologic assessment of primary hyperparathyroidism and its impact on therapy. A prospective evaluation of 50 cases with oil-red-O stain. *Ann. Surg. 190:*671–675, 1979.

22. Dufour, D. R., Marx, S. J., and Spiegel, A. M. Parathyroid gland morphology in nonparathyroid hormone-mediated hypercalcemia. *Am. J. Surg. Pathol. 9:*43–51, 1985.

23. Dufour, D. R., and Wilkerson, S. Y. The normal parathyroid revisited: Percentage of stromal fat. *Hum. Pathol. 13:*717–721, 1982.

24. Dufour, D. R., and Wilkerson, S. Y. Factors related to parathyroid weight in normal persons. *Arch. Pathol. Lab. Med. 107:*107–172, 1983.

25. Esselstyn, C. B., Levin, H. S., Eversman, J. J., Schumacher, O. D., and Skillern, P. G. Reappraisal of parathyroid pathology in hyperparathyroidism. *Surg. Clin. North Am. 54:*443–447, 1974.

26. Fitko, R., Roth, S. I., Hines, J. R., Roxe, D. M., and Cahill, E. Parathyromatosis in hyperparathyroidism. *Hum. Pathol. 21:*234–237, 1990.

27. Gilmour, J. R. The embryology of the parathyroid glands, the thymus and certain associated rudiments. *J. Pathol. 45:*507–522, 1937.

28. Gilmour, J. R., and Martin, W. J. The weight of the parathyroid glands. *J. Pathol. 44:*431–462, 1937.

29. Harlow, S., Roth, S. I., Bauer, K., and Marshall, R. B. Flow cytometric DNA analysis of normal and pathologic parathyroid glands. *Mod. Pathol. 4:*310–315, 1991.

30. Harness, J. K., Ramsburg, S. R., Nishiyama, R. H., and Thompson, N. W. Multiple adenomas of the parathyroids: Do they exist? *Arch. Surg. 114:*468–474, 1979.

31. Heath, H., III, Hodgson, S. F., and Kennedy, M. A. Primary hyperparathyroidism. Incidence, morbidity, and potential economic impact in a community. *N. Engl. J. Med. 302:*189–193, 1980.

32. Jackson, C. E., Norum, R. A., Boyd, S. B., Talpos, G. B., Wilson, S. D., Taggart, T., and Mallette, I. E. Hereditary hyperparathyroidism and multiple ossifying jaw fibromas: A clinically and genetically distinct syndrome. *Surgery 108:*1006–1013, 1990.

33. Joensuu, H., and Klemi, P. J. DNA aneuploidy in adenomas of endocrine organs. *Am. J. Pathol. 132:*145–151, 1988.

34. Krause, M. W., and Hedinger, C. E. Pathologic study of parathyroid glands in tertiary hyperparathyroidism. *Hum. Pathol. 16:*772–784, 1985.

35. Law, W. M., Jr., Carney, J. A., and Heath, H., III. Parathyroid glands in familial benign hypercalcemia (familial hypocalciuric hypercalcemia). *Am. J. Med. 76:* 1021–1026, 1989.

36. Mallette, L. E., Malini, S., Rappaport, M. P., and Kirkland, J. L. Familial cystic parathyroid adenomatosis. *Ann. Intern. Med. 107:*54–60, 1987.

37. Mandl, F. Hyperparathyroidism. A review of historical developments and the present state of knowledge of the subject. *Recent Adv. Surg. 21:*394–440, 1947.

38. Muller, H. True recurrence of hyperparathyroidism: Proposed criteria of recurrence. *Br. J. Surg. 62:*556–559, 1975.

39. Ordoñez, N. G., Samaan, N. A., Ibañez, M. L., and Hickey, R. C. Immunoperoxidase study of uncommon parathyroid tumors. Report of two cases of nonfunctioning parathyroid carcinoma and one intrathyroid parathyroid tumor-producing amyloid. *Am. J. Surg. Pathol. 7:*535–542, 1983.

40. Palmer, J. A., Brown, W. A., Kerr, W. H., Rosen, I. B., and Walters, N. A. The surgical aspects of hyperparathyroidism. *Arch. Surg. 110:*1004–1007, 1975.

41. Paloyan, E., Lawrence, A. M., and Strauss, F. M. *Hyperparathyroidism.* New York, Grune & Stratton, 1973.

42. Pearse, A. G. E., and Takor, T. T. Neuroendocrine embryology and the APUD concept. *Clin. Endocrinol. (Oxf.) [Suppl] 5:*2293–2445, 1976.

43. Powell, D., Singer, F. R., Murray, T. M., Minkin, C., and Potts, J. T. Nonparathyroid humoral hypercalcemia in patients with neoplastic disease. *N. Engl. J. Med. 289:*170–181, 1973.

44. Prinz, R. A., Barbato, A. L., Braithwaite, S. S., Brooks, M. H., Emanuele, M. A., Gordon, D. L., Lawrence, A. M., and Paloyan, E. Simultaneous primary hyperparathyroidism and nodular thyroid disease. *Surgery 93:*454–458, 1982.

45. Purnell, D. C., Scholz, D. A., and Beahrs, O. H. Hyperparathyroidism due to single gland enlargement. Prospective postoperative study. *Arch. Surg. 112:*369–372, 1977.

46. Rattner, D. W., Marrone, G. C., Kasdon, E., and Silen, W. Recurrent hyperparathyroidism due to implantation of parathyroid tissue. *Am. J. Surg. 149:*745–748, 1985.

47. Reddick, R. L., Costa, J. C., and Marx, S. J. Parathyroid hyperplasia and parathyromatosis. *Lancet* (Letter) *1:*549, 1977.

48. Roth, S. I. Recent advances in parathyroid gland pathology. *Am. J. Med. 50:*612–622, 1971.

49. Roth, S. I., and Gallagher, M. J. The rapid identification of "normal" parathyroid glands by the presence of intracellular fat. *Am. J. Pathol. 84:*521–528, 1976.

50. Silverberg, S. G. Imprints in the intraoperative evaluation of parathyroid disease. *Arch. Pathol. 100:*375–378, 1975.

51. Steiner, A. L., Goodman, A. D., and Powers, A. R. Study of a kindred with pheochromocytoma, medullary thyroid carcinoma, hyperparathyroidism and Cushing's disease: Multiple endocrine neoplasia, type 2. *Medicine (Baltimore) 47:*371–409, 1968.

52. van Heerden, J. A., Weiland, L. H., ReMine, W. H., Walls, J. T., and Purnell, D. C. Cancer of the parathyroid glands. *Arch. Surg. 114:*475–480, 1979.

53. Wang, C.-A. The anatomic basis of parathyroid surgery. *Ann. Surg. 183:*271–275, 1976.

54. Wang, C.-A., and Rieder, S. V. A density test for the intraoperative differentiation of parathyroid hyperplasia from neoplasia. *Ann. Surg. 187:*63–67, 1978.

55. Weiland, L. H., Garrison, R. C., ReMine, W. H., and Scholz, D. A. Lipoadenoma of the parathyroid gland. *Am. J. Surg. Pathol. 2:*3–7, 1978.

56. Wermer, P. Genetic aspects of adenomatosis of endocrine glands. *Am. J. Med. 31:*103–166, 1954.

57. Wilder, R. M. Hyperparathyroidism: Tumor of the parathyroid glands associated with osteitis fibrosa. *Endocrinology 13:*231–244, 1929.

Chapter 3

Pathobiology of the C-Cells

STEPHEN B. BAYLIN, ANDRÉE C. DE BUSTROS,
DOUGLAS W. BALL, AND BARRY D. NELKIN

The pathobiology of the thyroid C-cells principally involves the neoplasm, medullary thyroid carcinoma (MTC), which can arise from these neuroendocrine cells on a genetic or sporadic basis. This tumor was first described in 1959[13] and has since proven to be a formidable management problem for clinicians and an object of fascination for investigators of multiple disciplines. An understanding of the evolution of MTC and related disorders depends upon basic knowledge of the embryogenesis of the C-cells, of the molecular determinants for the neuroendocrine differentiation features of these cells, and of the genetic alterations responsible for the familial forms of MTC and the progression of this tumor. In this chapter, we will review, briefly, current knowledge about each of these areas.

ORIGINS OF THE C-CELLS

The calcitonin-secreting C-cells of the thyroid gland stand as the prototype of a small polypeptide hormone-producing cell of neural crest origin. Although some controversy still exists, all data point to embryologic derivation of C-cells from neural crest elements which migrate to the developing thyroid gland during early development (for review, see Ref. 33). This origin then closely ties these cells to other peripheral neural crest derivatives such as the chromaffin cells of the adrenal medulla and ganglionic cells of the gastrointestinal tract and elsewhere. This linkage is emphasized by a disease process, the multiple endocrine neoplasia syndromes, in which simultaneous lesions of C-cells and these other peripheral neural crest-derived structures occur.

In the context of its proposed neural crest derivation, much remains to be determined about the precise neural molecular pathways which drive thyroid C-cells to reach their full neuroendocrine phenotype. It has become apparent that embryologic neural crest stem cells have a development potential which is guided by a complex interaction between a family of neurotrophic hormones and their receptors (for review, see Ref. 6). During development, these neural crest cells demonstrate considerable plasticity as evidenced by the ability of adrenal medullary precursors to manifest either chromaffin or ganglionic properties dependent upon hormonal milieu (for review, see Ref. 1). Presumably, C-cells have a similar developmental history, and it will be important to clarify which neuro-

63

prophins and receptors are most important for their development. Some of the distinct relationships between adrenal medullary and C-cells will be further apparent in the discussion of regulation of MTC differentiation to follow.

CELLULAR AND MOLECULAR ORIGINS OF MTC

It is now well established that the calcitonin-secreting cancer, MTC, has its origins in the thyroid C-cells.[41] Definition of the series of autosomal dominant genetic syndromes involving MTC has offered an unparalleled view of how a human neoplasm evolves from an initial stage of multifocal hyperplasia, through clonal evolution, to a cancer, and through progression of the cancer to varying degrees of virulence (for review, see Refs. 4 and 30). The histology of these evolving lesions is discussed in Chapter 4, and we will focus on the latest understanding of the molecular events that underlie this process.

The molecular basis for the first steps in the evolution of MTC from C-cells must be viewed in the context of the genetic forms of this cancer. Three distinct syndromes have now been described (see Table 4.1) which all involve virtually 100% penetrance of MTC, but a different spectrum of associated neural and neuroendocrine lesions. Each of these syndromes has now been genetically linked to the pericentromeric region of chromosome 10.[19,23,37] The aggregation of three related syndromes to one chromosome region raises the possibility that either multiple genes influencing peripheral neural crest development reside in this region or different genetic alterations in a single gene have somewhat different pathologic consequences.

Definition of the precise gene(s) responsible for genetic MTC, and of the dynamics relating its structural alterations to development of the tumor, has remained elusive. Mapping the immediate centromeric region of a chromosome can prove difficult with respect to using reverse genetics to delineate genes responsible for disease processes. Classic relationships between combination frequencies for markers and chromosome distances may not be operative in areas contiguous to centromeric satellite DNA. Nevertheless, due to work of several groups, a detailed map of the region harboring the MTC region is emerging. The closest flanking markers cluster in chromosome region 10q11.2 (for example, Refs. 24 and 40). Multiple DNA probes, which are tightly linked to the disease, have emerged from these studies (for example, Refs. 19 and 40). Many of these are already proving useful for accurate prediction of gene carriers in kindreds afflicted with the MTC gene.[24,38]

In terms of candidate genes for MTC which reside in the pericentromeric area of chromosome 10, only the *ret* proto-oncogene, to date, has serious credentials. This gene, located at 10q11.2 and tightly linked to genetic MTC, encodes for a membrane receptor with potential for tyrosine kinase activity.[39] It is consistently rearranged in papillary, non-MTC, forms of thyroid cancer.[10] An intriguing aspect of its potential involvement with MTC is the fact that *ret* oncogene expression, at the steady-state mRNA level, is high in human neural tumors, such as neuroblastoma, MTC, and pheochromocytoma.[35] Nevertheless, no structural alterations of the *ret* oncogene have been reported for MTC DNA, and no definitive evidence now exists for directly designating this gene as important to the origins of MTC from the C-cell.

Definition of the gene(s) for MTC may help resolve important questions about the actual contribution of initial genetic alterations to the first steps in tumor development. Classically, as originally outlined for genetic retinoblastoma,[12,18] Knudson's "two hit" hypothesis has been thought to be operative for most inherited forms of cancer. In this theory, one allelic copy of a gene contains inherited structural alterations, such as a point mutation. However, no phenotypic consequences result from this until the opposite allelic copy is lost or altered by a somatic event. This second step, for tumors such as retinoblastoma, usually manifests as an allelic loss which is detected by Southern hybridizations as a reduction to homozygosity for a polymorphic DNA restriction site.

For MTC, our group[31] and others[15,20] have found no consistent reduction to homozygosity in MTC DNA for any chromosome 10 probes tested to date. As we have previously outlined,[31] this finding raises the possibility that disruption of a single allele of the MTC gene by a germline event may be sufficient to initiate the first stage of genetic MTC, C-cell hyperplasia. Subsequent evolution of a clonal tumor may then result from a second genetic event, possibly involving another chromosome. To date, the other candidate locus that has emerged is the short arm of chromosome 1. This region is known to show allelic reduction to homozygosity in MTC DNA[15,25,26] and very consistently in DNA from pheochromocytomas of patients with genetic MTC.[26]

Alternatively, genetic MTC is initiated by alterations of two allelic copies of a gene on chromosome 10, but the second somatic event is not visible in routine searches for locus reduction to homozygosity. Very small deletions or point mutations in the allele opposite to that bearing the initial germline defect would not be detectable by these strategies. Such genetic abnormalities may only be resolved when the actual gene(s) for MTC has been isolated.

CELLULAR AND MOLECULAR DETERMINANTS OF PROGRESSION FOR MTC: RELATIONSHIPS TO NEUROENDOCRINE DIFFERENTIATION

Studies of patients with all stages of genetic MTC have allowed mapping of biochemical characteristics of MTC cells at different points in tumor progression (for review, see Ref. 4). The findings have facilitated the development of model systems for MTC to relate changes observed in tumor progression to molecular determinants of neuroendocrine cell maturation. As we have reviewed in the past,[30] the progressive virulence of MTC is associated with loss of, or diminution in, the capacity of the tumor cells to synthesize and/or store calcitonin (CT). This results in a heterogeneous cell distribution for CT content in tumors from patients who die from MTC (for review, see Refs. 4 and 30). We have characterized a cell culture model for MTC which manifests this heterogeneous CT pattern.[5] Studies in this model have revealed a complex interaction between growth of the cells,[28] the signal transduction events which may guide differentiation of normal and neoplastic C-cells, and regulation of CT gene expression (Fig. 3.1). Understanding the molecular steps entailed may teach us much about the normal regulation of neural crest-derived endocrine cells, as well as the abnormalities responsible for multiple stages of MTC progression.

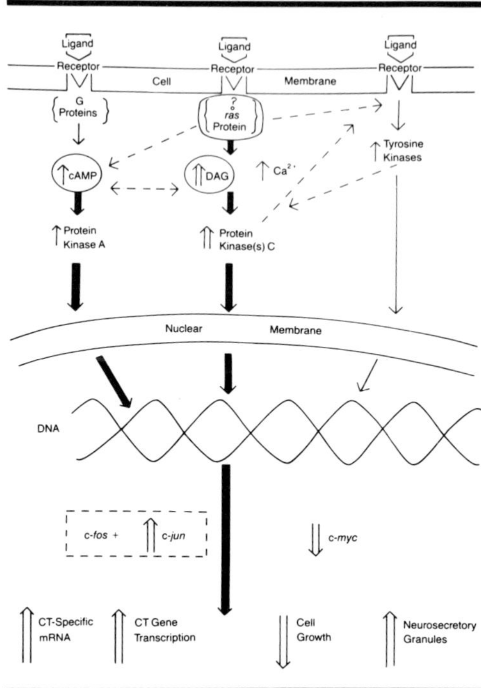

FIG. 3.1. Signal transduction in MTC cells. Three of the major pathways for signal transduction from cell membrane receptors to the nucleus are portrayed schematically. In the protein kinase A system, binding of a ligand to its cell membrane receptor results in activation of a G protein complex. This, in turn, activates adenylate cyclase, increasing intracellular cAMP, which in turn activates protein kinase A. Protein kinase A phosphorylates specific proteins, some of which result in changes in gene expression. In the protein kinase C pathway, ligand binding to a receptor activates a pathway of phosphoinositide breakdown, resulting in activation of protein kinase C by generation of diacylglycerol (DAG). Protein phosphorylation via the protein kinase C pathway can result in changes in gene expression; some of these changes are dependent on nuclear transcription factors c-*jun*/AP-1 and AP-2. *Question mark* indicates that *ras* function at this step in the pathway has not been conclusively determined. In the tyrosine kinase system, it is not yet established which nuclear transcription factors are responsible for the change in gene expression observed. *Dashed lines* indicate that there is evidence for cross-communication among these pathways, *downward arrows* show direction of pathways, and *solid thick arrows* indicate pathways we have shown to differentiate MTC cells. The potential for the tyrosine kinase pathway to induce MTC cell differentiation is suggested by the fact that activation of the *src* tyrosine kinase pathway has been shown to drive the differentiation of the closely related PC12 pheochromocytoma cell line. *CT* indicates calcitonin; *upward thick arrows*, steps activated in each pathway; *circles*, steps in these pathways modulated in MTC cells; *hollow thick arrows*, changes measured at the time of differentiation of MTC cells as reported herein. (Reprinted by permission from Nelkin, B. D., de Bustros, A. C., Mabry, M., and Baylin, S. B. The molecular biology of medullary thyroid carcinoma: A model for cancer development and progression. *JAMA 261*:3130–3135, 1989. Copyright 1989, American Medical Association.)

Our findings, to date, may be briefly summarized as follows (see also Fig. 3.1). Stimulation in cultured MTC cells of signal transduction pathways, including those mediated by protein kinases A and C, results in increased transcription of the CT gene.[7-9] An event which appears to coordinate these pathways, and results in potent differentiation of cultured MTC cells, is mimicked by insertion of the viral Harvey *ras* oncogene.[27] As shown in Fig. 3.1, this maneuver may heavily involve protein kinase C activation and eventual increase in expression of the c-*jun* oncogene.[28] Presumably, nuclear events activated downstream from increases in this general transcription factor mediate increased MTC differentiation. The differentiation includes increased CT gene transcription and restoration of the CT gene mRNA splicing pattern toward that seen in normal thyroid C-cells[27,30] (Fig. 3.1).

It is important to note that the above response of cultured MTC cells to the *ras* oncogene closely parallels responses seen in neural crest-derived rodent pheochromocytoma cells[3,11,32,36] and cultured neoplastic lung endocrine cells.[22] In the pheochromocytoma cells, the activation of *ras* gene expression seems to be an integral part of a differentiation pathway also triggered by interaction of the important neurtrophin, nerve growth factor, with its high-affinity receptor, the *trk* oncogene.[11,16,17,21] Whether this or the multiple closely related pathways mediated by the *trk* family of genes (for review, see Refs. 6 and 17) modulate differentiation of normal or neoplastic C-cells is an important question in neurobiology and for understanding of C-cell pathobiology. Culture models of MTC should help resolve these issues and could identify key molecular steps important to both normal and neoplastic neural crest differentiation.

Just as the above interactions between neurotrophic receptors and MTC differentiation may be critical to understanding C-cell pathobiology, so may elucidating the events that link activation of signal transduction to modulation of CT gene expression. We have used the MTC culture system to define regions of the CT gene which regulate both its tissue-specific basal and signal transduction-induced transcription. A complex series of interactive events between multiple DNA regulatory sequences and *cis*-acting transcription factors is being defined (Fig. 3.2). The findings can be summarized as follows.

Our group[2] and others[34] have found that tissue-specific basal transcription of the human CT gene requires a 5′ regulatory region located approximately 1 kilobase upstream from the transcription start site (Fig. 3.2). This area contains three consensus DNA motifs for recognition by the helix-loop-helix (HLH) family of transcription factors. Through a series of mutation and deletion studies, we have shown that these HLH recognition elements are required for maintenance of basal CT gene transcription.[2]

Signal transduction-induced transcription of the CT gene appears to require a series of DNA regulatory areas located within a region 130–200 base pairs upstream from the transcription start site.[9] Although characterization of this region is still in progress, consensus recognition motifs for homeodomain, cyclic adenosine monophosphate (cAMP) response elements, and a C-rich octamer all reside in the region of interest. Both cAMP- and Ha-*ras* gene-induced increases

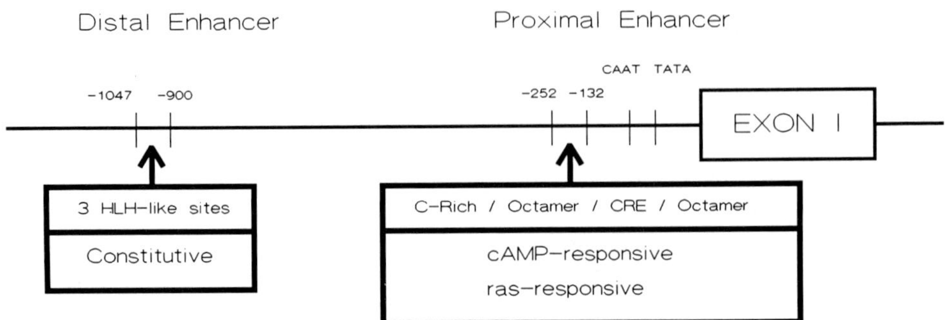

FIG. 3.2.   Schematic diagram of the 5′ regulatory region of the human CT gene. *Arrows* indicate regions discussed in the text which contain multiple DNA consensus sequences for known families of transcription factors. Each of these sites support basal or induced transcription of the CT gene in cultured human MTC cells as outlined in the *lower boxes. HLH*, helix-loop-helix; *CRE*, cAMP response element.

in CT gene transcription appear to involve interaction among these consensus motifs.

Elaboration of the specific transcription factors which interact with the above transcription regulatory areas of the CT gene could provide important information about C-cell development and the pathobiology of these cells. For example, the HLH and homeodomain transcription factors are now known to play critical roles for development of multiple cell systems, including the pituitary gland and various neural cells (for review, see Ref. 14). It is then a distinct possibility that one or more of the specific factors which interact with the CT gene could play a similar role in C-cell development. Abnormalities in structure of these genes, or in the gene products which signal their expression, could play pivotal roles in the genesis and progression of MTC.

SUMMARY

This brief review of the pathobiology of C-cells has stressed cellular and molecular aspects of MTC development. In the genetic forms of MTC, an alteration in one or more genes on chromosome 10, through an as yet unknown series of events, results in initial hyperproliferation of C-cells. Subsequent genetic steps, possibly at other chromosome loci, presumably result in selected clonal transformation of the hyperproliferative C-cells at risk for tumor development. Some of these same molecular events are probably operative in the development of sporadic MTC as well.

Once MTC has developed, it has the potential to undergo tumor progression events which result in loss of C-cell differentiation. Studies in a culture model of these events have revealed that activation of signal transduction pathways, similar to those active in differentiation of other neural crest-derived cells, can restore differentiation features of normal C-cells to MTC. Continued identification of the molecular factors mediating this restoration should teach us much about the relationships between general neural crest differentiation and that of normal C-cells. It will also reveal much about the pathobiology of C-cells contributing to each step of MTC development.

ACKNOWLEDGMENTS

Portions of cited studies were supported by National Institutes of Health Grants R01-CA47480 to B.D.N. and R01-CA49938 to A.d.B. and American Cancer Society Grant PDT-417H to S.B.B. D.W.B. is supported by Physician-Scientist Award K12-DK01298-07.

We thank our many collaborators over the years, including Drs. Geoffrey Mendelsohn, Bernie Roos, and Samuel Wells, for their contributions to the studies discussed in this review.

REFERENCES

1. Anderson, D. J. The neural crest cell lineage problem: Neuropoiesis? *Neuron 3:*1–12, 1989.
2. Ball, D. W., Compton, D., Nelkin, B. D., Baylin, S. B., and de Bustros, A. Human calcitonin gene regulation by helix-loop-helix recognition sequences. *Nucleic Acids Res. 20:*117–123, 1992.
3. Bar-Sagi, D., and Feramisco, J. R. Microinjection of the *ras* oncogene protein into PC12 cells induces morphological differentiation. *Cell 42:*841–848, 1985.
4. Baylin, S. B., and Mendelsohn, G. Medullary thyroid carcinoma: A model for the study of human tumor progression and cell heterogeneity. In: *Bristol-Myers Cancer Symposia,* Vol. 4, Tumor Cell Heterogeneity, edited by A. H. Owens, Jr., D. S. Coffey, and S. B. Baylin. Orlando, FL, Academic Press, Inc., 1982. pp. 9–27.
5. Berger, C. L., de Bustros, A., Roos, B. A., Leong, S. S., Mendelsohn, G., Gesell, M. S., and Baylin, S. B. Human medullary thyroid carcinoma in culture provides a model relating growth dynamics, endocrine cell differentiation, and tumor progression. *J. Clin. Endocrinol. Metab. 59:*338–343, 1984.
6. Bothwell, M. Keeping track of neurotrophin receptors. *Cell 65:*915–918, 1991.
7. de Bustros, A., Baylin, S. B., Berger, C. L., Roos, B. A., Leong, S. S., and Nelkin, B. D. Phorbol esters increase calcitonin gene transcription and decrease c-*myc* RNA levels in cultured human medullary thyroid carcinoma. *J. Biol. Chem. 260:*98–104, 1985.
8. de Bustros, A., Baylin, S. B., Levine, M. A., and Nelkin, B. D. Cyclic AMP and phorbol esters separately induce growth inhibition, calcitonin secretion and calcitonin gene transcription in cultured human medullary thyroid carcinoma. *J. Biol. Chem. 261:*8036–8041, 1986.
9. de Bustros, A., Lee, R. Y., Compton, D., Tsong, T. Y., Baylin, S. B., and Nelkin, B. D. Differential utilization of calcitonin gene regulatory DNA sequences in cultured lines of medullary thyroid carcinoma and small cell lung carcinoma. *Mol. Cell. Biol. 10:*1773–1778, 1990.
10. Fusco, A., Grieco, M., Santoro, M., Berlingieri, M. T., Pilotti, S., Pierotti, M. A., Della Porta, G., and Vecchio, G. A new oncogene in human thyroid papillary carcinomas and their lymph-nodal metastases. *Nature 328:*170–172, 1987.
11. Hagag, N., Halegoua, S., and Viola, M. Inhibition of growth factor-induced differentiation of PC12 cells by microinjection of antibody to ras p21. *Nature 319:*680–682, 1986.
12. Hansen, M. F., and Cavenee, W. K. Genetics of cancer predisposition. *Cancer Res. 47:*5518–5527, 1987.
13. Hazard, J. B. The C cells (parafollicular cells) of the thyroid gland and medullary thyroid carcinoma: A review. *Am. J. Pathol. 88:*214–250, 1977.
14. He, X., and Rosenfeld, M. G. Mechanisms of complex transcriptional regulation: Implications for brain development. *Neuron 7:*183–196, 1991.
15. Khosla, S., Patel, V. M., Hay, I. D., Schaid, D. J., Grant, C. S., vanHeerden, J. A., and Thibodeau, S. N. Loss of heterozygosity suggests multiple genetic alterations in pheochromocytomas and medullary thyroid carcinomas. *J. Clin. Invest. 87:*1691–1699, 1991.
16. Klein, R., Jing, S., Nanduri, V., O'Rourke, E., and Barbacid, M. The *trk* proto-oncogene encodes a receptor for nerve growth factor. *Cell 65:*189–197, 1991.

17. Klein, R., Nanduri, V., Jing, S., Lamballe, F., Tapley, P., Bryant, S., Cordon-Cardo, C., Jones, K. R., Reichardt, L. F., and Barbacid, M. The trkB tyrosine protein kinase is a receptor for brain-derived neurotrophic factor and neurotrophin-3. *Cell 66*:395–403, 1991.

18. Knudson, A. G. Hereditary cancer, oncogenes and antioncogenes. *Cancer Res. 45*:1437–1443, 1985.

19. Lairmore, T. C., Howe, J. R., Korte, J. A., Dilley, W. G., Aine, L., Aine, E., Wells, S. A., Jr., and Donis-Keller, H. Familial medullary thyroid carcinoma and multiple endocrine neoplasia type 2B map to the same region of chromcosome 10 as multiple endocrine neoplasia type 2A. *Genomics 9*:181–192, 1991.

20. Landsvater, R. M., Mathew, C. G. P., Smith, B. A., Marcus, E. M., te Meerman, G. J., Lips, C. J. M., Geerdink, R. A., Nakamura, Y., Ponder, B. A. J., and Buys, C. H. C. M. Development of multiple endocrine neoplasia type 2A does not involve substantial deletions of chromosome 10. *Genomics 4*:246–250, 1989.

21. Loeb, D. M., Maragos, J., Martin-Zanca, D., Chao, M. V., Parada, L. F., and Greene, L. A. The *trk* proto-oncogene rescues NGF responsiveness in mutant NGF-nonresponsive PC12 cell lines. *Cell 66*:961–966, 1991.

22. Mabry, M., Nakagawa, T., Baylin, S., Pettengill, O., Sorensen, G., and Nelkin, B. Introduction of the v-Ha-*ras* oncogene induces differentiation of calcitonin producing human small cell lung cancer. *J. Clin. Invest. 84*:194–199, 1989.

23. Mathew, C. G. P., Chin, K. S., Easton, D. F., Thorpe, K., Carter, C., Liou, G. I., Fong, S.-L., Bridges, C. D. B., Haak, H., Nieuwenhuijzen Kruseman, A. C., Schifer, S., Hansen, H. H., Telenius-Berg, M., and Ponder, B. A. J. A linked genetic marker for multiple endocrine neoplasia type 2A on chromosome 10. *Nature 328*:527–528, 1987.

24. Mathew, C. G. P., Easton, D. F., Nakamura, Y., and Ponder, B. A. J. The MEN2A international collaborative group. Presymptomatic screening for multiple endocrine neoplasia type 2A with linked DNA markers. *Lancet 1*:7–11, 1991.

25. Mathew, C. G. P., Smith, B. A., Thorpe, K., Wong, Z., Royle, N. J., Jeffries, A. J., and Ponder, B. A. J. Deletion of genes on chromosome 1 in endocrine neoplasia. *Nature 328*:524–526, 1987.

26. Moley, J. F., Brother, M. B., Fong, C. -T., White, P. S., Baylin, S. B., Nelkin, B., Wells, S. A., and Brodeur, G. M. Consistent association of 1p loss of heterozygosity with pheochromocytomas from patients with multiple endocrine neoplasia type 2 syndromes. *Cancer Res. 52*:770–774, 1992.

27. Nakagawa, T., Mabry, M., de Bustros, A., Ihle, J. N., Nelkin, B. D., and Baylin, S. B. Introduction of v-Ha-*ras* oncogene induces differentiation of cultured human medullary thyroid carcinoma cells. *Proc. Natl. Acad. Sci. USA 84*:5923–5927, 1987.

28. Nelkin, B. D., Borges, M., Mabry, M., and Baylin, S. B. Transcription factor levels in medullary thyroid carcinoma cells differentiated by Harvey *ras* oncogene: c-*jun* is increased. *Biochem. Biophys. Res. Commun. 170*:140–146, 1990.

29. Nelkin, B. D., Chen, K. Y., de Bustros, A., Roos, B. A., and Baylin, S. B. Changes in calcitonin gene RNA processing during growth of a human medullary thyroid carcinoma cell line. *Cancer Res. 49*:6949–6952, 1989.

30. Nelkin, B. D., de Bustros, A. C., Mabry, M., and Baylin, S. B. The molecular biology of medullary thyroid carcinoma: A model for cancer development and progression. *JAMA 261*:3130–3135, 1989.

31. Nelkin, B. D., Nakamura, Y., White, R. W., de Bustros, A. C., Herman, J., Wells, S. A., Jr., and Baylin, S. B. Low incidence of loss of chromosome 10 in sporadic and hereditary human medullary thyroid carcinoma. *Cancer Res. 49*:4114–4119, 1989.

32. Noda, M., Ko, M., Ogura, A., Liu, D., Amano, T., Takano, T., and Ikawa, Y. Sarcoma viruses carrying *ras* oncogenes induce differentiation-associated properties in a neuronal cell line. *Nature 318*:73–75, 1985.

33. Pearse, A. G. E. Common cytochemical and ultrastructural characteristics of cells producing polypeptide hormones (the APUD series) and their relevance to thyroid and ultimobranchial C-cells and calcitonin. *Proc. R. Soc. Lond. (Biol.) 170*:71–80, 1968.

34. Peleg, S., Abruzzese, R. V., Cote, G. J., and Gagel, R. F. Transcription of the human calcitonin

gene is mediated by a C-cell specific enhancer containing E-box-like elements. *Mol. Endocrinol.* 4:1750–1757, 1990.

35. Santoro, M., Rosati, R., Grieco, M., Berlingieri, M. T., D'Amato, G. L-C., de Frandiscis, V., and Fusco, A. The *ret* proto-oncogene is consistently expressed in human pheochromocytomas and thyroid medullary carcinomas. *Oncogene* 5:1595–1598, 1990.
36. Sassone-Corsi, P., Der, C. J., and Verma, I. M. Ras-induced neuronal differentiation of PC12 cells: possible involvement of fos and jun. *Mol. Cell. Biol.* 9:3174–3183, 1989.
37. Simpson, N. E., Kidd, K. K., Goodfellow, P. J., McDermid, H., Myers, S., Kidd, J. R., Jackson, C. E., Duncan, A. M. V., Farrer, L. A., Brasch, K., Castiglione, C., Genel, M., Gertner, J., Greenberg, C. R., Guserea, J. F., Holden, J. J. A., and White, B. N. Assignment of multiple endocrine neoplasia type 2A to chromosome 10 by linkage. *Nature* 328:528–530, 1987.
38. Sobol, H., Narod, S. A., Nakamura, Y., et al. Screening for multiple endocrine neoplasia type 2A with DNA-polymorphism analysis. *N. Engl. J. Med.* 321:996–1001, 1989.
39. Takahashi, M., Burma, Y., Iwamoto, T., Inaguma, Y., Ikeda, H., and Hiai, H. Cloning and expression of the *ret* proto-oncogene encoding a tyrosine kinase with two potential transmembrane domains. *Oncogene* 3:571–578, 1988.
40. Tokino, T., Imai, T., Tanigami, A., Takiguchi, S., and Nakamura, Y. Physical mapping of a 950-kb region surrounding a locus (D10S102) tightly linked to the MEN2A gene. *Genomics* 12:394–400, 1992.
41. Williams, E. D. Histogenesis of medullary carcinoma of the thyroid. *J. Clin. Pathol.* 19:114–118, 1966.

Chapter 4

The Pathology of Medullary Thyroid Carcinoma and Its Precursors

RONALD A. DeLELLIS

In 1951, R. C. Horn[48] reported a series of seven cases of a distinctive form of thyroid cancer characterized by the presence of sharply defined, rounded or ovoid, compact cell groups of moderate size in a background of hyalinized, connective tissue. He further stated that "while not pursuing the rapid course characteristic of the giant cell, spindle cell and small cell thyroid carcinoma, these tumors have, by no means, the favorable prognosis of malignant adenoma and papillary tumors." Subsequent studies by Hazard, Hawk, and Crile[45] established this variant of thyroid carcinoma as a distinct clinicopathologic entity characterized by a solid nonfollicular histologic pattern, the presence of amyloid in the stroma, and a high incidence of lymph node metastases. Hazard and associates chose the name "medullary carcinoma" to reflect the predominantly solid pattern of growth and the intermediate degree of malignancy, as compared to the papillary/follicular neoplasms, on the one hand, and the anaplastic carcinomas on the other.

Although the association of thyroid carcinoma and pheochromocytoma had been recognized since the 1930s, Sipple's report in 1961[90] focused attention on the fact that this association was more than coincidental. The patient described by Sipple was a 33-year-old man who was hypertensive after having had surgery for an arteriovenous brain malformation. At autopsy, the patient proved to have large bilateral pheochromocytomas, bilateral thyroid masses, and nodular enlargement of one parathyroid gland.

Subsequent studies by Williams and associates[103,105] and by Schmike and Hartmann[81] demonstrated that the thyroid tumors associated with pheochromocytomas were of Hazard's medullary type. Further studies established that the association of medullary carcinomas and pheochromocytomas occurred with an autosomal dominant pattern of inheritance and that parathyroid abnormalities also occurred frequently in affected individuals. Steiner and associates[95] suggested that this triad of endocrine tumors should be termed type 2 multiple endocrine neoplasia (MEN) or MEN 2A.[21]

A second, genetically distinct syndrome characterized by medullary carcinoma, pheochromocytoma, and ocular, gastrointestinal, and oral ganglioneuromatosis was subsequently termed MEN 2B.[38] Patients with the latter syndrome also commonly exhibit a Marfanoid habitus, pes cavus, and a variety of other skeletal abnormalities including talipes equinovarus, slipped capital femoral epiphysis, kyphosis, scoliosis, lordosis, increased joint laxity, and weakness of the proximal musculature. Megacolon has also been found in association with the type 2B phenotype.[18,60]

Although the major histologic features of medullary carcinoma were clearly delineated by the mid-1960s, the origin of this tumor remained unknown. Williams suggested in 1966[104] that these tumors might arise from the parafollicular cells of the thyroid since their cytologic characteristics resembled parafollicular cell-derived tumors in the canine and rodent thyroid. Williams further suggested that the parafollicular cells might be the source of the hormone, calcitonin. This hypothesis was subsequently substantiated by studies which demonstrated that calcitonin was a product of the normal parafollicular cells (C-cell) and that this hormone was present in high concentrations in tumor extracts and serum of patients with medullary thyroid carcinoma.[11,12,76,97]

CLINICAL FEATURES AND PATHOGENESIS

Medullary carcinomas account for 5–10% of thyroid malignancies in most large series. In addition to their association with the dominantly inherited MEN 2 syndromes, the tumors may also occur sporadically. In fact, in most large series, sporadic tumors account for approximately 70% of all cases. Sporadic tumors apparently occur with equal frequency in different parts of the world.[45,60,62]

Sporadic medullary carcinomas are principally tumors of middle-aged adults with a slight female predominance. Generally, patients are seen with unilateral involvement of the gland with or without associated nodal metastases. Rarely, they may have evidence of distant metastases. The tumors generally pursue an indolent course with 5-year survivals in the range of 70–80%.[91]

There are few data relating to the pathogenesis of the sporadic tumors. The incidence of medullary carcinoma is not apparently increased in human subjects treated by irradiation to the head and neck area. However, data in experimental animals suggest that rats treated with low doses of ^{131}I have an increased incidence of C-cell tumors.[99]

There are some data to support the view that chronic hypercalcemia may be associated with an increased incidence of these tumors.[63,64] In contrast to their relative rarity in humans, medullary carcinomas occur commonly in rodents, particularly after the age of 2 years,[22,57] and they are common in bulls, where they have been called ultimobranchial tumors.[9,50] The chronic administration of vitamin D_3 has been reported to increase the incidence of medullary carcinoma in the rat,[98] and it has been suggested that the high frequency of these tumors in bulls (in contrast to cows) may be related to a relatively higher calcium concentration in the blood.[14]

There is considerable variation in the incidence of medullary carcinoma in different strains of rat.[98] The tumors occur in approximately 50% of old WAG/ Rij rats but in only 5–10% of Wistar rats. In comparison to the Wistar strain, WAG/Rij rats have higher levels of calcitonin synthesis and secretion in addition to a genetically transmitted loss of calcitonin binding sites in the outer renal medulla.[20] Experimental studies suggest that an enhanced expression of the calcitonin gene is genetically transmitted, possibly as a consequence of the first mutation involved in the loss or renal calcitonin-binding sites.

The familial forms of medullary carcinoma are summarized in Table 4.1. In addition to their association with adrenal medullary and parathyroid abnormalities, these tumors may also occur alone as autosomal dominant traits.

The laboratory diagnosis of medullary carcinoma is dependent upon the demonstration of increased levels of calcitonin in the serum.[32,36,91,102] Since most patients with the sporadic disease have nodular thyroid glands, workup most commonly includes a thyroid scan with or without a fine needle aspiration biopsy. A diagnosis of medullary carcinoma can be confirmed by the demonstration of calcitonin by immunohistochemistry and by analysis of plasma levels of calcitonin.

The observation that calcitonin secretion could be augmented by the administration of secretagogues such as calcium gluconate or pentagastrin has formed the basis of large-scale screening studies aimed at the early diagnosis of C-cell neoplasia and hyperplasia.[32,91] Generally, those patients with higher basal and stimulated levels of calcitonin had larger tumors than those patients with low levels. Sequential increments of basal and stimulated calcitonin levels have been predictive of the development and spread of C-cell tumors.

In patients with the MEN 2A phenotype, the mean age at diagnosis of the thyroid tumors is 20.[32] Affected patients often show evidence of multicentric tumors involving both lobes of the gland. The tumors tend to be slow growing, and the prognosis is similar to that observed in patients with sporadic tumors. With the use of prospective screening studies in patients at high risk for the development of the syndrome, the mean age at diagnosis has become progressively younger. Thyroid tumors in patients with the type 2B syndrome occur at a mean age of 15 years. In addition to the younger age at onset, the tumors tend to be more aggressive than those seen in the type 2A syndrome.

The pheochromocytomas in patients with both the MEN 2A and 2B syndromes are typically bilateral and multicentric and are often preceded by phases of adrenal medullary hyperplasia.[19,26]

Rarely, hyperparathyroidism may mask the signs and symptoms of thyroid neoplasms in patients with MEN 2A. Generally, however, hyperparathyroidism is an uncommon presentation of MEN 2A and does not occur at all in association with the type MEN 2B syndrome.[18,32]

TABLE 4.1. FAMILIAL MEDULLARY THYROID CARCINOMA SYNDROMES

Isolated Medullary Carcinoma
Type 2A Multiple Endocrine Neoplasia[a]
  C-cell hyperplasia—medullary carcinoma
  Adrenal medullary hyperplasia—pheochromocytoma
  Parathyroid hyperplasia—Adenoma
Type 2B Multiple Endocrine Neoplasia
  C-cell hyperplasia—medullary carcinoma
  Adrenal medullary hyperplasia—pheochromocytoma
  Gastrointestinal and ocular ganglioneuromas
  Skeletal abnormalities

[a] Rarely, type 2A men may be associated with hereditary cutaneous lichen amyloidosis.

MEN 2A may rarely be associated with cutaneous lichen amyloidosis.[40] The dermal amyloid in this disorder is caused by a deposition of keratin-like peptides rather than by calcitonin-related peptides.

MOLECULAR APPROACHES TO DIAGNOSIS

A major advance in the early detection of the MEN 2 syndromes has occurred directly as a result of advances in molecular diagnostics. Linkage analyses have been successful in assigning the disease-associated gene to the centromeric region of chromosome 10.[69,89,92,93] This type of analysis is based on the concept that a DNA marker that is localized close to a disease-associated gene is more likely to be inherited with that gene through multiple recombinant events as compared to one which is located at a more distant site. The availability of polymorphic DNA probes for the centromeric region of chromosome 10 has now permitted the use of restriction fragment length polymorphisms to identify carriers of the gene for this disorder before the development of thyroid, adrenal medullary, and parathyroid abnormalities.[69,78,92,93]

The use of restriction fragment length polymorphisms analysis for the identification of the carrier state has, however, several potential problems.[40] First, the currently available markers cannot provide more than 90–98% certainty of correctly predicting gene carrier status. Second, a closely linked marker for MEN 2 may not be informative in a particular family.

Recent studies have mapped the site of the *ret* protooncogene to chromosome 10q11.2, close to the site of the MEN2 gene.[41] Increased expression of normal-sized transcripts of the *ret* proto-oncogene has been found in medullary carcinomas of both familial and sporadic types and in pheochromocytomas.[31,79]

PATHOLOGIC FEATURES

Medullary carcinomas vary in size from those which are just barely visible to those which replace the entire thyroid gland.[45] The larger tumors are generally sharply circumscribed lesions that are not usually encapsulated (Fig. 4.1). On cross-section, the tumors are pink to tan with a generally soft consistency. Some tumors, however, are quite sclerotic with areas of granular yellow discoloration. The small tumors commonly occur at the junction of the upper and middle thirds of the lateral lobes, corresponding to areas where C-cells normally predominate.[25] Such tumors are typically firm and yellow to white and have indistinct borders which appear to infiltrate the adjacent thyroid parenchyma. As the tumors become very large, they may replace the entire lobe and extend into the perithyroidal soft tissues. While the sporadic tumors most commonly present as unilateral lesions, the familial tumors characteristically involve both lobes of the gland.[10,30]

HISTOLOGIC FEATURES

The protypic medullary carcinoma shows lobular, trabecular, insular, or sheet-like growth patterns (Fig. 4.2).[45,105] Although many of the tumors appear sharply circumscribed grossly, microscopic examination often reveals extension of the tumor into the adjacent thyroid parenchyma. Individual tumor cells may be round, polygonal, or spindle-shaped, and most tumors show admixtures of these

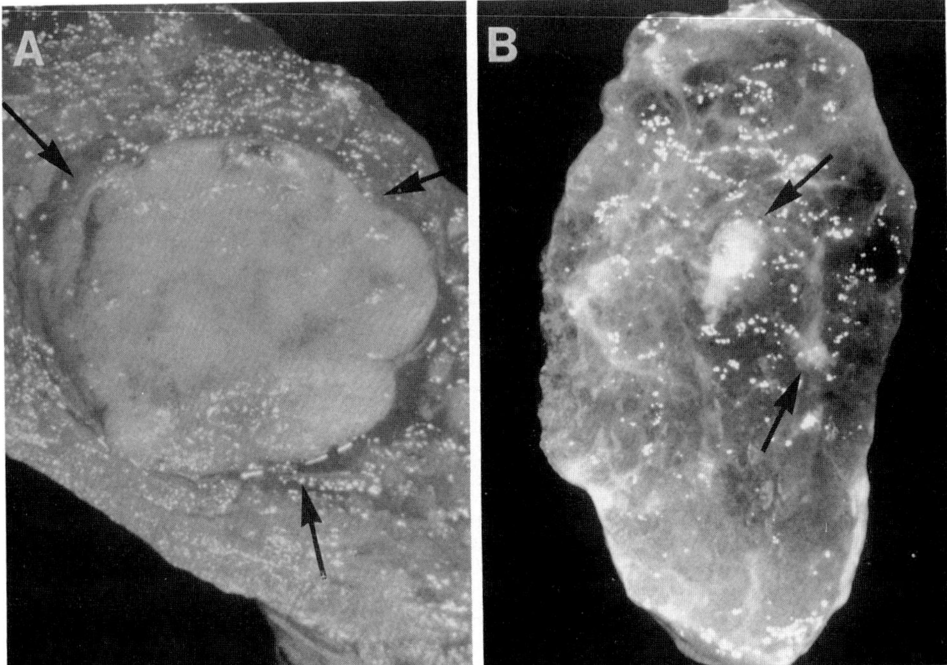

FIG. 4.1.   *A*, familial medullary thyroid carcinoma. The tumor, which measures 1.5 cm in diameter, is sharply circumscribed (*arrows*) but is not encapsulated. *B*, familial medullary thyroid carcinoma. Two separate tumor nodules (*arrows*) are evident. The upper nodule measures approximately 5 mm in diameter.

cell types. The nuclei are round to ovoid with speckled chromatin and inconspicuous nucleoli. Occasional nuclei may contain cytoplasmic pseudoinclusions resembling those seen in papillary carcinomas.

Foci of necrosis, hemorrhage, and mitotic activity are uncommon in small medullary carcinomas; however, these features become more apparent in larger tumors, particularly in those measuring more than 1.5 cm in diameter.[8] Lymphatic and vascular invasion is seen typically in the advancing front of the tumor. In very advanced cases, foci of lymphatic invasion may be seen in the contralateral lobe.

The cytoplasm is generally eosinophilic or amphophilic and finely granular. Argyrophilia, as demonstrated with the Grimelius stain, has been reported in more than 90% of medullary carcinomas. Although the argentaffin stain is usually negative, occasional tumors may contain isolated argentaffin cells.

Ultrastructural analyses have revealed that medullary carcinoma cells are characterized by the presence of membrane-bound secretory granules which represent the storage sites of calcitonin and other secretory products (Fig. 4.3 and 4.4).[4,13,23] At least two types of secretory granules have been identified within the tumor cells. The larger granules (type I) have an average diameter of 280 nm with moderately electron-dense, finely granular contents that are closely applied to the limiting membranes of the granules. Smaller granules (type II) have an

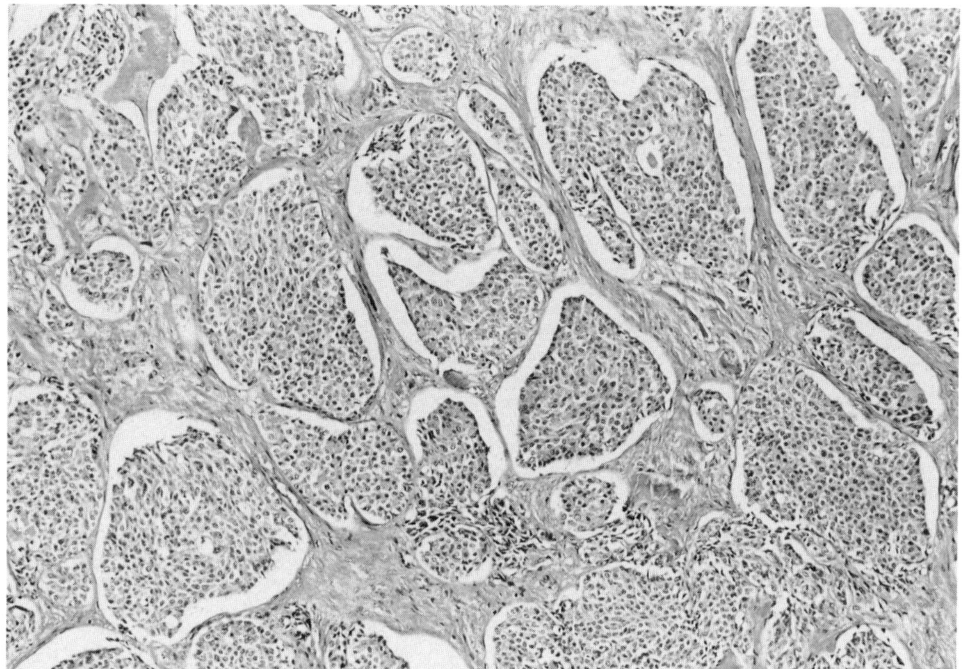

FIG. 4.2. Medullary thyroid carcinoma. This tumor shows a typical lobular growth pattern.

average diameter of 130 nm with more electron-dense contents, which are separated from the limiting membranes by a narrow electron lucent space (Fig. 4.3).[23] Some tumor cells may exhibit considerably more heterogeneity in the appearance of the secretory granules. For example, Capella and co-workers[13] have described cells with the ultrastructural features of serotonin, somatostatin, and adrenocorticotropin-containing cells.

Neoplastic C-cells commonly show morphologic evidence of active protein synthesis including the presence of prominent Golgi regions, abundant stacks of granular endoplasmic reticulum, and frequent cytoplasmic polyribosomes.

Occasional tumor cells may contain conspicuous mucin droplets.[108] Receptors for *Ulex europaeus* I, concanavalin A, *Ricinus communis* (RCA-I), wheat germ agglutinin, and soybean agglutinin have been identified in many cases, but there are considerable differences in lectin binding patterns among different cases.[37,54]

Amyloid deposits have been identified in up to 80% of cases of medullary carcinoma.[45,74,105] Typically, the amyloid deposits show green birefringence in polarized light and have a fibrillar ultrastructure. The amyloid is of tumor cell origin and most likely represents altered calcitonin or one or more of its precursors.

Histologic characteristics of sporadic and familial medullary carcinomas are identical; however, a number of other features may distinguish the two groups. As noted earlier, familial tumors occur at a young age and may be associated with adrenal medullary, parathyroid, and neural abnormalities. The familial

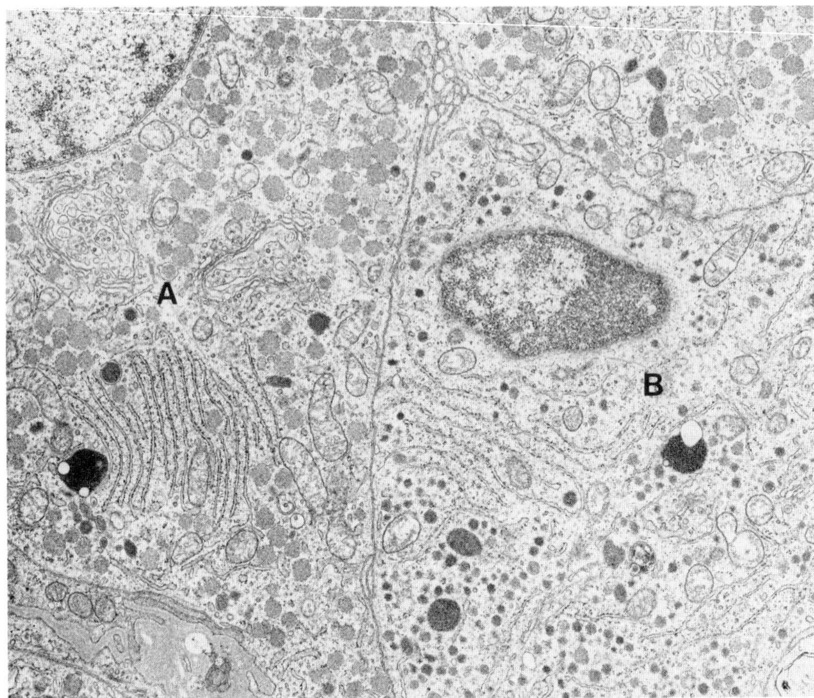

FIG. 4.3.   Medullary thyroid carcinoma. Some cells contain a predominance of type I granules (*A*) while others contain a predominance of type II granules (*B*). Original magnification, ×12,300. (From DeLellis and Wolfe[25] with permission of Appleton Century Crofts.)

tumors are typically multicentric and bilateral. In the series of cases reported by Block and co-workers,[10] bilateral tumors were found in 40 of 41 familial cases. In contrast, all 24 of the sporadic tumors were unilateral. It should be noted, however, that patients with large sporadic tumors may have metastases to the contralateral lobe.

An important feature which distinguishes familial and sporadic medullary carcinoma is the presence of C-cell hyperplasia in the former group (Fig. 4.5).[10] In cases of familial disease, foci of C-cell hyperplasia and early carcinoma are often apparent in sections away from the main tumor mass.[25] Early medullary carcinomas are characterized by the extension of C-cells through the follicular basal lamina into the interstitial tissue of the thyroid.[23] The finding of C-cell hyperplasia in an individual with apparent sporadic disease should alert both the pathologist and the clinician to the possibility of familial disease and appropriate clinical testing should be performed in family members.

In some instances, it may be extremely difficult to distinguish intrathyroidal metastases of medullary carcinoma from foci of C-cell hyperplasia or early carcinoma. In cases of metastatic disease, tumor emboli are found within vascular or lymphatic channels. When the tumor has extended beyond the confines of the vessel, it may infiltrate the thyroid in a manner similar to that observed in small

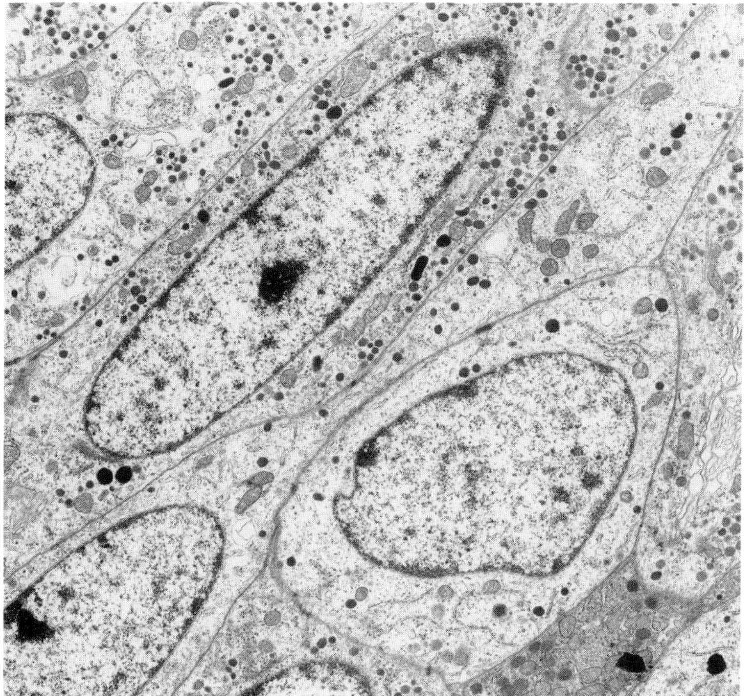

FIG. 4.4. Medullary thyroid carcinoma. This tumor shows a predominantly spindle cell pattern of growth. Original magnification, ×6,600. (From DeLellis and Wolfe[25] with permission of Appleton Century Crofts.)

primary carcinomas. The presence of C-cell hyperplasia adjacent to such a focus is highly suggestive of primary rather than metastatic tumor.

MARKERS FOR MEDULLARY CARCINOMA

HORMONES

The major secretory product of the normal and neoplastic C-cell is calcitonin, and this hormone has been used extensively as a marker for medullary carcinoma in tissue sections and as a serum marker (Fig. 4.6).[91,97,102] Calcitonin has been identified immunohistochemically in approximately 80% of medullary carcinomas. While many cases show extensive calcitonin immunoreactivity, occasional tumors may show small foci of staining. Approximately 20% of the tumors may be negative for calcitonin by immunohistochemistry, but in many of these cases, messenger RNA encoding calcitonin may be demonstrated with *in situ* hybridization techniques.[28,66,109] This finding suggests that in some cases, newly synthesized calcitonin may be released directly into the circulation without significant intracellular storage.

The cloning of the calcitonin gene has led to the discovery of several other peptides including the calcitonin gene-related peptide (CGRP) and katacalcin.[67] The CGRP is produced by alternative splicing of the primary RNA transcript of

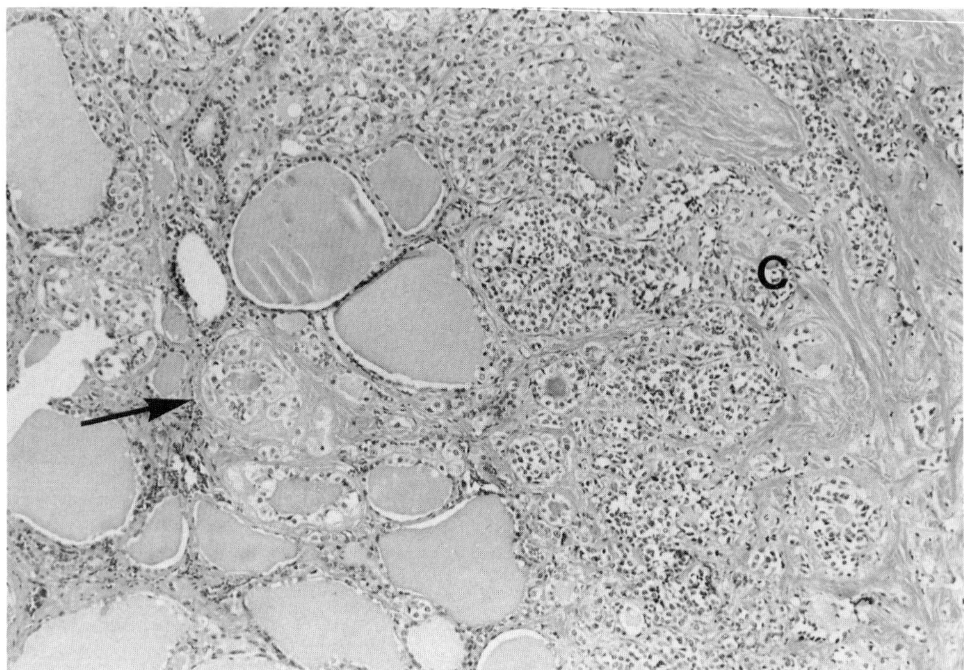

FIG. 4.5.   Familial medullary thyroid carcinoma. Foci of C-cell hyperplasia (*arrow*) are present adjacent to the carcinoma (*C*).

the calcitonin gene. The process is tissue-specific in that the normal C-cell will splice the primary transcript to produce calcitonin messenger RNA, while neural cells use the same transcript to produce CGRP. While normal C-cells produce calcitonin predominantly, neoplastic C-cells may process the primary transcript to produce both calcitonin and CGRP. Katacalcin is produced by proteolytic cleavage of the C-terminal portion of the calcitonin precursor protein.

Many other peptides have been localized by immunohistochemistry within medullary carcinomas, and their presence has been confirmed by radioimmuno-assays of tumor extracts.[25,94,100] Both somatostatin and bombesin (gastrin-releasing peptide) are present in subpopulations of normal C-cells, and both of these peptides are also commonly found in medullary carcinomas.[87,96] Generally, somatostatin is present in single cells or in small cell groups which often represent less than 5% of the total tumor cell population.[87] Other peptides that have been demonstrated in medullary carcinoma include adrenocorticotropin, other pro-opiomelanocortin-related peptides, Leu-enkephalin, neurotensin, substance P, vasoactive intestinal peptide, chorionic gonadotropin, and prolactin-stimulating factors. Rarely, these tumors may contain subpopulations of cells immunoreactive for glucagon, gastrin, or insulin. Both serotonin and catecholamines are also present in medullary carcinomas.[46,100]

In some species, the C-cells also contain thyrotropin-releasing hormone (TRH) as determined by immunohistochemistry. Northern analysis of total thyroid

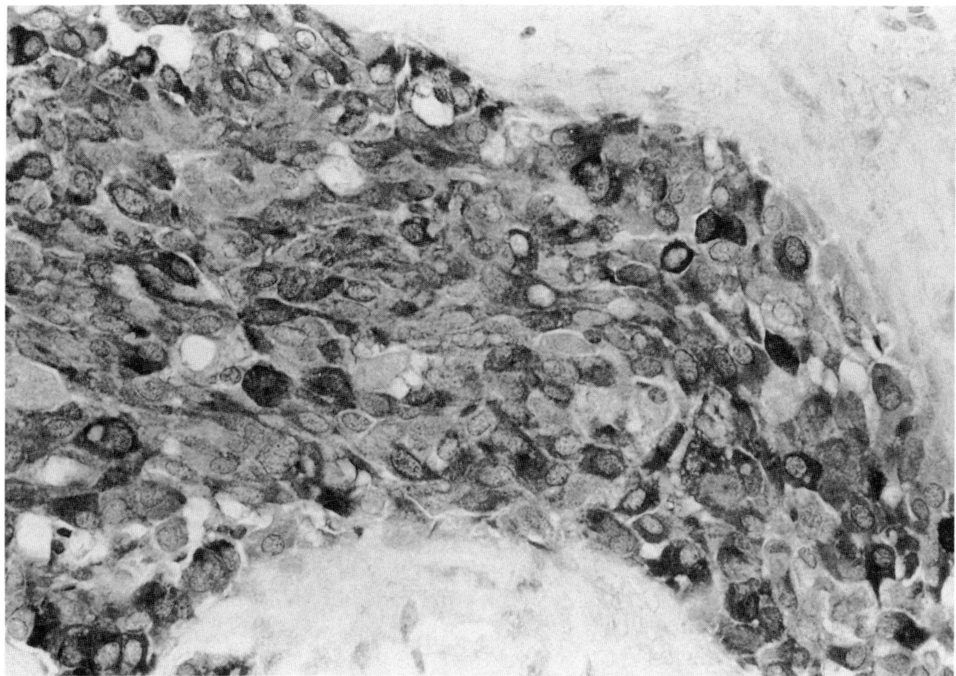

FIG. 4.6.   Medullary thyroid carcinoma. Immunoperoxidase stain for calcitonin. Staining intensity varies in individual cells. (From DeLellis and Wolfe[25] with permission of Appleton Century Crofts.)

RNA with a prepro-TRH-specific RNA probe has identified a single hybridizing band which is the same size as authentic TRH found in the hypothalamus. These results support a potential paracrine role for TRH gene products directly within the thyroid.[34]

NonHormonal Markers

Medullary carcinomas demonstrate positive staining with antibodies directed to a variety of nonhormonal constituents of neuroendocrine cells.[88] The tumors are commonly positive for neuron-specific enolase, histaminase, DOPA decarboxylase, synaptophysin, and chromogranins. Neuron-specific enolase, however, is also expressed in a variety of non-C-cell neoplasms and should not be used as the only marker to distinguish medullary carcinomas from other thyroid malignancies.[101] Chromogranin, on the other hand, is a more specific marker for medullary carcinoma and may be more sensitive than calcitonin.[80] Synaptophysin is also commonly expressed in these tumors.[39] Several reports have suggested that the presence of histaminase may be used to distinguish carcinomas, which are usually positive, from hyperplastic areas, which are typically negative.

Medullary carcinomas are positive for low molecular weight keratins; however, there may be considerable variation in staining intensity in different areas of the same tumor. Vimentin is variably expressed within the tumor cells, while some medullary carcinomas may be positive for neurofilament proteins in contrast to normal C-cells which are negative.

Carcinoembryonic antigen (CEA) levels are typically increased in the plasma of patients with medullary thyroid carcinoma, as compared to patients with other primary thyroid malignancies.[24,83] Correlative immunohistochemical studies have revealed that virtually all medullary carcinomas contain immunoreactive CEA. In some instances, medullary carcinomas may lose their capability to synthesize calcitonin while maintaining their capacity for CEA production.[72] Correlative immunohistochemical studies have shown that calcitonin negative areas in such tumors frequently exhibit CEA positivity. In patients with medullary carcinoma, the finding of persistently high CEA levels in the face of declining calcitonin levels may predict aggressive disease.[72]

High levels of histaminase have also been demonstrated in the tumor extracts and plasma of patients with medullary carcinoma.[71]

Variants of Medullary Thyroid Carcinoma

Medullary thyroid carcinomas often exhibit a remarkable degree of diversity in their histologic features. While many medullary carcinomas may show scattered follicular structures admixed with more typical solid areas, occasional tumors may show a pure *follicular* or *tubular* growth pattern (Fig. 4.7).[44] The lumina may appear empty or may contain an eosinophilic material that is indistinguishable from colloid. Immunohistochemical studies have revealed that

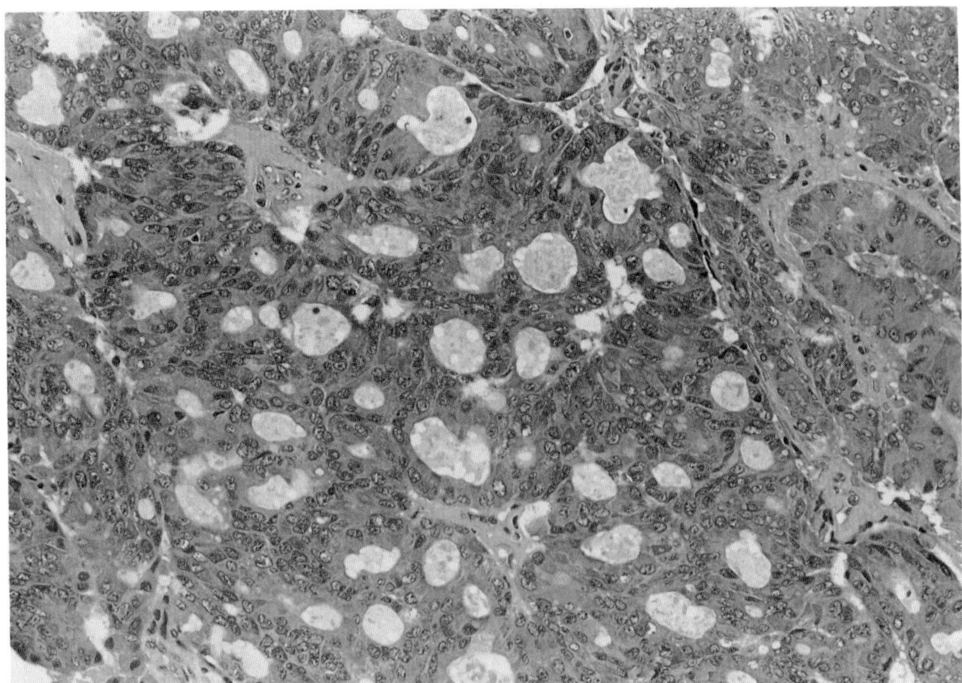

Fig. 4.7. Medullary thyroid carcinoma, follicular variant.

this material is negative for thyroglobulin but shows variable degrees of staining for calcitonin. Very rarely, medullary carcinomas may exhibit a true *papillary* growth pattern.[52] The pseudopapillary variant is considerably more common, and this appearance most likely results from a fixation artefact in which groups of tumor cells appear to be attached to the stromal compartments with intervening empty areas.

The *small cell* variant is characterized by the presence of cells with high nuclear cytoplasmic ratios, which most closely resemble the intermediate variant of small cell bronchogenic carcinoma.[20,62,70] This variant may exhibit compact, trabecular, or diffuse growth patterns (Fig. 4.8). Overall mitotic activity is often high and foci of necrosis may be frequent. Eusebi and co-workers[29] have reported two cases of small cell carcinoma of the thyroid which were positive for chromogranin and synaptophysin but negative for calcitonin by immunohistochemistry. Both tumors were negative for calcitonin messenger RNA when studied by *in situ* hybridization methods. These results suggest that such tumors may represent primary small cell carcinomas of the thyroid and that they should be separated from the small cell variant of medullary carcinoma.

Isolated tumor giant cells may be found in occasional medullary carcinomas of both familial and nonfamilial types (Fig. 4.9). Rarely, the tumors may contain a predominance of giant cells, and such cases have been classified as *giant cell* variants.[51] Although some authors[73] have suggested that C-cell differentiation

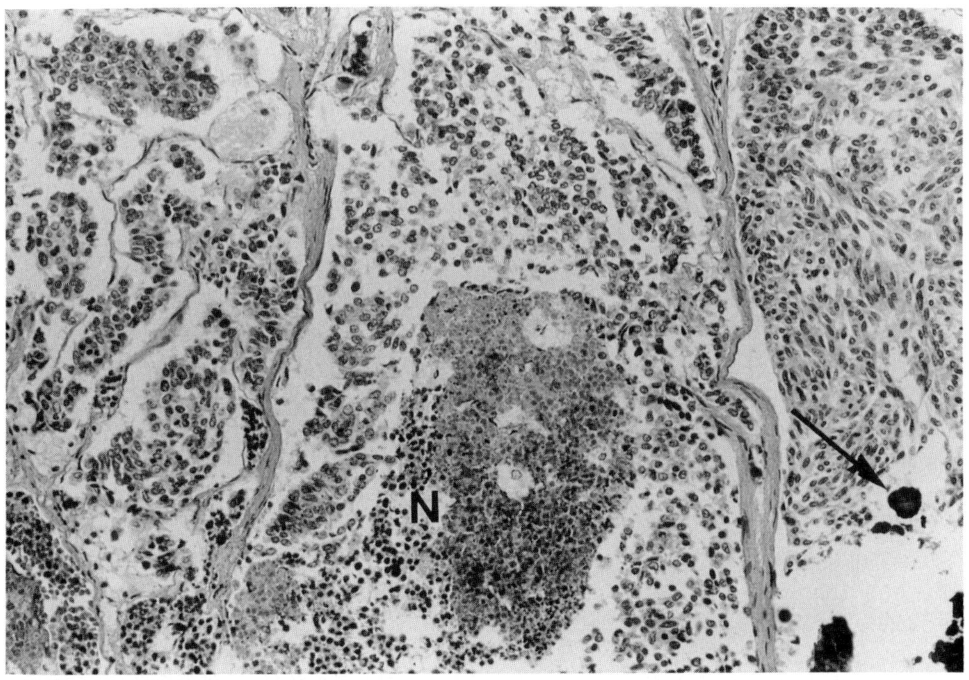

Fig. 4.8. Medullary thyroid carcinoma, small cell type. Foci of necrosis (*N*) and calcification (*arrow*) are evident.

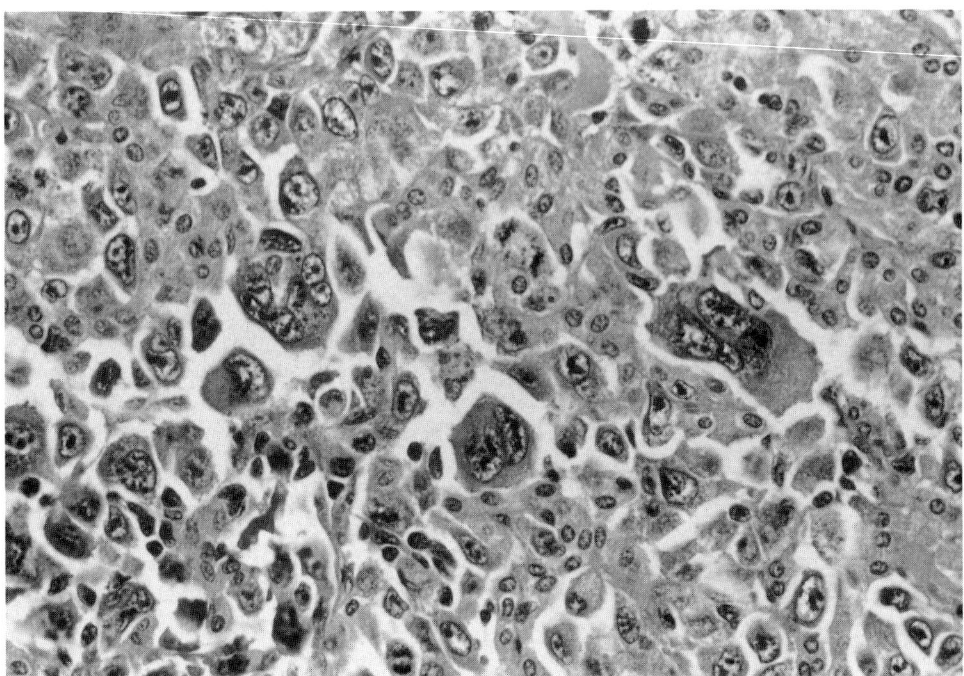

FIG. 4.9. Medullary thyroid carcinoma, giant cell type. This tumor also contained melanin pigment.

occurs relatively commonly in anaplastic thyroid carcinomas, this observation has not been substantiated by other studies.[15] Occasional medullary carcinomas may show a predominant spindle cell growth pattern (Fig. 4.10).

Other rare forms of medullary carcinoma include oncocytic, clear cell, melanocytic squamous, and amphicrine variants.[3,27,35,43,55,68] The latter type represents a composite calcitonin- and mucin-producing neoplasm in which the cells have a signet ring appearance (Fig. 4.11).[35]

Occasional medullary carcinomas may be encapsulated and may be arranged in a broad trabecular pattern with an amyloid negative hyalinized stroma.[49] These tumors may bear a striking similarity to the hyalinizing trabecular adenoma or paraganglioma-like adenoma.

Although C-cell adenomas have been described,[53] these lesions most likely represent encapsulated carcinomas rather than true benign C-cell neoplasms.

MIXED FOLLICULAR AND C-CELL TUMORS

The existence of tumors composed of C-cells and follicular cells has been a hotly debated issue.[3,47,61,65,77] The cellular origins of such neoplasms are unknown, but several studies have noted their similarities to the ultimobranchial neoplasms of bulls. It has been suggested that mixed tumors could arise from uncommitted stem cells of the ultimobranchial body which would have the potential to differentiate either into C-cells or into follicular cells.[65] Alternatively, this phe-

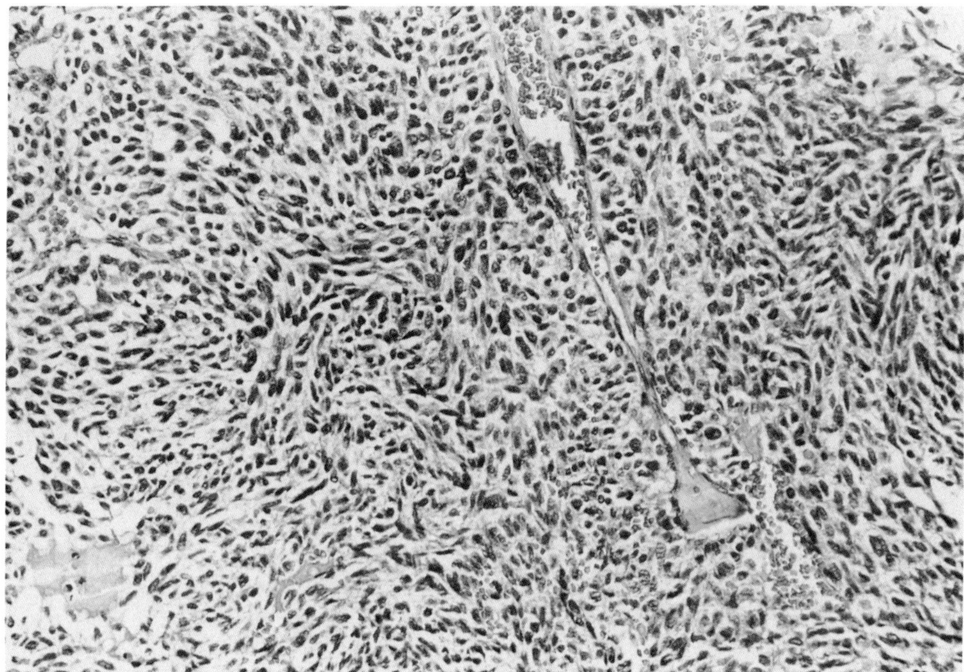

FIG. 4.10. Medullary thyroid carcinoma, spindle cell type.

nomenon might result from activation of neuropeptide genes in neoplastic follicular cells or thyroid hormone genes in C-cell tumors. It is also possible, although unlikely, that mixed follicular and C-cell tumors represent collision neoplasms.

When strictly defined as neoplasms composed of cells showing both follicular and C-cell differentiation as manifested by the presence of thyroglobulin and calcitonin or other peptides, mixed tumors are rare.[3] They have also been referred to as intermediate carcinomas in some studies (Figs. 4.12 and 4.13).[65] These tumors must be distinguished from medullary carcinomas with entrapped normal follicles (Fig. 4.14) and from the follicular variant of medullary carcinoma. The existence of such mixed tumors may explain the rare cases of medullary carcinoma which have the capacity to incorporate radioactive iodine.

Microscopically, mixed follicular and C-cell tumors are solid or follicular and may or may not show foci of cribriform tumor growth. The solid areas resemble typical medullary carcinomas and are characterized by the presence of polyhedral cells arranged in compact lobules and trabecula. The stroma may be devoid of amyloid. Most of the follicles are arranged in a microfollicular pattern.

In contrast to medullary carcinomas with entrapped follicles, the nuclei of the follicular areas of mixed tumors have features similar to those of the solid areas. Rarely, some of the tumors have a component of indifferent cells with tubules and cystic structures reminiscent of ultimobranchial elements.[65]

Albores-Saavedra and co-workers[2] have described a variant of medullary carcinoma in which there is an admixture of cells with the characteristic clear nuclei

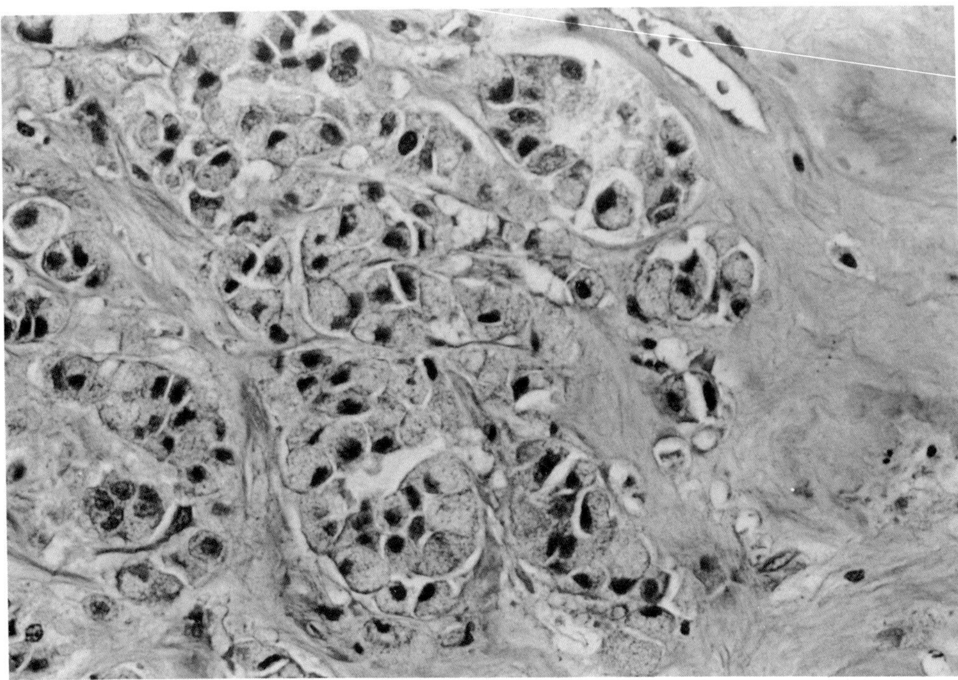

FIG. 4.11. Medullary thyroid carcinoma, amphicrine type. The vacuolated appearance of the tumor cells is due to the presence of mucin deposits. (Courtesy of Dr. Vincenzo Eusebi.)

of papillary carcinoma. Cells with clear nuclei were thyroglobulin-positive and CEA-negative. Cells of the medullary component, on the other hand, were thyroglobulin-negative but CEA- and calcitonin-positive. Admixtures of the papillary and medullary elements were present both in the primary tumors and in nodal metastases.

DIFFERENTIAL DIAGNOSIS

Medullary carcinomas may mimic a wide variety of benign and malignant thyroid neoplasms. Although true papillary variants of medullary carcinoma are rare, the pseudopapillary variants are relatively common. Papillary carcinomas of follicular cell origin are characterized by alignment of tumor cells on fibrovascular cores. The nuclei are usually irregular and overlapping with pseudoinclusions and grooves, and a ground glass nuclear appearance is common. The nuclei of medullary carcinomas, on the other hand, tend to have coarsely punctate chromatin, and pseudoinclusions are considerably less common than in papillary carcinomas. The frequent solid growth pattern of sclerosing papillary carcinomas together with the abundant collagenous stroma may present considerable diagnostic confusion. However, sclerosing papillary carcinomas are negative for amyloid, lack calcitonin, and exhibit positive staining for thyroglobulin. Although foci of calcification are relatively common within the stroma of medullary carcinomas, true psammoma bodies are rare.

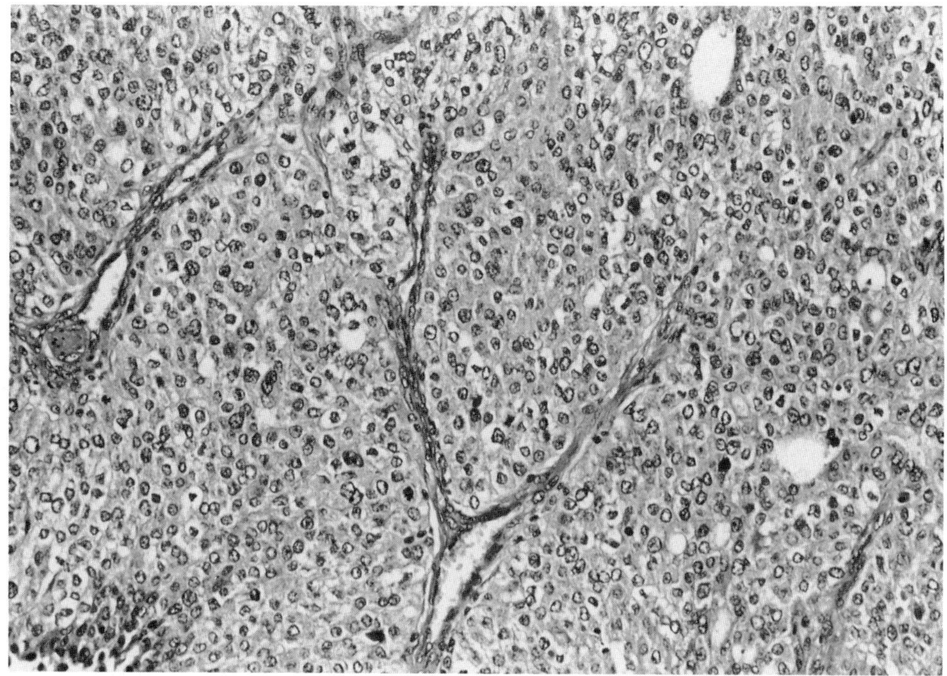

FIG. 4.12.   Mixed medullary and follicular carcinoma. This tumor shows a solid pattern of growth. (Courtesy of Dr. Otto Ljungberg.)

Medullary carcinomas often contain follicular structures and must, therefore, be distinguished from follicular carcinomas. Entrapped normal follicles are frequently encountered in medullary carcinomas; however, both the follicles and the colloid are typically positive for thyroglobulin. Rarely, medullary carcinomas may exhibit a completely follicular structure; however, immunoperoxidase studies reveal calcitonin positivity, while thyroglobulin stains are negative. The true mixed follicular C-cell tumors are positive both for thyroglobulin and calcitonin.

The hyalinizing trabecular adenoma is typically encapsulated as are occasional variants of medullary carcinoma.[47] Both lesions may show hyalinization and focal calcification, but the presence of amyloid is typical of medullary carcinoma. Follicle formation may be apparent in both tumors, but the presence of papillae is more typical of trabecular adenomas. Medullary carcinomas are calcitonin-positive but thyroglobulin-negative, while the reverse pattern is true of hyalinizing trabecular adenoma.

Medullary carcinomas must also be distinguished from poorly differentiated or insular carcinomas.[16] The latter tumors are characterized by the presence of solid islands of tumor cells containing occasional small follicles. The stroma of insular carcinomas is typically negative for amyloid, while the tumor cells are thyroglobulin-positive but calcitonin-negative.

Since medullary carcinomas often exhibit a solid pattern of growth, they have in the past been classified as undifferentiated or anaplastic carcinomas. Medul-

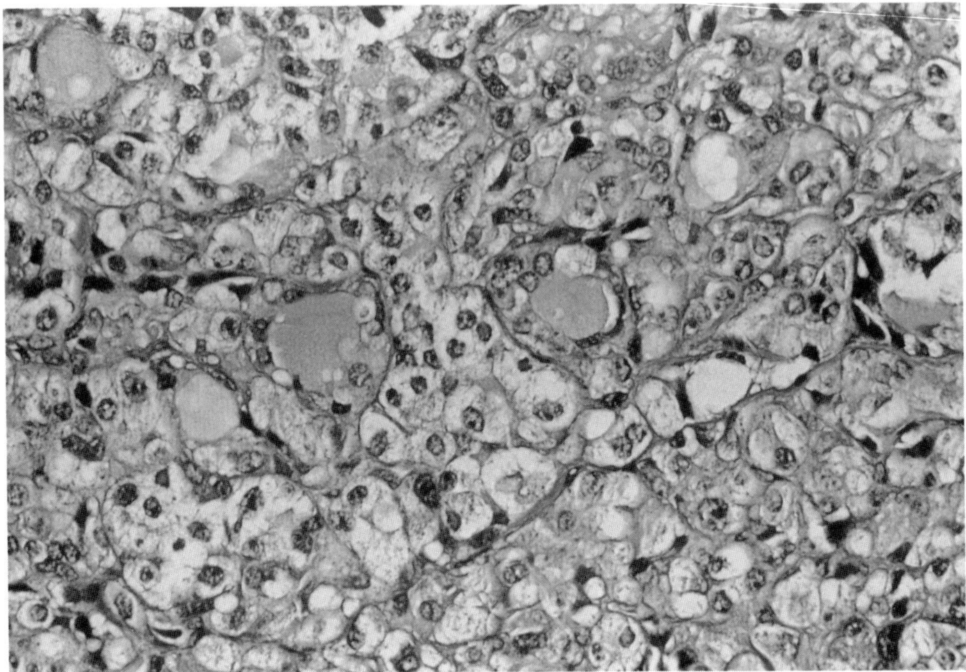

FIG. 4.13.   Mixed medullary and follicular carcinoma. This case shows scattered microfollicles. (Courtesy of Dr. Otto Ljungberg.)

lary carcinomas of spindle and giant cell types may be distinguished from undifferentiated carcinomas and sarcomas on the basis of their calcitonin immunoreactivity. Moreover, spindle and giant cell variants of medullary carcinoma may show more typical patterns of growth on extensive sectioning.

Most small cell malignant tumors in the thyroid represent lymphomas, as demonstrated by positivity for leukocyte common antigen and other lymphoid markers. Small cell variants of medullary carcinoma are typically positive for calcitonin by immunohistochemistry or give positive signals for calcitonin messenger RNA when *in situ* hybridization procedures are performed. The so-called primary oat cell carcinoma of the thyroid is typically negative for calcitonin and calcitonin messenger RNA.[29]

As noted in the previous section, medullary carcinomas may show clear cell or oxyphilic features. In contrast to clear cell and oxyphilic variants of follicular carcinoma which are positive for thyroglobulin, these variants of medullary carcinoma are positive for calcitonin but negative for thyroglobulin.

Rarely, parathyroid adenomas may present as intrathyroidal masses which simulate thyroid carcinomas. Such tumors are typically encapsulated and are composed of cords and nests of chief cells with small centrally placed nuclei and relatively clear or vacuolated cytoplasm. The chief cells are negative for calcitonin, but may exhibit weak reactivity for chromogranin and parathyroid hormone.

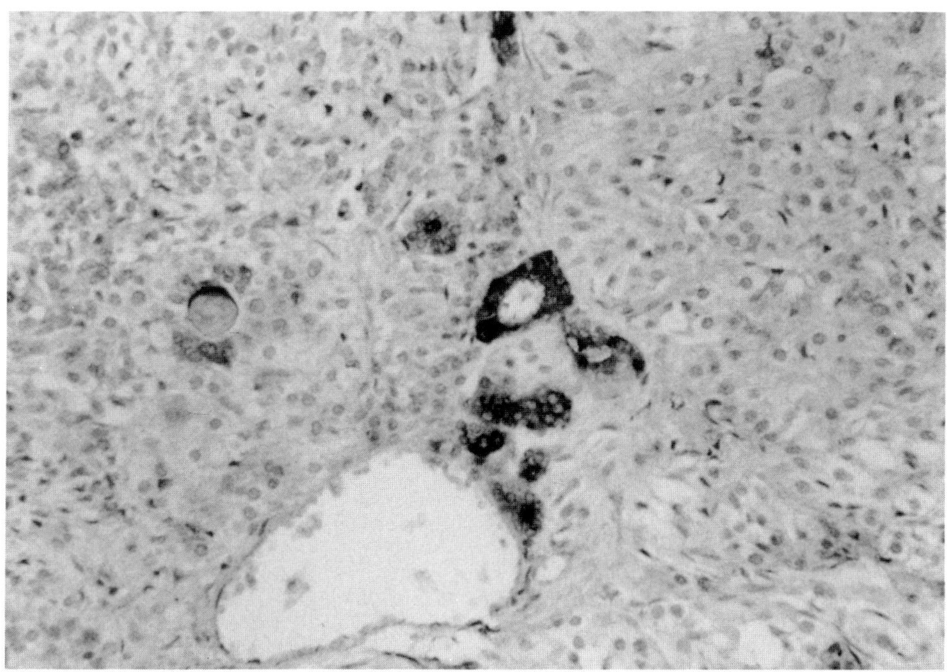

FIG. 4.14. Medullary thyroid carcinoma with entrapped normal follicles. Immunoperoxidase stain for thyroglobulin. The tumor cells are negative, while the normal follicular cells are stained intensely.

TREATMENT AND PROGNOSIS

The definitive treatment of both sporadic and familial medullary carcinoma is total thyroidectomy with removal of the lymph nodes in the central compartment of the neck.[40,82,91]

In most large series, the 5-year survival rates are 60–70%, while 10-year survivals have ranged from 40–50%. Survival is correlated significantly with age, sex, and tumor stage.[40] Patients less than 40 years of age at the time of diagnosis have a significantly better prognosis than older patients even when individuals with the familial form of the disease are considered. Women generally have a better prognosis than men.

The probability of nodal metastasis is positively correlated with the size of the primary neoplasm. The studies of Bigner and co-workers[8] on familial medullary carcinomas have demonstrated that approximately 20% of patients with tumors measuring less than 0.7 cm had nodal metastases. In contrast, nodal metastases were found in 80% of patients whose tumors were greater than 1.5 cm, while 30% of patients whose tumors measured between 0.7 and 1.5 cm had nodal metastases.

Schroder and associates[82] have reported no differences in survival when comparing different histologic patterns of primary tumors. Prominent mitotic activity, however, was shown to have an adverse influence on prognosis.

The amount of immunoreactive calcitonin within the tumor also has been shown to have an impact on prognosis.[58] In a study of 249 medullary carcinomas,

TABLE 4.2. SPECTRUM OF C-CELL HYPERPLASIA

Isolated (Familial) Medullary Carcinoma
Type 2A Multiple Endocrine Neoplasia
Type 2B Multiple Endocrine Neoplasia
Hypercalcemia (*e.g.*, hyperparathyroidism)
Hypergastrinemia (*e.g.*, Zollinger-Ellison syndrome)
Hashimoto's disease
Goitrous hypothyroidism
Peritumoral (adjacent to non-C-cell neoplasms)

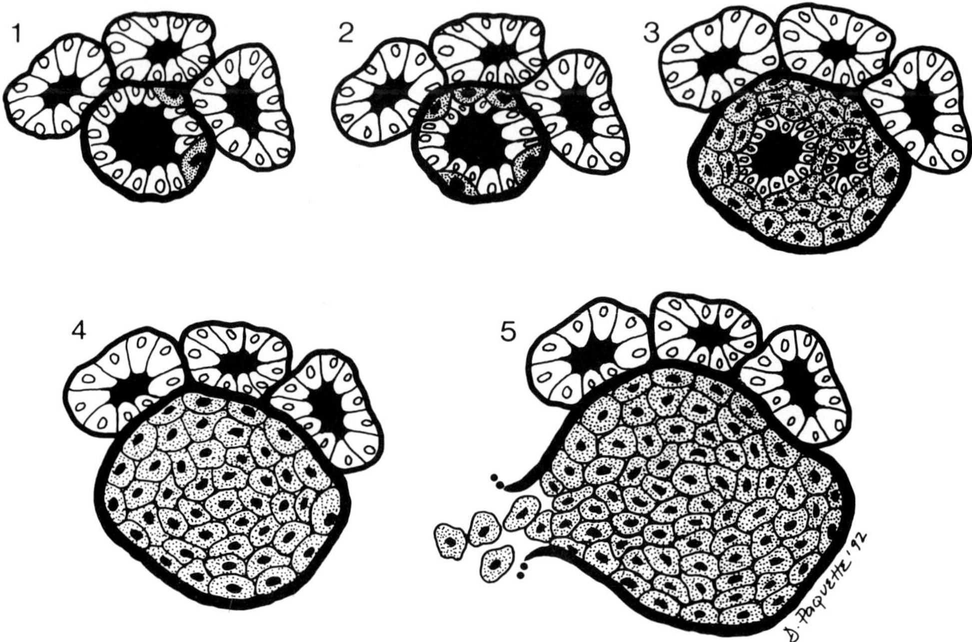

FIG. 4.15. Stages in the development of familial medullary thyroid carcinoma. C-cells are depicted with stippled cytoplasm and closed nuclei. Follicular cells have opened nuclei with clear cytoplasm. *1*, normal C-cell topography; *2*, mild diffuse C-cell hyperplasia; *3* and *4*, nodular C-cell hyperplasia; *5*, medullary thyroid carcinoma.

Bergholm and co-workers[6] have noted that tumors with less than 10% of cells immunoreactive for calcitonin were more aggressive than tumors containing more than 50% calcitonin immunoreactive cells. These findings support the earlier studies of Lippman and co-workers[58] who noted a worse prognosis in calcitonin-poor tumors.

The presence of peptides including bombesin, somatostatin, and neurotensin does not appear to affect prognosis.[82] Similarly, the numbers of S-100 positive dendritic cells do not have an impact on prognosis. The presence of Leu M1, on the other hand, appears to correlate with prognosis. In a study of 39 medullary carcinomas, local recurrences were three times more common in tumors containing more than 15% Leu-M1-positive cells as compared to tumors that were Leu-M1-negative or weakly positive.[84]

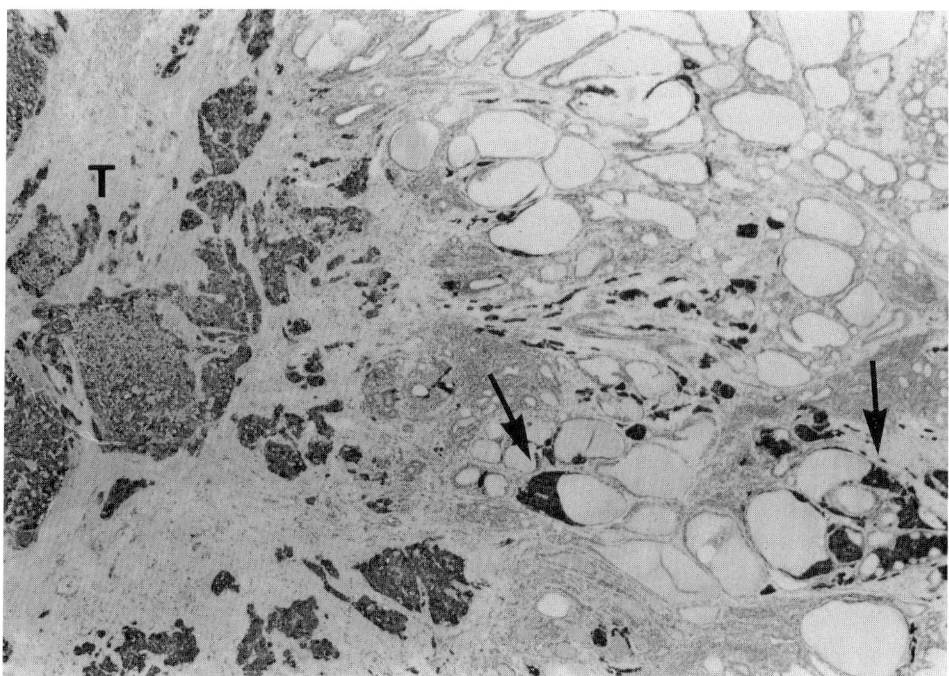

FIG. 4.16. Familial medullary thyroid carcinoma with C-cell hyperplasia. A small focus of tumor (*T*) is surrounded by areas of diffuse and nodular (*arrows*) C-cell hyperplasia. Immunoperoxidase stain for calcitonin.

The impact of amyloid content on prognosis has been controversial. Schroder and co-workers[82] concluded that amyloid-free tumors did not differ prognostically from amyloid-rich tumors. Bergholm and co-workers,[6] on the other hand, concluded that amyloid-rich tumors had a better prognosis.

C-CELL HYPERPLASIA

C-cell hyperplasia is an uncommon entity characterized by an increased mass of C-cells within the follicles of the thyroid. Although C-cell hyperplasia was first described in patients with familial medullary carcinoma, a similar increase in C-cell mass has now been recognized in a variety of other conditions[107] (Table 4.2).

In patients with the MEN 2 syndromes, C-cell hyperplasia was first recognized on the basis of abnormal calcitonin secretory responses following the administration of calcium gluconate or pentagastrin.[32] Subsequent studies suggested that C-cell hyperplasia is a preneoplastic condition that precedes the development of the multifocal medullary carcinomas characteristic of MEN 2 syndromes. The presence of C-cell hyperplasia has also been used as a histologic marker to distinguish sporadic from familial forms of the tumor, as discussed previously.[10] C-cell hyperplasia occurs spontaneously in many rat strains in an age-dependent manner, and it is frequently associated with multifocal medullary carcinomas, particularly after the age of 2 years.[57,104] Many of the affected animals also have

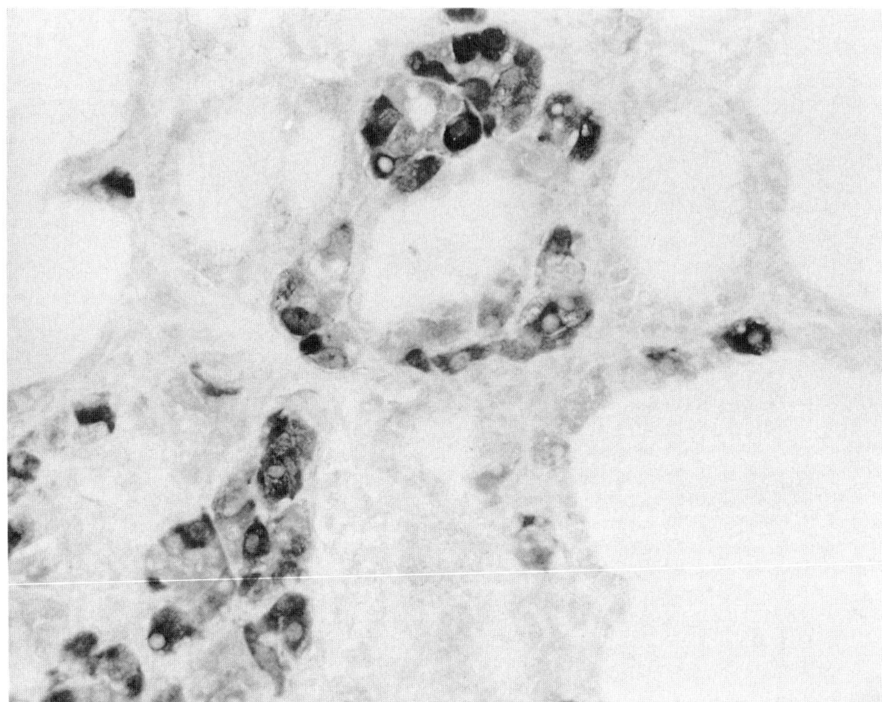

FIG. 4.17.   Areas of predominantly diffuse C-cell hyperplasia in a patient with MEN 2A. Immunoperoxidase stain for calcitonin.

evidence of pheochromocytomas, pituitary adenomas, and pancreatic endocrine tumors.

Experimental studies have suggested that the chronic administration of calcitonin secretagogues leads to the development of C-cell hyperplasia.[14] C-cell hyperplasia has been recognized in human thyroid glands from occasional patients with nonfamilial hyperparathyroidism, other hypercalcemic states, and hypergastrinemia.[64]

C-cell hyperplasia has also been recognized in occasional patients with Hashimoto's thyroiditis.[7,56] Albores-Saavedra and Libby and associates[1,56] have suggested that C-cell hyperplasia in patients with goitrous hypothyroidism and Hashimoto's disease could result from chronic thyrotropin stimulation. In this regard, several experimental studies have suggested that both follicular cells and C-cells might be under the control of thyrotropin.[1]

C-cell hyperplasia has also been recognized adjacent to both follicular and papillary carcinomas.[4,86] In one patient with C-cell hyperplasia adjacent to a papillary carcinoma, both basal and stimulated calcitonin levels were increased. C-cell hyperplasia in these cases occurred only in the tumor-bearing lobe in contrast to the typical bilaterality of C-cell changes in patients with MEN 2.[4,86]

PATHOLOGIC FEATURES

The thyroid glands from patients with C-cell hyperplasia associated with MEN 2 are grossly unremarkable.[25,107] Each lobe of the thyroid should be blocked in its

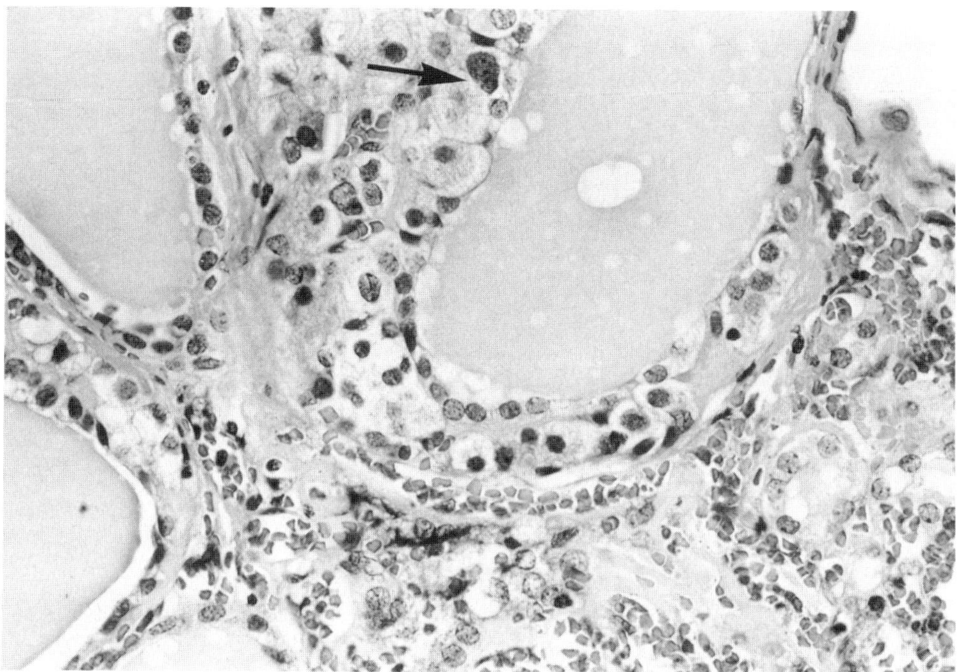

FIG. 4.18. C-cell hyperplasia in a patient with MEN 2A. C-cells completely surround the follicle. An occasional C-cell has an enlarged hyperchromatic nucleus.

entirety for histologic sampling.[25] If C-cell hyperplasia is present, it will most likely be found in sections corresponding to the middle thirds of the lateral lobes.

The earliest phases of C-cell proliferative disease are characterized by increased numbers of C-cells in both thyroid lobes, as compared to age- and sex-matched controls (Figs. 4.15, 4.16, and 4.17).[23,107] In view of the recent studies that have shown considerable variations in C-cell densities in normal glands, a diagnosis of C-cell hyperplasia should be made with caution. The process should involve both lobes, with at least 50 C-cells per single low-power field. Occasional C-cells in this disorder may also be enlarged and hyperchromatic. As in normal glands, hyperplastic C-cells occupy an exclusively intrafollicular position and are separated from the interstitium by the follicular basal lamina and from the luminal colloid by the follicular cell cytoplasm. In some instances, C-cells may appear to lie directly within the interstitium; however, electron microscopy invariably reveals continuity of the C-cells within the follicular basal lamina. C-cells in diffuse hyperplasia generally exhibit intense immunoreactivity for calcitonin.

The proliferation of C-cells within the follicle may completely encircle the more centrally located follicular cells to produce a circumferential collar (Figs. 4.18, 4.19, and 4.20).[4,23,85] Nodular hyperplasia of C-cells is characterized by the complete obliteration of the follicular space by C-cells. Since C-cell nodules may be found in occasional normal glands, a definite diagnosis of nodular C-cell hyperplasia should be made only when the change is extensive, bilateral, and multifocal. Similar to the C-cells in diffuse hyperplasia, foci of nodular hyperplasia typically exhibit intense calcitonin immunoreactivity.

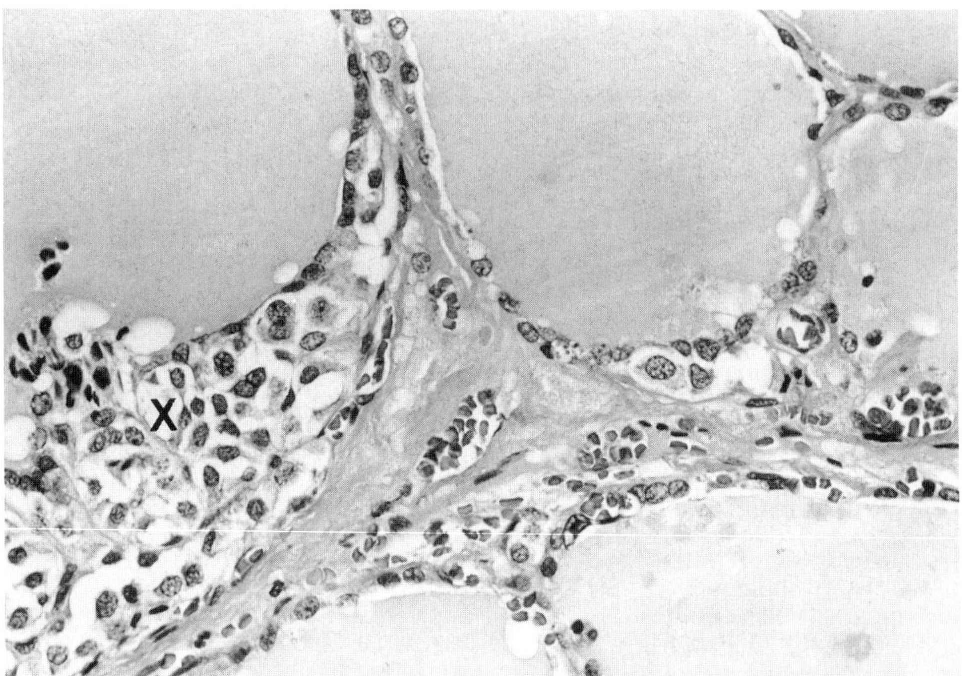

FIG. 4.19.   C-cell hyperplasia in a patient with MEN 2A. In one follicle, the C-cells are proliferating toward the center of the follicle (*X*).

Early microscopic carcinomas are diagnosed when C-cells extend through defects in the follicular basal lamina into the interstitium.[23] Invasion in this setting is characterized by the presence of fibrosis around the infiltrating tumor cell nests. At the ultrastructural level, occasional tumor cells in early carcinomas may be devoid of basal lamina. The majority of infiltrating tumor cells, however, are surrounded at least focally by basal lamina.

Although early studies suggested that normal adult thyroids contained less than 10 C-cells per single low-power field, more recent studies indicate that up to 50 C-cells may be found in some low-power fields.[1,75,86] Moreover, occasional nodules composed of C-cells have been identified in some normal glands, particularly from older individuals.[33] The observed variations in C-cell density in normal glands have important implications with respect to the diagnosis of early C-cell proliferative disease in patients with MEN 2.

In this regard, Lips and co-workers[59] identified five patients from a large MEN 2A kindred who had thyroidectomies because of slightly increased calcitonin levels following provocative testing. Although the resected glands showed evidence of mild C-cell hyperplasia, these authors concluded that these individuals did not have MEN 2A, since none of them subsequently developed pheochromocytoma or hyperparathyroidism. Moreover, all of their children have had repeatedly normal calcitonin levels on provocative testing. These findings indicate that it may be difficult, if not impossible, to distinguish mild forms of C-cell hyperplasia from occasional normal glands.

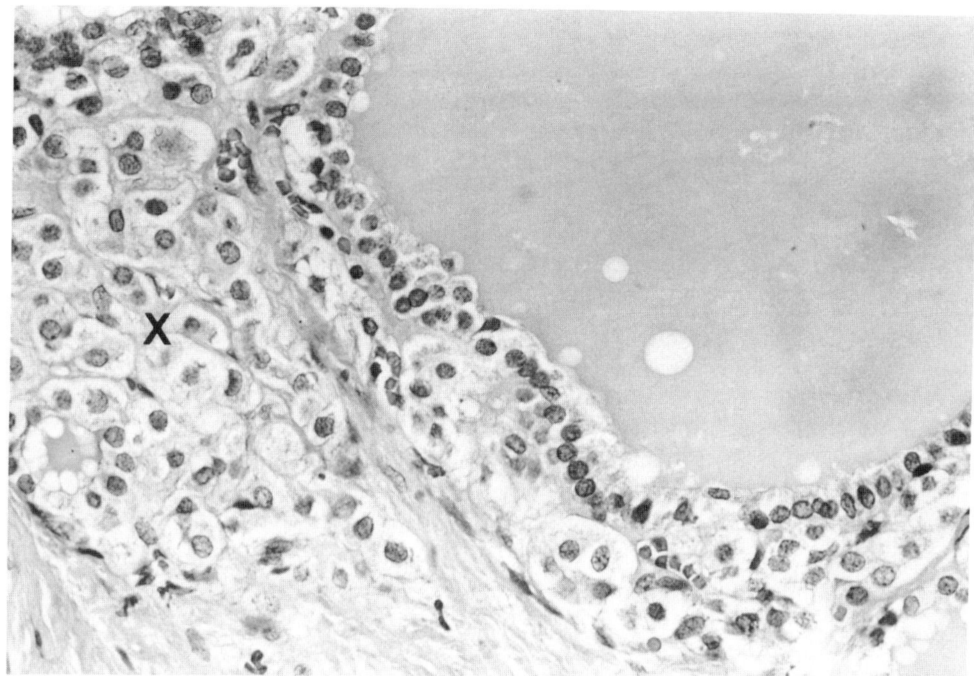

FIG. 4.20. Microscopic focus (*X*) of medullary carcinoma in a patient with MEN 2A.

The localization of the MEN 2A gene to chromosome 10 now offers the opportunity to study the direct correlation of C-cell hyperplasia with the genetic abnormality. Members of a large MEN 2A kindred followed for 20 years were studied using six different pericentromeric markers for chromosome 10.[40] The probes used were 14–34, B14–34, MEN203, TBQ16, RBP9, and MEN203W-1.[106] Excellent correlations were found between the presence of C-cell proliferative disease identified histopathologically and the carrier state for this disorder detected by genetic linkage analysis. However, in two cases of mild diffuse C-cell hyperplasia, genetic linkage analyses were negative.[106]

DIFFERENTIAL DIAGNOSIS

Foci of C-cell hyperplasia, particularly of the nodular type, may be difficult to distinguish from a variety of other changes including squamous metaplasia, solid cell nests, intrathyroidal thymic or parathyroid tissue, palpation thyroiditis (multifocal granulomatous folliculitis), and tangential cuts of normal follicles[17,42,62] (Table 4.3).

Squamous metaplasia has been noted in a variety of inflammatory and neoplastic conditions of the thyroid.[62] Foci of squamous metaplasia are common in nodular goiter and Hashimoto's thyroiditis. Additionally, foci of squamous change are common in papillary carcinomas of the thyroid.

Solid cell nests correspond to remnants of the ultimobranchial bodies, and they are found most commonly in the midportions of the lateral lobes along their

TABLE 4.3.　DIFFERENTIAL DIAGNOSIS OF NODULAR C-CELL HYPERPLASIA

Squamous metaplasia
Solid cell nests
Multifocal granulomatous folliculitis (palpation thyroiditis)
Intrathyroidal thymus/parathyroid
Tangential cuts of follicles
Intrathyroidal metastasis of medullary carcinoma

central axes.[42] The component cells are polygonal to oval with nuclei having finely granular chromatin. Ultrastructurally, the solid cell nests have tonofilaments, desmosomes, and intraluminal cytoplasmic projections. The cells are positive for high and low molecular weight keratins. Some solid cell nests are connected to follicles with the formation of so-called mixed follicles, which may exhibit focal reactivity for thyroglobulin.

Palpation thyroiditis refers to a trauma-induced change characterized by accumulations of intrafollicular histiocytes, lymphocytes, plasma cells, and giant cells.[17] In some cases, the histiocytes encircle the innermost aspect of the follicle in a pattern reminiscent of early phases of C-cell hyperplasia. In contrast to C-cells, however, other histiocytes are typically positive for lysozyme and may give positive reactions for iron.

Tangential cuts of follicles may occasionally be difficult to distinguish from foci of nodular C-cell hyperplasia; however, tangential cuts of follicles generally are composed of polyhedral cells with well defined cell borders and centrally placed nuclei. The cytologic characteristics are identical to those of the adjacent follicular cells.

CONCLUSIONS

The four decades that have elapsed since the original descriptions of medullary thyroid carcinoma in the 1950s have witnessed an extraordinary series of advances in our understanding of this tumor and its precursor lesions. Many of these advances have occurred as a direct result of a close working relationship between clinical and basic scientists. Originally regarded as a pathologic curiosity, medullary carcinoma has served as a model system for the understanding of inherited neoplastic disease.

Most recently, linkage analyses have resulted in the assignment of the MEN 2 gene to chromosome 10. With the specific identification of the gene, which is likely to occur over the next several years, genetic diagnosis of the MEN 2 syndromes will become a reality. The identification and cloning of the gene will also undoubtedly provide a means to study the interactions of other genetic and environmental influences on the development of these dominantly inherited tumor syndromes.

REFERENCES

1. Albores-Saavedra, J. C-cell hyperplasia. *Am. J. Surg. Pathol.* *13*:987, 1989.
2. Albores-Saavedra, J., De la Mora, T. G., De la Torre-Rendon, F., and Gould, E. Mixed medullary

papillary carcinoma of the thyroid: A previously unrecognized variant of thyroid carcinoma. *Hum. Pathol. 21:*1151–1155, 1990.

3. Albores-Saavedra, J., LiVolsi, V. A., and Williams, E. D. Medullary carcinoma. *Semin. Diagn. Pathol. 2:*137–146, 1985.

4. Albores-Saavedra, J., Monforte, H., Nadji, M., and Morales, A. R. C-cell hyperplasia in thyroid tissue adjacent to follicular cell tumors. *Hum. Pathol. 19:*795–799, 1988.

5. Al Saadi, A. A. Ultrastructure of C-cell hyperplasia in asymptomatic patients with hypercalcitoninemia and a family history of medullary thyroid carcinoma. *Hum. Pathol. 12:*617–622, 1981.

6. Bergholm, U., Adami, H-O., Auer, G., Bergström, R., Bäckdahl, M., Grimelius, L., Hansson, G., Ljungberg, D., and Wilander, E. Histopathologic characteristics and nuclear DNA content as prognostic factors in medullary thyroid carcinoma. *Cancer 64:*135–142, 1989.

7. Biddinger, P. W., Brennan, M. F., and Rosen, P. P. Symptomatic C-cell hyperplasia associated with chronic lymphocytic thyroiditis. *Am. J. Surg. Pathol. 15:*599–604, 1991.

8. Bigner, S. H., Cox, E. B., Mendelsohn, G., Baylin, S. B., Wells, S. A., and Eggleston, J. Medullary carcinoma of the thyroid in the multiple endocrine neoplasia IIA syndrome. *Am. J. Surg. Pathol. 5:*459–472, 1981.

9. Black, H. E., Capen, C. C., and Young, D. M. Ultimobranchial thyroid neoplasms in bulls. *Cancer 32:*865–878, 1973.

10. Block, M. A., Jackson, C. E., Greenwald, K. A., Yott, J. B., and Tashjian, A. H. Jr. Clinical characteristics distinguishing hereditary from sporadic medullary thyroid carcinoma: Treatment implications. *Arch. Surg. 115:*142–148, 1980.

11. Bussolati, G., Foster, G. V., Clark, M. B., and Pearse, A. G. E. Immunofluorescent localization of calcitonin in medullary (C-cell) thyroid carcinoma using antibody to the pure porcine hormone. *Virchows Arch. [B] 2:*234–238, 1969.

12. Bussolati, G., and Pearse, A. G. E. Immunofluorescent localization of calcitonin in the C-cells of the pig and dog thyroid. *J. Endocrinol. 37:*205–210, 1967.

13. Capella, C., Bordi, C., Monga, G., Buffa, R., Fontana, P., Bonfanti, S., Bussolati, G., and Solcia, E. Multiple endocrine cell types in thyroid medullary carcinoma. Evidence for calcitonin, ACTH, 5-HT and small granule cells. *Virchows Arch [A] 377:*111–128, 1978.

14. Capen, C. C., and Young, D. M. Fine structural alterations in thyroid parafollicular cells in cows in response to experimental hypercalcemia induced by vitamin D. *Am. J. Pathol. 57:*365–382, 1969.

15. Carcangiu, M. L., Steeper, T., Zampi, G., and Rosai, J. Anaplastic thyroid carcinoma. A study of 70 cases. *Am. J. Clin. Pathol. 83:*135–158, 1985.

16. Carcangiu, M. L., Zampi, G., and Rosai, J. Poorly differentiated (insular) thyroid carcinoma. *Am. J. Surg. Pathol. 8:*655–668, 1984.

17. Carney, J. A., Moore, S. B., Northcutt, R. C., Woolner, L. B., and Stillwell, G. K. Palpation thyroiditis (multifocal granulomatous folliculitis). *Am. J. Clin. Pathol. 64:*639–647, 1975.

18. Carney, J. F., Sizemore, G. W., and Hales, A. B. Multiple endocrine neoplasia type 2b. *Pathobiol. Annu. 8:*105–153, 1978.

19. Carney, J. F., Sizemore, G. W., and Sheps, S. G. Adrenal medullary disease in multiple endocrine neoplasia type 2b. *Am. J. Clin. Pathol. 66:*279–290, 1976.

20. Delehaye, M. C., Bouizar, Z., Minvielle, S., Pidoux, E., Segond, N., Treilhou-Lahille, F., Milhaud, G., and Moukhtar, M. S. Increase in calcitonin mRNA levels in rats at high risk of C-cell tumors is genetically determined. *Biochem. Biophys. Res. Commun. 167:*232–237, 1990.

21. DeLellis, R. A., Dayal, Y., Tischler, A. S., Lee, A. K., and Wolfe, H. J. Multiple endocrine neoplasia syndromes. Cellular origins and interrelationships. *Int. Rev. Exp. Pathol. 28:*136–215, 1968.

22. DeLellis, R. A., Nunnemacher, G., Bitman, W. R., Gagel, R. F., Tashjian, A. H., Blount, M., and Wolfe, H. J. C-cell hyperplasia and medullary thyroid carcinoma in the rat. An immunohistochemical and ultrastructural study. *Lab. Invest. 40:*140–154, 1989.

23. DeLellis, R. A., Nunnemacher, G., and Wolfe, H. J. C-cell hyperplasia: An ultrastructural analysis. *Lab. Invest. 36:*237–248, 1977.

24. DeLellis, R. A., Rule, A. H., Spiler, F., Nathanson, L., Tashjian, A. H., and Wolfe, H. J. Calcitonin and carcinoembryonic antigen as tumor markers in medullary thyroid carcinoma. *Am. J. Clin. Pathol. 70:*587–594, 1978.

25. DeLellis, R. A., and Wolfe, H. J. The pathobiology of the human calcitonin (C) cell. *Pathol. Annu. 16* (part 2):25–52, 1981.

26. DeLellis, R. A., Wolfe, H. J., Gagel, R. F., Feldman, Z. T., Miller, H. H., Gang, D. L., and Reichlin, S. Adrenal medullary hyperplasia. *Am. J. Pathol. 83:*177–196, 1976.

27. Dominquez-Malagon, H., Delgado-Chavez, R., Torres-Najera, M., Gould, E., and Albores-Saavedra, J. Oxyphil and squamous variants of medullary thyroid carcinoma. *Cancer 63:*1183–1188, 1989.

28. Driman, D., Murray, D., and Kovacs, K. Encapsulated medullary carcinoma of the thyroid. A morphological study including immunocytochemistry, electron microscopy, flow cytometry and *in situ* hybridization. *Am. J. Surg. Pathol. 15:*1089–1095, 1991.

29. Eusebi, V., Damiani, S., Riva, C., Lloyd, R. V., and Capella, C. Calcitonin free oat cell carcinoma of the thyroid gland. *Virchows Arch [A] 417:*267–271, 1990.

30. Franc, B., Cillou, B., Carrier, A. M., Dutrieux-Berger, N., Floquet, J., Houcke, M., Justrabo, E., Lange, F., Pages, A., and Rigaud, C. Immunohistochemistry in medullary thyroid carcinoma: Prognosis and distinction between hereditary and sporadic tumors. *Henry Ford Hosp. Med. J. 25:*139–142, 1987.

31. Frauman, A. G., and Moses, A. C. Oncogenes and growth factors in thyroid carcinogenesis. *Endocrinol. Metab. Clin. North Am. 19:*479–493, 1990.

32. Gagel, R. F., Tashjian, A. H., Jr., Cummings, T., Papathanasopoulos, N., Kaplan, M. M., DeLellis, R. A., Wolfe, H. J., and Reichlin, S. The clinical outcome of prospective screening for multiple endocrine neoplasia type 2a. *N. Engl. J. Med. 318:*478–484, 1988.

33. Gibson, W. C. H., Peng, T-C., and Croker, B. P. C-cell nodules in adult human thyroid. A common autopsy finding. *Am. J. Clin. Pathol. 75:*347–350, 1981.

34. Gkonos, P. J., Tavianini, M. A., Liu, C-C., and Roos, B. A. Thyrotropin releasing hormone gene expression in normal thyroid parafollicular cells. *Mol. Endocrinol. 3:*2101–2109, 1989.

35. Golough, R., Us-Krasovec, M., Auersperg, M., Jancar, J., Bondi, A., and Eusebi, V. Amphicrine composite calcitonin and mucin producing carcinoma of the thyroid. *Ultrastruct. Pathol. 8:*197–206, 1985.

36. Goltzman, D., Potts, J. T., Ridgway, E. C., and Maloof, F. Calcitonin as a tumor marker. *N. Engl. J. Med. 290:*1035–1039, 1974.

37. Gonzalez-Campora, R., Sanchez-Gallego, F., Martin Lacave, I., Mora-Marin, J., Montero-Linares, C., and Galera-Davidsohn, H. Lectin histochemistry of the thyroid gland. *Cancer 62:*2354–2362, 1988.

38. Gorlin, R. J., Sedano, H. O., Vickers, R. A., and Cervenka, J. Multiple mucosal neuromas pheochromocytoma and medullary carcinoma of the thyroid. A syndrome. *Cancer 22:*293–299, 1968.

39. Gould, V. E., Wiedemann, B., Lee, I., Schwechheimer, K., Dockhorn-Dworniczak, B., Radosevich, J. A., Moll, R., and Franke, W. W. Synaptophysin expression in neuroendocrine neoplasms as determined by immunohistochemistry. *Am. J. Pathol. 126:*243–257, 1987.

40. Grauer, A., Raue, F., and Gagel, R. F. Changing concepts in the management of hereditary and sporadic medullary thyroid carcinoma. *Endocrinol. Metab. Clin. North Am. 19:*613–635, 1990.

41. Grieco, M., Santoro, M., Berlingieri, M. T., Mellilo, M., Donghi, R., Bongarzone, I., Pierotti, M. A., Della Porte, G., Fusco, A., and Vecchio, G. PTC is a novel rearranged form of the *ret* proto-oncogene and is frequently detected in human papillary thyroid carcinomas. *Cell 60:*557–563, 1990.

42. Harach, H. R. Solid cell nests in the thyroid. *J. Pathol. 155:*191–200, 1988.

43. Harach, H. R., and Bergholm, V. Medullary (C-cell) carcinoma of the thyroid with features of follicular oxyphilic tumors. *Histopathology 13:*645–656, 1988.

44. Harach, H. R., and Williams, E. D. Glandular (tubular and follicular) variants of medullary carcinoma of the thyroid. *Histopathology 7:*83–97, 1983.

45. Hazard, J. B., Hawk, W. A., and Crile, G., Jr. Medullary (solid) carcinoma of the thyroid: A clinicopathologic entity. *J. Clin. Endocrinol. Metab. 19:*152–161, 1959.

46. Holm, R., Sobrinho-Simões, M., Nesland, J. M., Gould, V. E., and Johannessen, J. V. Medullary carcinoma of the thyroid gland. An Immunocytochemical study. *Ultrastruct. Pathol.* 8:25–41, 1985.

47. Holm, R., Sobrinho-Simões, M., Nesland, J. M., and Johannesson, J. V. Concurrent production of calcitonin and thyroglobulin by the same neoplastic cells. *Ultrastruct. Pathol.* 10:241–251, 1986.

48. Horn, R. C. Carcinoma of the thyroid. Description of a distinctive morphological variant and report of 7 cases. *Cancer* 4:697–707, 1951.

49. Huss, L. J., and Mendelsohn, G. Medullary carcinoma of the thyroid gland: An encapsulated variant resembling the hyalinizing trabecular (paraganglioma-like) adenoma of the thyroid. *Mod. Pathol.* 3:581–585, 1990.

50. Jubb, K. V., and McEntee, K. The relationship of ultimobranchial remnants and derivatives to tumor of the thyroid gland in cattle. *Cornell. Vet.* 49:41–50, 1959.

51. Kakudo, K., Miyauchi, A., Ogihara, T., Takai, S. I., Kitamura, H., Kosaki, G., and Kuma-Hara, Y. Medullary carcinoma of the thyroid. Giant cell type. *Arch. Pathol. Lab. Med.* 102:445–447, 1978.

52. Kakudo, K., Miyauchi, A., Takai, S. I., Katayama, S., Kuma, K., and Kitamura, H. C-cell carcinoma of the thyroid, papillary type. *Acta. Pathol. Jpn.* 29:633–659, 1979.

53. Kodama, T., Okamoto, T., Fujimoto, Y., Obara, T., Ito, Y., Aiba, M., and Hirayama, A. C-cell adenoma of the thyroid. A rare but distinct clinical entity. *Surgery* 104:997–1003, 1988.

54. Lacave, I. M., Gonzalez-Campora, R., Fernandez, A. M., Gallego, S. F., Montero, C., and Gallera-Davidsohn, H. Mucosubstances in medullary carcinoma of the thyroid. *Histopathology* 13:55–66, 1988.

55. Landon, G., and Ordonez, N. G. Clear cell variant of medullary carcinoma of the thyroid. *Hum. Pathol.* 16:844–847, 1985.

56. Libbey, N. P., Nowakowski, K. J., and Tucci, J. R. C-cell hyperplasia of the thyroid in a patient with goitrous hypothyroidism and Hashimoto's thyroiditis. *Am. J. Surg. Pathol.* 13:71–77, 1989.

57. Lindsay, S., Nichols, C. W., and Chaikoff, I. L. Naturally occurring thyroid carcinoma in the rat. Similarities to human medullary thyroid carcinoma. *Arch. Pathol.* 86:353–364, 1968.

58. Lippman, S. M., Mendelsohn, G., Trump, D. L., Wells, S. A., and Baylin, S. B. The prognostic and biological significance of cellular heterogeneity in medullary thyroid carcinoma. *J. Clin. Endocrinol. Metab.* 54:233–244, 1982.

59. Lips, C. J. M., Leo, J. R., and Berends, M. J. H. Thyroid C-cell hyperplasia and micronodules in close relatives of MEN-2A patients: Pitfalls in early diagnosis and re-evaluation of criteria for surgery. *Henry Ford Hosp. Med. J.* 35:133–138, 1987.

60. Lips, C. J. M., Vasen, H. F. A., and Lamers, C. B. H. W. Multiple endocrine neoplasia syndromes. *CRC Crit. Rev. Oncol. Hematol.* 2:117–184, 1988.

61. LiVolsi, V. A. Mixed thyroid tumors: A real entity? *Lab. Invest.* 57:237–239, 1987.

62. LiVolsi, V. A. *Surgical Pathology of the Thyroid.* Philadelphia, W.B. Saunders, 1990, pp. 213–252.

63. LiVolsi, V. A., and Feind, C. R. Incidental medullary thyroid carcinoma in sporadic hyperparathyroidism. *Am. J. Clin. Pathol.* 71:595–599, 1979.

64. LiVolsi, V. A., Feind, C. R., LoGerfo, P., and Tashjian, A. H. Demonstration by immunoperoxidase staining of hyperplasia of parafollicular cells in the thyroid gland in hyperparathyroidism. *J. Clin. Endocrinol. Metab.* 37:550–559, 1973.

65. Ljungberg, O., Bondeson, L., and Bondeson, A. G. Differentiated thyroid carcinoma, intermediate type: A new tumor entity with features of follicular and parafollicular carcinoma. *Hum. Pathol.* 15:218–228, 1984.

66. Lloyd, R. V. Use of molecular probes in the study of endocrine disease. *Hum. Pathol.* 18:1199–1121, 1987.

67. MacIntyre, I. Calcitonin, physiology, biosynthesis, secretion, metabolism and mode of action. In: *Endocrinology*, 2nd edition, edited by L.J. DeGroot. Philadelphia, W.B. Saunders, 1989, vol. 2, pp. 892–901.

68. Marcus, J. N., Dise, C. A., and LiVolsi, V. A. Melanin production in a medullary thyroid carcinoma. *Cancer 49:*2518–2526, 1982.

69. Mathew, C. G. P., Chin, K. S., Easton, D. F., Thorpe, K., Carter, C., Liou, G. I., Fong, S. L., Bridges, C. D., Haak, H., and Kruseman, A. C. A linked genetic marker for multiple endocrine neoplasia type 2A on chromosome 10. *Nature 328:*527–528, 1987.

70. Mendelsohn, G., Baylin, S. B., Bigner, S. H., Wells, S. A., and Eggleston, J. C. Anaplastic variants of medullary thyroid carcinoma. A light microscopic and immunohistochemical study. *Am. J. Surg. Pathol. 4:*333–341, 1980.

71. Mendelsohn, G., Eggleston, J. C., Weisburger, W. R., Gann, D. S., and Baylin, S. B. Calcitonin and histaminase in C-cell hyperplasia and medullary thyroid carcinoma. A light microscopic and immunohistochemical study. *Am. J. Pathol. 92:*35–52, 1978.

72. Mendelsohn, G., Wells, S. A., and Baylin, S. B. Relationship of tissue carcinoembryonic antigen and calcitonin to tumor virulence in medullary thyroid carcinoma. An immunohistochemical study in early, localized and virulent disseminated stages of disease. *Cancer 54:*657–662, 1984.

73. Nieuwenhuizjen-Kruseman, A. C., Bosman, F. T., van Bergen Henegouw, J. C., Cramer-Knijnenburg, G., and Brutel Dela Riviere, G. Medullary differentiation of anaplastic thyroid carcinoma. *Am. J. Clin. Pathol. 77:*541–547, 1982.

74. Normann, T., Johannessen, J. V., Gautvik, K. M., Olsen, B. R., and Brennhovd, I. O. Medullary carcinoma of the thyroid. Diagnostic problems. *Cancer 38:*366–377, 1976.

75. O'Toole, K., Fenoglio-Preiser, C. M., and Pushparaj, N. Endocrine changes associated with the human aging process. III. Effect of age on the number of calcitonin reactive cells in the thyroid gland. *Hum. Pathol. 16:*991–1000, 1985.

76. Pearse, A. G. E. Common cytochemical and ultrastructural characteristics of cells producing polypeptide hormones (the APUD series) and their relevance to thyroid and ultimobranchial C-cells and calcitonin. *Proc. R. Soc. Lond. [Biol.] 170:*71–80, 1968.

77. Pfaltz, M., Hedinger, C. E., and Muhlethaler, J. P. Mixed medullary and follicular carcinoma of the thyroid. *Virchows Arch. [A] 400:*53–59, 1983.

78. Ponder, B. A. J., Ponder, M. A., Coffey, R., Pembrey, M. E., Gagel, R. F., Telenius-Berg, M., Semple, P., and Easton, D. F. Risk estimation and screening in families of patients with medullary carcinoma. *Lancet 1:*397–400, 1988.

79. Santoro, M., Rosati, R., Grieco, M., Berlingieri, M. T., D'Amato, G. L., De Franciscis, V., and Fusco, A. The *ret* protooncogene is consistently expressed in human pheochromocytomas and thyroid medullary carcinomas. *Oncogene 5:*1595–1598, 1990.

80. Schmid, K. W., Fischer-Colbrie, J., Hagn, C., Jasani, B., Williams, E. D., and Winkler, H. Chromogranin A and B and secretogranin II in medullary carcinomas in the thyroid. *Am. J. Surg. Pathol. 11:*551–556, 1987.

81. Schimke, R. N., and Hartmann, W. H. Familial amyloid producing medullary thyroid carcinoma and pheochromocytoma. A distinct genetic entity. *Ann. Intern. Med. 63:*1027–1039, 1965.

82. Schroder, S., Bocker, W., Baisch, H., Burk, C. G., Arps, H., Meiners, I., Kastendieck, H., Heitz, P. U., and Kloppel, G. Prognostic factors in medullary thyroid carcinoma. Survival in relation to age, sex, stage, histology, immunocytochemistry and DNA content. *Cancer 61:*806–816, 1988.

83. Schroder, S., and Kloppel, G. Carcinoembryonic antigen and non-specific cross reacting antigen in thyroid cancer. *Am. J. Surg. Pathol. 11:*100–108, 1987.

84. Schroder, S., Schwarz, W., Rehpenning, W., Dralle, H., Bay, Y., and Bocker, W. Leu M1 immunoreactivity and prognosis in medullary carcinoma of the thyroid gland. *J. Cancer Res. Clin. Oncol. 114:*291–296, 1988.

85. Schurch, W., Babai, F., Boivin, Y., and Verdy, M. Light, electron microscopic and cytochemical studies on the morphogenesis of familial medullary thyroid carcinoma. *Virchows Arch. [A] 376:*29–46, 1977.

86. Scopsi, L., DiPalma, S., Ferrari, C., Holst, J. J., Rehfeld, J. H., and Rilke, F. C-cell hyperplasia accompanying thyroid diseases other than medullary thyroid carcinoma: An immunocytochemical study by means of antibodies to calcitonin and somatostatin. *Mod. Pathol. 4:*297–304, 1991.

87. Scopsi, L., Ferrari, C., and Pilotti, S. Immunocytochemical localization and identification of prosomatostatin gene products in medullary carcinoma of human thyroid gland. *Hum. Pathol.* 21:820–830, 1990.
88. Sikri, K. L., Varndell, I. M., Hamid, Q. A., Wilson, B. S., Kameya, T., Ponder, B. A., Lloyd, R. V., Bloom, S. R., and Polak, J. M. Medullary carcinoma of the thyroid. An immunocytochemical and histochemical study of 25 cases using eight separate markers. *Cancer 56*:2481–2491, 1985.
89. Simpson, N. E., Kidd, K. K., Goodfellow, P. J., McDermid, H., Myers, S., Kidd, J. R., Jackson, C. E., Duncan, A. M., Farrer, L. A., and Brasch, K. Assignment of multiple endocrine neoplasia type 2A to chromosome 10 by linkage. *Nature 328*:528–529, 1987.
90. Sipple, J. H. The association of pheochromocytoma with carcinoma of the thyroid gland. *Am. J. Med. 31*:163–166, 1961.
91. Sizemore, G. W. Medullary of the carcinoma of the thyroid gland. *Semin. Oncol. 14*:306–314, 1987.
92. Sobol, H., Narod, S. A., Nakamura, T., Boneu, A., Calmettes, C., Chadenas, D., Charpantier, G., Chatal, J. F., Delepine, N., and Delisle, M. J. Screening for multiple endocrine neoplasia type 2A with DNA polymorphism analysis. *N. Engl. J. Med. 321*:996–1001, 1989.
93. Sobol, H., Narod, S. A., Schuffenecher, I., Amos, C., Ezekowitz, R. A., and Lenoir, G. M. Hereditary medullary thyroid carcinoma: Genetic analysis of 3 related syndromes. *Henry Ford Hosp. Med. J. 37*:109–111, 1989.
94. Stanta, G., Carcangiu, M. L., and Rosai, J. The biochemical and immunohistochemical profile of thyroid neoplasia. *Pathol. Annu. 23* (part 1):129–157, 1988.
95. Steiner, A. L., Goodman, A. D., and Powers, S. R. Study of a kindred with pheochromocytoma, medullary thyroid carcinoma, hyperparathyroidism and Cushing's disease. Multiple endocrine neoplasia type 2. *Medicine (Baltimore) 47*:371–409, 1968.
96. Sunday, M. E., Wolfe, H. J., Roos, B. A., and Spindel, E. R. Gastrin releasing peptide gene expression in developing hyperplastic and neoplastic human thyroid C-cells. *Endocrinology 122*:1551–1558, 1988.
97. Tashjian, A. H., Jr., and Melvin, K. E. W. Medullary carcinoma of the thyroid gland. *N. Engl. J. Med. 279*:279–283, 1968.
98. Thurston, V., and Williams, E. D. Experimental induction of C-cell tumors in thyroid by increased content of vitamin D3. *Acta Endocrinol. (Copenh.) 100*:41–45, 1982.
99. Triggs, S. M., and Williams, E. D. Experimental carcinogenesis in the rat follicular and C-cells. *Acta Endocrinol. (Copenh.) 85*:84–92, 1977.
100. Uribe, M., Fenoglio-Preiser, C. M., Grimes, M., and Feind, C. Medullary carcinoma of the thyroid gland: Clinical, pathological and immunohistochemical features with review of the literature. *Am. J. Surg. Pathol. 9*:577–594, 1985.
101. Vinores, S. A., Bonnin, J. M., Rubinstein, L. J., and Marangos, P. J. Immunohistochemical demonstration of neuron specific enolase in neoplasms of the CNS and other tissues. *Arch. Pathol. Lab. Med. 108*:536–540, 1984.
102. Wells, S. A., Jr., Baylin, S. B., Leight, G. S., Dale, J. K., Dilley, W. G., and Farndon, J. R. The importance of early diagnosis in patients with hereditary medullary thyroid carcinoma. *Ann. Surg. 195*:595–599, 1982.
103. Williams, E. D. A review of 17 cases of carcinoma of the thyroid and pheochromocytoma. *J. Clin. Pathol. 18*:288–292, 1965.
104. Williams, E. D. Histogenesis of medullary carcinoma of the thyroid. *J. Clin. Pathol. 19*:114–118, 1966.
105. Williams, E. D., Brown, C. L., and Doniach, I. Pathological and clinical findings in a series of 67 cases of medullary carcinoma of the thyroid. *J. Clin. Pathol. 19*:103–113, 1966.
106. Wolfe, H. J., Delellis, R. A., Kaplan, M., Cummings, T., Ponder, B. A. J., Ponder, M., Gardner, E., Papi, L., and Reichlin, S. Re-evaluation of histological criteria for C-cell hyperplasia in MEN 2A using genetic recombinant DNA markers. *Lab. Invest. 66*:39A, 1992.
107. Wolfe, H. J., Melvin, K. E. W., Cervi-Skinner, S. J., Saadi, A. A., Juliar, J. F., Jackson, C. E.,

and Tashjian, A. H. Jr. C-cell hyperplasia preceding medullary thyroid carcinoma. *N. Engl. J. Med. 289:*437–441, 1973.

108. Zaatari, G. S., Saigo, P. E., and Huvos, A. G. Mucin production in medullary carcinoma of the thyroid. *Arch. Pathol. Lab. Med. 107:*70–74, 1983.

109. Zajac, J. D., Penschow, J., Mason, T., Tregear, G., Coghlan, J., and Martin, T. J. Identification of calcitonin and calcitonin gene related peptide messenger RNA in medullary thyroid carcinoma by hybridization histochemistry. *J. Clin. Endocrinol. Metab. 62:*1037–1043, 1986.

Chapter 5

Mechanisms of Human Autoimmune Thyroid Disease—1992*

TERRY F. DAVIES AND DAVID L. KENDLER

The group of human thyroid diseases associated with immunologic abnormalities, the autoimmune thyroid diseases (AITD), encompasses both thyroid overactivity and underactivity: hyperthyroid Graves' disease and its ophthalmic manifestations and autoimmune thyroiditis of goitrous and nongoitrous types including thyroiditis presenting in the postpartum period. Only when autoimmune thyroiditis is associated with goiter formation should it be referred to as Hashimoto's disease.

THYROIDAL AUTOANTIGENS

THE THYROID-STIMULATING HORMONE

Thyroid-stimulating hormone (TSH) binds to a defined TSH receptor (TSHR) on the surface of the thyroid epithelial cell which is G-protein linked and uses cyclic adenosine monophosphate and the phosphoinositol pathways for signal transduction.[60] Although the TSHR is present at low density on the thyroid cell surface, with 10^3 to 10^4 sites per cell, it is the primary autoantigen of Graves' disease. Putative extrathyroidal TSH binding sites on adipose and other tissues are of undefined function.[8,14,15]

The geography of the human TSHR gene has now been fully defined and localized to chromosome 14.[25,39] TSHR-specific mRNA consists of at least two major transcripts of 4.6 and 4.4 kilobases (kb), suggesting that alternate splicing may occur. Two distinct regions of the extracellular domain of the TSHR differentiate it from the luteinizing hormone and follicle-stimulating hormone receptor structures. These regions are, therefore, a potential focus for autoimmune epitopes since the gonadotropin receptors are much less commonly involved in autoimmune disease. Recombinant human TSHR has now been expressed in Chinese hamster ovary cells (Fig. 5.1).[37]

The TSHR was thought to consist of a 120 kD, 744 amino acid sequence made up of two subunits, A and B, linked by a disulfide bond.[28,29] This structure has recently been refined following the derivation of the protein sequence and could also be a single protein in its natural state and only present artifactually in subunits.[64] Nevertheless, the putative 55-kD A subunit is water-soluble and

103

contains the TSH binding site (forming so-called long-acting thyroid stimulator absorbing activity).[18,19] The 35-kD B fragment is insoluble and contains the membrane-spanning domain.

Short synthesized peptides have recently been used to identify immunogenic regions of the TSHR. Two peptides spanning residues 14–29 of the extracellular domain reacted with Graves' disease sera, suggesting not just the region of an epitope but also the lack of conformational requirements for TSHR antibody (Ab) recognition.[50] Whether such preliminary reports imply interactions of sufficient affinity to be important requires further study. This is particularly relevant to determine in view of the failure of such an approach to detect TSHR clones in λ gt11 expression libraries.[54] Another recent study has suggested different binding sites for TSH receptor antibodies, which are antagonists rather than agonists, and this approach is likely to provide important information on the TSHR epitopes involved.[51]

Although solubilized TSHR has been shown to induce T-cell activation as measured by cytokine release,[42] there have been no studies to date of the TSHR T-cell epitopes in human autoimmune thyroid disease or in animals immunized with recombinant TSHR.

Human Thyroglobulin

Thyroglobulin (Tg) is the principal constituent of the follicular colloid, produced by the thyroid epithelial cells and stored in the gland. Thyroid peroxidase (TPO) is responsible for the iodination of specific tyrosine residues on Tg to monoiodotyrosine and diiodotyrosine.

Genomic DNA encoding Tg is a 200-kb sequence located on chromosome 8 which transcribes both 9.0- and 0.9-kb mRNAs (termed Tg1 and Tg2).[24] The

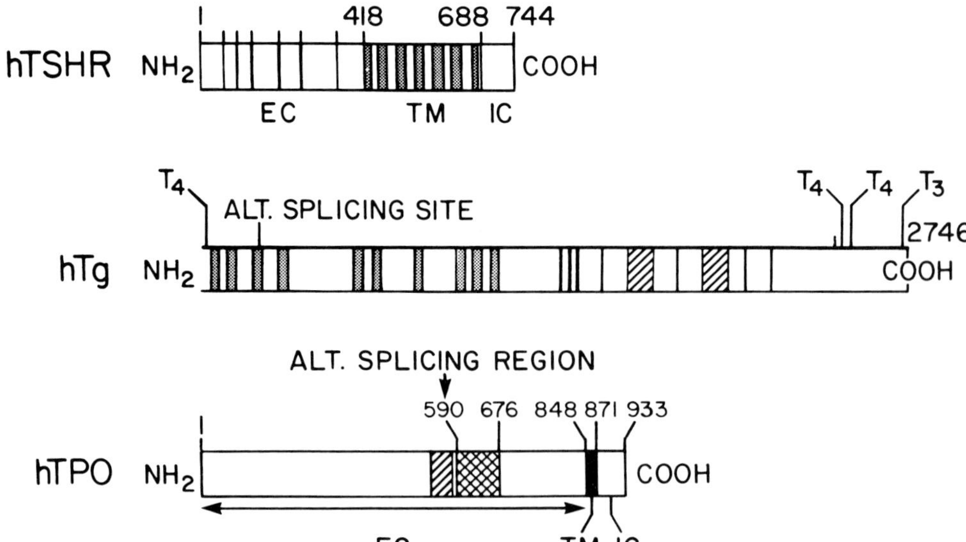

Fig. 5.1.   The structure of the TSHR, hTg, and hTPO antigens.

transcription of Tg mRNAs is induced by TSH via a series of thyroid-specific *trans*-activating factors (TTF1 and TTF2). TSH-stimulated Tg gene transcription is also regulated by a variety of thyroid cell-secreted growth factors (such as insulin-like growth factor-1) and cytokines.

Tg is a large, water-soluble glycoprotein dimer, with each subunit being approximately 330 kD (Fig. 5.1). Although about 45 specific tyrosine residues of a total of 72 in the molecule are accessible to iodination by TPO, only a few act as primary iodine acceptors and donor sites *in vitro* and these are located in defined polypeptide sequences near the amino- and carboxy-terminal ends of the molecule.

Immunization of laboratory animals with Tg induces the formation of thyroglobulin autoantibodies (Tg Ab) which recognize conformational Tg epitopes. There are 4–6 principal epitopes as shown by reactivity of Tg antisera to fragments prepared by enzymatic digestion of Tg, heat or chemically denatured Tg, and Tg of differing iodine content. It has also been shown that these conformational B-cell epitopes depend on the integrity of the disulfide bonds which maintain the structure of Tg. The epitopes recognized by antisera and monoclonal antibodies (MAb) have been compared to the epitopes recognized in patients with autoimmune thyroid disease.[58,62] Human autoantibodies were inhibited by some, but not all, murine Tg MAb and the pattern of inhibition by patient sera was distinct from sera with Tg Ab obtained from individuals without disease, suggesting the presence of disease-specific epitopes. However, the structure of hTg epitopes have not been defined to date. Up to 70% of Tg autoantibodies have been reported to be directed against thyroxine (T_4)-containing regions of the Tg molecule while others have found that the tyrosine residues do not significantly contribute to B-cell epitopes.

As expected, T-cells from animals immunized with Tg react to smaller, presumably more linear, Tg fragments than recognized by autoantibodies. Recently a murine Tg peptide sequence (a 9mer beginning at Asp 2551) has been characterized which is a potent T-cell epitope only when hormone (T_4)-containing.[9] This suggests that T-cell reactive epitopes, while not conformational, are likely to be iodine-dependent, at least in an animal model. The evidence that the iodine content of Tg endows greater immunogenicity[59] would agree with such data. However, to date, the epitopes operative in human Tg antigen-specific T-cells have not been fully explored.

HUMAN THYROIDPEROXIDASE

TPO is situated on the luminal surface of the microvilli of the thyroid epithelial cell in the appropriate location to catalyze intrafollicular reactions on stored Tg. TPO is the major "microsomal" antigen of autoimmune thyroid disease.[65]

TPO transcription and translation are closely regulated by TSH. The genomic DNA for hTPO is located on the short arm of chromosome 2, although its geography has not yet been fully elucidated.[33] Two different human TPO cDNA sequences differing by 171 bases have been isolated and proposed as the reason for the 100 and 107 kD protein doublet often seen on Western blotting. There is also evidence for alternative splicing of TPO message with at least two distinct mRNAs of 3.0 and 3.2 kb.[74] TPO polymorphisms have been reported.[43]

The deduced amino acid sequence of human TPO is 933 amino acids (Fig. 5.1). It is a 107-kD glycoprotein with 10% glycosylation and a membrane-spanning region close to the carboxy terminus. TPO iodinates tyrosine residues on Tg and couples iodinated tyrosines to form triiodothyronine (T_3) (monoiodotyrosine + diiodotyrosine) and T_4. Antithyroid drugs, such as methimazole or propylthiouracil, act by competing for substrate with TPO.

At least 6 epitopes have been described on TPO including one or both of the enzyme catalytic sites. Some autoantigenic epitopes have been identified through competition with anti-TPO MAb and human sera containing anti-TPO Ab of differing subclasses.[63] There is evidence that the intrachain loop of amino acids formed by a disulfide bridge is essential to immunogenicity, suggesting that conformational epitopes may be important. The poor binding of anti-TPO to reduced and denatured TPO antigen also reflects the destruction of such conformational epitopes. Studies with tryptic fragments of TPO have suggested that one major epitope is associated with TPO enzyme activity, but such studies were performed with a relatively large fragment. Of interest, an 85-amino acid fragment of TPO (amino acids 590–675) was recognized in a nonglycosylated state by 63% of human sera positive for anti-TPO whereas other nonglycosylated fragments have not been immunoreactive.[22,36] The relative importance of these different epitopes remains unclear. Recombinant glycosylated human TPO has been shown to be antigenically similar to natural TPO and can be used as an immune target.[31]

Data are now available defining human TPO T-cell epitopes using peripheral blood mononuclear cells and T-cell clones from patients with autoimmune thyroid disease interacting with a series of synthesized TPO peptides.[30] These studies have defined short linear epitopes within the TPO molecule. However, many different peptides have been shown to be reactive in different patients, and this may be secondary to HLA restriction as well as to technical differences in the studies reported. Of additional interest has been the homology of TPO and Tg. There is a common 8-amino acid sequence with 6 identical and 2 conserved amino acids which may also represent a linear cross-reactive T-cell epitope.[47]

RETRO-ORBITAL ANTIGENS

Cross-reacting epitopes between thyroid tissue and retro-orbital tissue have been sought to explain the orbital manifestations of Graves' disease. Antigens (64 and 73 kD) in porcine extraocular muscle are, however, recognized by sera from patients with Graves' disease with or without ophthalmopathy.[2] The recent cloning of a 64-kD extraocular muscle antigen, claimed not to be present in skeletal muscle and recognized by antibodies in serum from patients with Graves' ophthalmopathy may, however, confirm the potential for this tissue epitope cross-reactivity.

Retro-orbital and dermal fibroblasts are morphologically and functionally distinct *in vitro*. For example, dexamethasone and T_3 inhibit synthesis of glycosaminoglycans in dermal but not retro-orbital fibroblast cultures.[66] A 23-kD soluble human fibroblast antigen appears not to be specific for retro-orbital fibroblasts and may also be recognized by patients with Graves' disease with or without ophthalmopathy.

T-CELL FUNCTION IN AUTOIMMUNE THYROID DISEASE

T-cell surface markers in the peripheral blood of patients with Graves' disease have been influenced by the sensitivity and specificity of antibodies and detection techniques used and by the differing selection of patients and their clinical status.[6] However, from a large and confusing body of literature a number of general conclusions can be drawn. Firstly, relatives of patients with autoimmune thyroid disease have normal peripheral blood T-cell subset phenotypic markers, indicating a lack of easily detectable familial abnormalities (related to HLA or non-HLA influences). Secondly, the consistent finding of decreased numbers of CD8[+] T-cells in hyperthyroid patients appears primarily to be secondary to hyperthyroidism since such abnormalities, where they have been detected, may be corrected with antithyroid drug treatment and can be seen in hyperthyroidism not secondary to autoimmune thyroid disease.[5] However, some patients with Graves' disease show not just a decrease in suppressor-cytotoxic (CD8[+]) T-cells but also a fall in "naive" (suppressor-inducer, CD4[+]CD45RA[+]) T-cells even when rendered euthyroid. Similar observations have been made in patients with multiple sclerosis and systemic lupus erythematosus.[48,49] Those patients who retain lower circulating numbers of CD8[+] T-cells are likely to have more severe disease, an observation that originally suggested a suppressor T-cell "defect" in autoimmune thyroid disease.[3]

The intrathyroidal T-cell population has been shown to exhibit highly specific phenotypic changes when compared to the peripheral circulation. It should be noted that a number of suppressor-cytotoxic (CD8[+]) cells predominantly localize to the follicles but only form a small percentage of the infiltrate (3–4%). When thyroid tissues from patients with Graves' or Hashimoto's diseases are examined histologically, the intrathyroidal interstitial lymphocytes are more than 80% T-cells with suppressor-cytotoxic cells predominating. Although the suppressor/cytotoxic (CD8[+]) and suppressor-inducer (CD4[+]CD45RA[+]) T-cell content of the peripheral blood may be depressed in certain patients with Graves' disease, particularly those requiring surgery, there is a relative excess of such cells within the intraepithelial compartment of the thyroid gland in Graves' disease, as evidenced both by flow cytometry and immunocytochemistry[44] (Fig. 5.2). This accumulation of CD8[+] cells may be secondary to changes in the CD4[+] T-cell subsets which may influence intrathyroidal CD8[+] T-cell development and function. An attractive explanation for the observed accumulation of CD8[+] T-cells in Graves' thyroid tissue might be a "homing" mechanism involving tissue-specific molecules on lymphocytes (such as LFA-1) as well as molecules expressed by tissues themselves including the expression of ICAM-1 by thyroid epithelial cells.[45,70]

Migration inhibition factor assays originally provided data on thyroid antigen responsiveness of peripheral blood T-cells but have largely been replaced by more specific assays. These early studies, using a crude thyroid antigenic extract and lacking HLA-matched controls, suggested that an antigen-specific T-cell defect

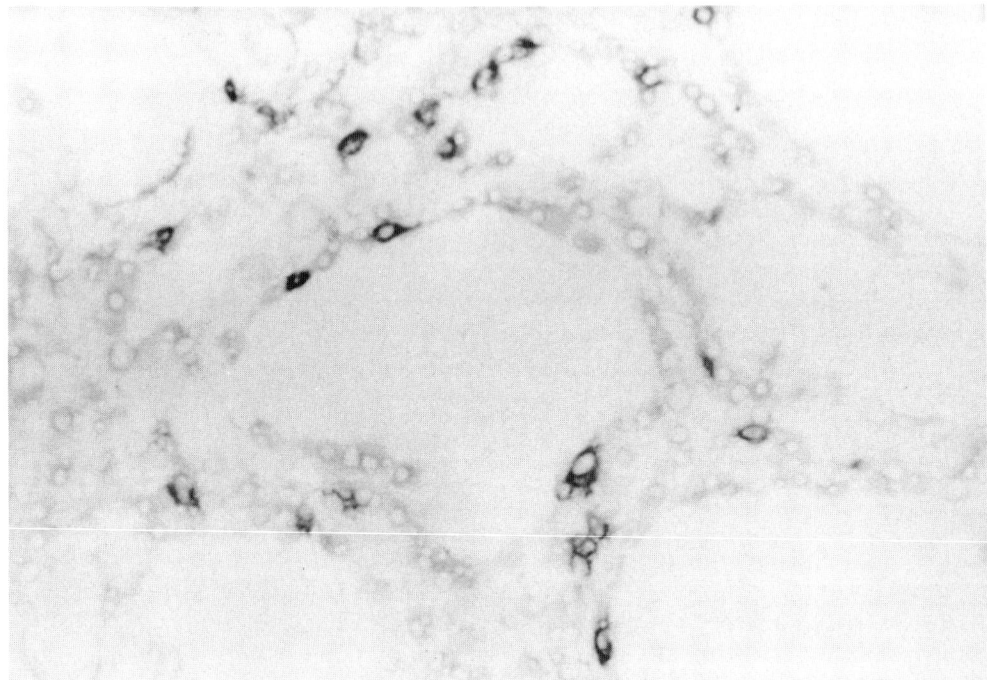

FIG. 5.2. Intraepithelial accumulation of CD8+ cells in the thyroid of a patient with Graves' disease.

was present in patients with autoimmune thyroid disease.[69] Although other workers were sometimes unable to show such a defect,[38] using newer techniques, Volpe *et al.*[26,27] have continued to generate data in favor of a thyroid antigen-specific defect in T-cell function, thus allowing autoantibody secretion. How such a thyroid-specific defect could encompass many different thyroid antigens is unclear and would require the presence of a common epitope on each of the three major thyroid antigens.

HLA class II antigen-positive thyroid epithelial cells are effective simulators of T-cell proliferation in patients with AITD on the basis of a mixed cell reaction which is HLA-restricted and which may or may not be thyroid antigen-dependent[11,34] while thyroid cells may also act as antigen-presenting cells. The influence of such activated T-cells on B-cell function is assumed to enhance autoantibody (Tg Ab, TPO Ab, and TSHR Ab) secretion and cytotoxic T-cell activity. While non-TSHR antigen interactions are unlikely to be etiologic in Graves' disease, in autoimmune thyroiditis these T-cells are likely to be cytotoxic for thyroid cells and of major importance in thyroid destruction. Animal models of thyroiditis have shown clear evidence of the importance of cytotoxic T-cells[10] and a thyroid cell-specific cytotoxic clone has been described in human disease.[40]

The conditions used for cloning T-cells may favor the growth of certain subpopulations, giving a biased view of lymphocyte subset frequencies. However, we estimate that up to 10% of activated T-cells infiltrating the thyroid gland in patients with AITD proliferate in response to autologous thyroid cells or thyroid cell antigens.[41] Intrathyroidal lymphocytes reacting with self-major histocompatability complex (MHC) (autologous mixed lymphocyte reactors) may comprise up to 50% of T-cells, probably secondary to such bias in the selection conditions. In Graves' disease the intrathyroidal lymphocytes from T-cell cloning are up to 75% memory T-cells (helper-inducer, $CD4^+CD29^+$) while in thyroiditis there is a much lower prevalence of such cells.[41] There have been no antigen-specific cytotoxic T-cell clones obtained from the glands of patients with Graves' disease as compared to those with Hashimoto's disease.[4,40] Some investigators have, however, found a high prevalence of natural killer cell clones in glands from patients with Graves' disease when selected with mitogen.[20]

The detailed characterization of thyroid antigen-specific human T-cell lines and clones is presently being undertaken in a number of laboratories. $CD4^+$ antigen-reactive T-cells are known to be HLA class II restricted, but their helper and suppressor activities have not yet been extensively explored. We found more than 60% of intrathyroidal T-cell hybridomas to secrete helper factors which enhanced IgG secretion compared with only 10% of peripheral blood T-cell control hybridomas. Such data provide additional evidence for a mechanistic basis for autoantibody secretion within the thyroid.

The human T-cell receptor (hTcR) V genes code for the antigen-MHC recognition site on the hTcR, affording antigen specificity. Restricted heterogeneity of hTcR V gene receptor families implicates T-cell immunity as etiologic in the disease as well as identifying potential sites for immune modulation. In order to examine the T-cell receptor V gene usage of intrathyroidal T-lymphocytes we have recently used the polymerase chain reaction and multiple oligonucleotide amplimers to test for V gene families utilized by intrathyroidal T-cells from patients with autoimmune thyroid disease. Our data demonstrated a marked bias in hTcR V α gene utilization by T-cells from within the thyroid when compared to peripheral blood from the same individuals.[12] However, the predominant V α genes differed from patient to patient with no clear disease-related preference. Such information, however, supports the concept of restricted T-cell heterogeneity in human autoimmune thyroid disease and points to the primacy of T-cells in the etiology of Graves' and Hashimoto's thyroid dysfunction.

ANTIGEN-PRESENTING POTENTIAL OF THE THYROID CELL

Human T-cells recognize thyroid antigen complexed with HLA antigen. Normal thyroid cells constitutively express HLA class I antigen but do not express class II antigen. Cytokines such as interferon-γ (INF-γ) and tumor necrosis factor-α are capable of influencing HLA class II antigen expression in thyroid epithelial cells, both *in vitro* and *in vivo*, and may be relevant to the pathophysiology of AITD.[7,57] Mice treated with INF-γ develop widespread MHC class II antigen expression and a thyroiditis and INF-γ-treated thyroid tissue is lysed when returned to syngeneic hosts.[23] INF-γ induces MHC class II antigen expression in cultured human and rodent thyrocytes, an effect potentiated by TSH. Once a thyroid cell is induced to express MHC class II antigens, it will present viral antigen to cloned antigen-specific T-cells[35] or thyroid-antigen specific T-cells,[32] suggesting that thyroid cells have true antigen-presenting capacity and can provide the second signal necessary for T-cell activation. The question remains of whether cytokines arising from the immune cells themselves indirectly initiate MHC class II antigen expression or whether direct expression of class II antigens on the thyroid cells themselves could initiate the immune response. Of particular interest, therefore, has been the direct modulation and induction of thyroid cell MHC class II antigens by viral infection.[52] However, *in situ* hybridization studies showed that HLA-DR gene expression was greatest in Graves' disease in areas of thyroid glands associated with lymphocytic infiltrate (Fig. 5.3). Such observations that HLA class II antigen expression was localized to areas of the thyroid gland infiltrated with lymphocytes but not present in normal thyroid tissue caused great interest in the potential of the thyroid cell to act as a classical antigen-presenting cell *in vivo.*[35,56] Most of the evidence to date suggests that such a reaction is secondary to the presence of activated T-cells releasing local cytokines but more needs to be learned about viral regulation of human thyroid cell HLA genes.

THYROID AUTOANTIBODIES

TSHR Ab are detectable only in patients with autoimmune thyroid disease and, therefore, are disease-specific and absent in the normal population. Furthermore, TSHR Ab are unique human autoantibodies; there are no animal models that secrete TSHR Ab. Eighty to 100% of untreated hyperthyroid patients with Graves' disease have detectable TSHR Ab which is biologically thyroid-stimulating. These TSHR Ab are altered by treatment of the disease and may predict relapse after withdrawal of antithyroid drug treatment.[13,17] TSHR Ab are also detectable in 10–15% of patients with autoimmune thyroiditis but are TSHR-blocking Ab on further analysis.[21]

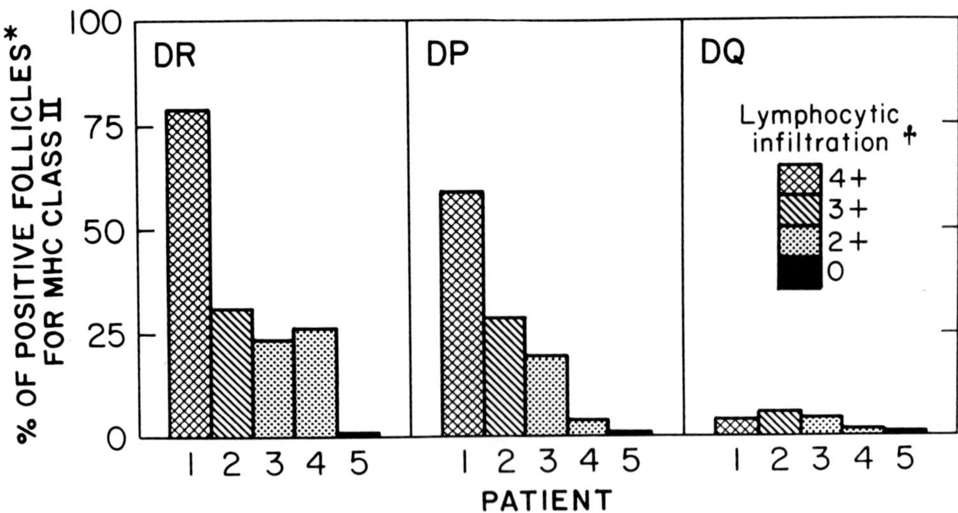

FIG. 5.3. Correlation between lymphocytic infiltration and degree of HLA class II antigen expression in thyroid tissues from patients with Graves' disease.

The original self-infusion of serum from patients with Graves' disease by Adams and colleagues[1] and the resulting thyroid stimulation was the first example of the role of TSHR Ab in the induction of human hyperthyroidism. Another early demonstration of the *in vivo* effects of TSHR Ab came from neonatal studies demonstrating the transplacental stimulation of the fetal thyroid in mothers with high titers of TSHR Ab.[67] TSHR Ab demonstrate light chain restriction in many patients with Graves' disease[73] and a restriction to the IgG_1 subclass.[72] These data are supportive evidence for oligoclonality and a V gene etiology for Graves' disease on the basis of a forbidden clone.

Tg Ab are found in 50–60% of patients with Graves' disease compared to 10–30% of normal subjects and over 75% of patients with autoimmune thyroiditis. Tg Ab are most commonly IgG and polyclonal, demonstrating only partial restriction to IgG_1 and IgG_4 subclasses depending on the monoclonal antibodies utilized.[16,46] Such lack of severe restriction in Tg Ab indicates that these auto-antibodies are most likely secondary in the immune response of human autoimmune thyroid disease. Although human monoclonal Tg Ab have been reported, extensive V gene characterization is not yet available. Passive transfer of Tg Ab in animal models does not cause thyroiditis and human Tg Ab are not commonly complement fixing. However, circulating Tg-anti-Tg immune complexes have been demonstrated, as well as thyroid gland basement membrane deposition of Tg immune complexes. In rare cases, Graves' disease may be associated with glomerulonephritis and nephrotic syndrome. There is cross-over specificity of Tg with acetylcholinesterase based on sequence analysis and Western blotting. Anti-human red blood cell acetylcholinesterase was found in 21% of patients with autoimmune thyroid disease and 4% of normal subjects, but there was no correlation with Tg Ab titer and antigen inhibition experiments showed limited binding inhibition.[71] Such cross-over specificity is of uncertain significance.

Human TPO Ab are found in up to 20% of normal subjects, 75% of patients with Graves' disease, and over 90% of patients with autoimmune thyroiditis. As with Tg Ab, TPO Ab are also polyclonal with only partial restriction to IgG_1 and IgG_4 subclasses indicating their lack of primary involvement in disease etiology.[16,46] However, TPO Ab, unlike Tg Ab, can mediate complement-dependent cytotoxicity. There is also a strong correlation between TPO Ab and the presence of histologic thyroiditis. Furthermore, the TPO Ab IgG_1 (complement fixing) subclass has been correlated with higher anti-TPO titers and thyroid failure including the postpartum period. However, the fetal human thyroid gland survives despite transplacental passage of maternal TPO Ab. This contrasts with the marked effects of transferred maternal TSHR Ab in neonates. Although hTPO is localized to the thyroid cell follicular membrane, isolated from the circulation, histologic studies show that TPO Ab are able to bind to TPO *in vivo* and may be capable of *in vitro* inhibition of TPO enzyme activity. Because this effect is independent of the titer of anti-TPO, the inhibiting antibody may be directed at specific TPO epitopes and inhibiting antibody is more frequent in Hashimoto's thyroiditis than in Graves' disease.

HLA Polymorphism and AITD

A genetic determinant of susceptibility to AITD was first suspected because of family clustering of AITD. Associations between AITD and the human major histocompatibility complex have since been revealed by many population studies, principally implicating the HLA-DR3 gene.[68] Furthermore, the observation that expression of HLA class II molecules on the surface of thyrocytes occurs in the thyroid tissue of patients with AITD suggested that these polymorphic molecules may be genetic determinants of disease susceptibility acting at the level of the thyroid cell itself. However, none of the reported risk ratios (of 3–5) associating AITD with HLA haplotypes have been high enough to suggest that MHC susceptibility genes, measured serologically, are of fundamental importance to the pathogenesis of AITD. While population associations of AITD and HLA antigens derived from cross-sectional data have been consistent, the demonstration of true linkage within families has only been suggested by one study of sib pair analysis.[55] We have recently been unable to confirm this evidence of linkage to the HLA region, using serologic markers, in families of patients with AITD despite a population association.[61] This finding questioned the importance of HLA-related susceptibility in AITD. Restriction fragment length polymorphisms obtained with specific restriction endonuclease-gene probe combinations correlate well with serologically and cellularly defined HLA specificities and have the additional advantage that novel specificities can be defined with fewer "blanks." The restriction fragment length polymorphism methodology has demonstrated that HLA-DQ β genes are associated with autoimmune diseases such as diabetes, rheumatoid arthritis, and multiple sclerosis, and such HLA-DQ β (DQB) polymorphisms showed stronger disease associations than previously known HLA-DR associations. We, and others, have therefore applied this methodology to patients with AITD. Such data have also failed to confirm linkage to the HLA region in within family studies[53] and have even questioned many of the reported population associations.[43] Nevertheless, most of the literature and our own experience do indicate a population association between HLA-DR3/DR5 and AITD, but in the absence of true linkage it is possible that such genes confer only a minor degree of enhanced susceptibility. Whether oligonucleotide typing will cast any further light on this relationship remains to be determined.

The Sequence of Events in AITD

AITD appears to occur in genetically susceptible patients after an unknown triggering event. Although the immunogenetics have been explored, it has been more difficult to quantify the many possible environmental insults that might serve as disease-triggering events. Susceptible individuals must have an immune repertoire containing T-cells and B-cells programmed for thyroid antigen recognition and their immune balance is maintained by a state of nondeletional tolerance. The high prevalence rate of autoantibody secretion in the general population suggests that if our techniques were sensitive enough we would also be able to detect anergized T-cells coded for thyroid antigen recognition as in animals.[32] Data are accumulating indicating a variety of trigger factors which may break this tolerant state and require further exploration including bacterial and viral (including retroviral) infections, environmental insults, and drugs and hormones. Hopefully, clarity will prevail in the near future.

ACKNOWLEDGMENTS

We thank Drs Andreas Martin, Peter Graves and Sheila Roman for their continuing support and helpful discussions.

This work was supported in part by Grants DK28243 and DK35674 from the National Institute of Diabetes and Digestive and Kidney Diseases.

REFERENCES

1. Adams, D. D., Faster, F. N., Howie, J. B., Kennedy, T. H., Kilpatrick, J. A., and Stewart, R. D. Stimulation of the human thyroid by infusions of plasma containing LATS protector. *J. Clin. Endocrinol. Metab. 39:*826–832, 1974.
2. Ahmann, A., Baker, J. R., Weetman, A. P., Wartofsky, L., Nutman, T. B., and Burman, K. D. Antibodies to porcine eye muscle in patients with Graves' ophthalmopathy: Identification of serum immunoglobulins directed against unique determinants by immunoblotting and enzyme-linked immunosorbent assay. *J. Clin. Endocrinol. Metab. 64:*454–460, 1987.
3. Aoki, M., Pinnamaneni, K. M., and DeGroot, L. J. Studies on suppressor cell function in thyroid diseases. *J. Clin. Endocrinol. Metab. 48:*803, 1979.
4. Bagnasco, M., Venuti, D., Prigione, I., Torre, G. C., Ferrini, S., and Canonica, G. W. Graves' disease: Phenotypic and functional analysis at the clonal level of the T-cell repertoire in peripheral blood and in thyroid. *Clin. Immunol. Immunopathol. 47:*230–239, 1988.
5. Bonnyns, M., Bentin, J., Devetter, G., and Duchateau, J. Heterogeneity of immunoregulatory T cells in human thyroid autoimmunity: Influence of thyroid status. *Clin. Exp. Immunol. 52:*629–634, 1983.
6. Burman, K. D., and Baker, J. R., Jr. Immune mechanisms in Graves' disease. *Endocr. Rev. 6:*183–232, 1985.
7. Burman, P., Totterman, T. H., Oberg, K., and Karlsson, F. A. Thyroid autoimmunity in patients on long-term therapy with leukocyte-derived interferon. *J. Clin. Endocrinol. Metab. 63:*1086–1090, 1986.
8. Chabaud, O., and Lissitzky, S. Thyrotropin-specific binding to human peripheral blood monocytes and polymorphonuclear leukocytes. *Mol. Cell. Endocrinol. 7:*79–87, 1977.
9. Champion, B. R., Page, K. R., Parish, N., Rayner, D. C., Dawe, K., Biswas-Hughes, G., Cooke, A., Geysen, M., and Roitt, I. M. Identification of a thyroxine-containing self-epitope of thyroglobulin which triggers thyroid autoreactive T cells. *J. Exp. Med. 174:*363–369, 1991.
10. Creemers, P., Rose, N. R., and Kong, Y. C. M. Experimental autoimmune thyroiditis: In vitro cytotoxic effects of T lymphocytes on thyroid monolayers. *J. Exp. Med. 157:*559–571, 1983.
11. Davies, T. F. Cocultures of human thyroid monolayer cells and autologous T cells: Impact of HLA class II antigen expression. *J. Clin. Endocrinol. Metab. 61:*418–422, 1985.
12. Davies, T. F., Martin, A., Concepcion, E. S., Graves, P., Cohen, L., and Ben-Nun, A. Evidence of limited variability of antigen receptors on intrathyroidal T-cells in autoimmune thyroid disease. *N. Engl. J. Med. 325:*238–244, 1991.
13. Davies, T. F., Platzer, M., Schwartz, A. E., and Friedman, E. Functionality of thyroid-stimulating antibodies assessed by cryopreserved human thyroid cell bioassay. *J. Clin. Endocrinol. Metab. 57:*1021–1028, 1983.
14. Davies, T. F., Rees Smith, B., and Hall, R. Binding of thyroid simulators to guinea pig testis, and thyroid. *Endocrinology 103:*6, 1978.
15. Davies, T. F., Teng, C. S., McLachlan, S. M., Rees Smith, B., and Hall, R. Thyrotropin receptors in adipose tissue, retro-orbital tissue and lymphocytes. *Mol. Cell. Endocrinol. 9:*303, 1978.
16. Davies, T. F., Weber, C. M., Wallack, P., and Platzer, M. Restricted heterogeneity and T-cell

dependence of human thyroid autoantibody immunoglobulin G subclasses. *J. Clin. Endocrinol. Metab. 62:*945–949, 1986.

17. Davies, T. F., Yeo, P. P. B., Evered, D. C., Clark, F., Rees Smith, B., and Hall, R. Value of thyroid-stimulating antibody determinations in predicting short-term thyrotoxic relapse in Graves' disease. *Lancet 1:*1181–1183, 1977.
18. Davies Jones, E., Hashim, F. A., Kajita, Y., Creagh, F. M., Buckland, P. R., Petersen, V. B., Howells, R. D., and Rees Smith, B. Interaction of autoantibodies to thyrotropin receptor with a hydrophilic subunit of the thyrotropin receptor. *Biochem. J. 228:*111–117, 1985.
19. Davies Jones, E., Hashim, F. A., Kajita, Y., Creagh, F. M., Buckland, P. R., Petersen, V. B., Howells, R. D., and Rees Smith, B. Photoaffinity labelling of the TSH receptor on FRTL5 cells. *FEBS Lett. 215:*316, 1987.
20. Del Prete, G. F., Mariotti, S., Tiri, A., Ricci, M., Pinchera, A., and Romagnani, S. Characterization of thyroid infiltrating lymphocytes in Hashimoto's thyroiditis: Detection of B and T cells specific for thyroid antigens. *Acta Endocrinol. [Suppl.] (Copenh). 281:*111–114, 1985.
21. Endo, K., Kasagi, K., Konishi, J., Ikekubo, K., Okuno, T., Takeda, Y., Mori, T., and Torikuza, K. Detection and properties of TSH-binding inhibitor immunoglobulins in patients with Graves' disease and Hashimoto's thyroiditis. *J. Clin. Endocrinol. Metab. 46:*734, 1978.
22. Finke, R., Seto, P., and Rapoport, B. Evidence for the highly conformational nature of the epitopes on human thyroid peroxidase that are recognized by sera from patients with Hashimoto's thyroiditis. *J. Clin. Endocrinol. Metab. 71:*53–59, 1990.
23. Frohman, M., Francfort, J. W., and Cowing, C. T-dependent destruction of thyroid isografts exposed to IFN-γ. *J. Immunol. 146:*2227–2234, 1991.
24. Graves, P. N., and Davies, T. F. A second thyroglobulin messenger RNA species (rTg-2) in rat thyrocytes. *Mol. Endocrinol. 4:*155–161, 1990.
25. Gross, B., Misrahi, M., Sar, S., and Milgrom, E. Composite structure of the human thyrotropin receptor gene. *Biochem. Biophys. Res. Commun. 177:*679, 1991.
26. Iitaka, M., Bernstein, J., Gerstein, H. C., Iwatani, Y., Row, V. V., and Volpe, R. Sensitization of T lymphocytes to thyroid antigen in autoimmune thyroid disease as demonstrated by the monocyte procoagulant activity test. *J. Endocrinol. Invest. 9:*471–478, 1986.
27. Iitaka, M., Iwatani, Y., Gerstein, H. C., Row, V. V., and Volpe, R. Immunomodulatory effect of the treatment of Graves' disease on antigen-specific monocyte procoagulant activity production. *Clin. Endocrinol. (Oxf.) 27:*321–330, 1987.
28. Kajita, Y., Rickards, C. R., Buckland, P. R., Howells, R. D., and Rees Smith, B. A structure for the porcine TSH receptors. *FEBS Lett. 181:*218, 1985.
29. Kajita, Y., Rickards, C. R., Buckland, P. R., Howells, R. D., and Rees Smith, B. Analysis of thyrotropin receptors by photoaffinity labelling: Orientation of receptor subunits in the cell membrane. *Biochem. J. 227:*413, 1985.
30. Kawakami, Y. et al. Proliferative responses of peripheral blood mononuclear cells from patients with autoimmune thyroid disease to synthetic peptide epitopes of human thyroid peroxidase. *Autoimmunity 13:*17, 1992.
31. Kendler, D. L., Martin, A., Magnusson, R. P., and Davies, T. F. Detection of autoantibodies to recombinant human thyroid peroxidase by sensitive enzyme immunoassay. *Clin. Endocrinol. (Oxf.) 33:*751–760, 1990.
32. Kimura, H., and Davies, T. F. Thyroid specific T cells in the normal Wistar rat. II. T cell clones interact with cloned Wistar rat thyroid cells and provide direct evidence for autoantigen presentation by thyroid epithelial cells. *Clin. Immunol. Immunopathol. 58:*195–206, 1991.
33. Kimura, S., Kotani, T., McBride, O. W., Umeki, K., Hirai, K., Nakayama, T., and Ohtaki, S. Human thyroid peroxidase: Complete cDNA and protein sequence, chromosome mapping, and identification of two alternately spliced mRNAs. *Proc. Natl. Acad. Sci. USA 84:*5555–5559, 1987.
34. Londei, M., Bottazzo, G. F., and Feldmann, M. Human T-cell clones from autoimmune thyroid glands: Specific recognition of autologous thyroid cells. *Science 228:*85–89, 1985.
35. Londei, M., Lamb, J. R., Bottazzo, G. F., and Feldmann, M. Epithelial cells expressing aberrant MHC class II determinants can present antigen to cloned human T cells. *Nature 312:*639–641, 1984.

36. Ludgate, M., Mariotti, S., Libert, F., Dinsart, C., Piccolo, P., Santini, F., Ruf, J., Pinchera, A., and Vassart, G. Antibodies to human thyroid peroxidase in autoimmune thyroid disease: Studies with a cloned recombinant complimentary deoxyribonucleic acid epitope. *J. Clin. Endocrinol. Metab. 68:*1091–1096, 1989.

37. Ludgate, M., Perret, J., Parmentier, M., Gerard, C., Libert, F., Dumont, J. E., and Vassart, G. Use of the recombinant human thyrotropin receptor (TSH-R) expressed in mammalian cell lines to assay TSH-R autoantibodies. *Mol. Cell. Endocrinol. 73:*R13–R18, 1990.

38. Ludgate, M. E., Ratanachaiyavong, S., Weetman, A. P., Hall, R., and McGregor, A. M. Failure to demonstrate cell-mediated immune responses to thyroid antigens in Graves' disease using in vitro assays of lymphokine-mediated migration inhibition. *J. Clin. Endocrinol. Metab. 60:*98–102, 1985.

39. Ludgate, M., and Vassart, G. The molecular genetics of three thyroid autoantigens: Thyroglobulin, thyroid peroxidase, and the thyrotropin receptor. *Autoimmunity 7:*210–211, 1990.

40. MacKenzie, W. A., and Davies, T. F. An intrathyroidal T-cell clone specifically cytotoxic for human thyroid cells. *Immunology 61:*101–103, 1987.

41. MacKenzie, W. A., Schwartz, A. E., Friedman, E. W., and Davies, T. F. Intrathyroidal T cell clones from patients with autoimmune thyroid disease. *J. Clin. Endocrinol. Metab. 64:*818–824, 1987.

42. Makinen, T., Wagar, G., Apter, L., von Willebrand, E., and Pekonen, F. Evidence that the TSH receptor acts as a mitogenic antigen in Graves' disease. *Nature 275:*314–315, 1978.

43. Mangklabruks, A., Cox, N., and DeGroot, L. J. Genetic factors in autoimmune thyroid disease analyzed by restriction fragment length polymorphisms of candidate genes. *J. Clin. Endocrinol. Metab. 73:*236–244, 1991.

44. Martin, A., Goldsmith, N. K., Friedman, E. W., Schwartz, A. E., Davies, T. F., and Roman, S. H. Intrathyroidal accumulation of T cell phenotypes in autoimmune thyroid disease. *Autoimmunity 6:*269–281, 1990.

45. Martin, A., Huber, G. K., and Davies, T. F. Induction of human thyroid cell ICAM-1 (CD54) antigen expression and ICAM-1-mediated lymphocyte binding. *Endocrinology 127:*651–657, 1990.

46. McLachlan, S. M., Feldt-Rasmussen, U., Young, E. T., Middleton, S. L., Dlichert-Toft, M., Siersboek-Nielson, K., Date, J., Carr, D., Clark, F., and Rees Smith, B. IgG subclass distribution of thyroid autoantibodies: A 'fingerprint' of an individual's response to thyroglobulin and thyroid microsomal antigen. *Clin. Endocrinol. (Oxf.) 26:*335–346, 1987.

47. McLachlan, S. M., and Rapoport, B. Evidence for a potential common T-cell epitope between human thyroid peroxidase and human thyroglobulin with implications for the pathogenesis of autoimmune thyroid disease. *Autoimmunity 5:*101–106, 1989.

48. Morimoto, C., Hafler, D. A., Weiner, H. L., Letvin, N., Hagan, M., Daley, J., and Schlossman, S. F. Selective loss of the suppressor-inducer T-cell subset in progressive multiple sclerosis. *N. Engl. J. Med. 316:*67–72, 1987.

49. Morimoto, C., Steinberg, A. D., Letvin, N. L., Hagan, M., Takeuchi, T., Daley, J., Levine, H., and Schlossman, S. F. A defect in immunoregulatory T-cell subsets in systemic lupus erythematosus patients demonstrated with anti-2H4 antibody. *J. Clin. Invest. 79:*762–768, 1987.

50. Murakami, M., and Mori, M. Identification of immunogenic regions in human thyrotropin receptor for immunoglobulin G of patients with Graves' disease. *Biochem. Biophys. Res. Commun. 171:*512–518, 1990.

51. Nagayama, Y., Wadsworth, H. L., Russo, D., Chazenbalk, G. D., and Rapoport, B. Binding domains of stimulatory and inhibitory TSH receptor autoantibodies determined with chimeric TSH-LH/CG receptors. *J. Clin. Invest. 88:*336–340, 1991.

52. Neufeld, D. S., Platzer, M., and Davies, T. F. Reovirus induction of MHC class II antigen in rat thyroid cells. *Endocrinology 124:*543–545, 1989.

53. O'Connor, G., Neufeld, D. S., Greenberg, D. A., Concepcion, L., Roman, S. H., and Davies, T. F. Lack of disease associated HLA-DQ restriction fragment length polymorphisms in families with autoimmune thyroid disease. *Autoimmunity* (in press).

54. Parmentier, M., Libert, F., Maenhaut, C., Lefort, A., Gerard, C., Perret, J., Van Sande, J.,

Dumont, J. E., and Vassart, G. Molecular cloning of the thyrotropin receptor. *Science 246:*1620–1623, 1989.

55. Payami, H., Joe, S., Farid, N. R., Stenszky, V., Aran, S. H., Yeo, P. P. B., Cheah, J. S., and Thomson, G. Relative predispositional effects of marker alleles with disease: HLA-DR alleles and disease susceptibility. *Am. J. Hum. Genet. 45:*541–546, 1989.

56. Piccinini, L. A., Goldsmith, N. K., Schachter, B. S., and Davies, T. F. Localization of HLA-DR alpha-chain messenger ribonucleic acid in normal and autoimmune human thyroid using in situ hybridization. *J. Clin. Endocrinol. Metab. 66:*1307–1315, 1988.

57. Piccinini, L. A., Mackenzie, W. A., Platzer, M., and Davies, T. F. Lymphokine regulation of HLA-DR gene expression in human thyroid cell monolayers. *J. Clin. Endocrinol. Metab. 64:*543–548, 1987.

58. Piechaczyk, M., Bouanani, M., Salhi, S. L., Baldet, L., Bastide, M., Pau, B., and Bastide, J. M. Antigenic determinants on the human thyroglobulin molecule recognized by autoantibodies in patients' sera and by natural autoantibodies isolated from the sera of healthy subjects. *Clin. Immunol. Immunopathol. 45:*114–121, 1987.

59. Pierce, C. J., Byfield, P. H. G., Edmonds, C. J., Lalloz, M. R. A., and Himsworth, R. L. Autoantibodies to thyroglobulin cross reacting with iodothyronines. *Clin. Endocrinol. (Oxf.) 15:*1, 1981.

60. Rees Smith, B., McLachlan, S. M., and Furmaniak, J. Autoantibodies to the thyrotropin receptor. *Endocr. Rev. 9:*106–121, 1988.

61. Roman, S. H., Greenberg, D., Rubinstein, P., Wallenstein, S., and Davies, T. F. Genetics of autoimmune thyroid disease: Lack of evidence for linkage to HLA within families. *J. Clin. Endocrinol. Metab. 74:*496–503, 1992.

62. Ruf, J., Carayon, P., Sarles-Philip, N., Kourilsky, F., and Lissitzky, S. Specificity of monoclonal antibodies against human thyroglobulin: Comparison with autoimmune antibodies. *EMBO J. 2:*1821–1826, 1983.

63. Ruf, J., Toubert, M.-E., Czarnocka, B., Durand-Gorde, J. M., Ferrand, M., and Carayon, P. Relationship between immunological structure and biochemical properties of human thyroid peroxidase. *Endocrinology 125:*1211–1218, 1989.

64. Russo, D., Chazenbalk, G. D., Nagayama, Y., Wadsworth, H. L., Seto, P., and Rapoport, B. A new structural model for the TSH receptor, as determined by covalent cross-linking of TSH to recombinant receptor in intact cells: Evidence for a single polypeptide chain. *Mol. Endocrinol. 5:*1607, 1991.

65. Seto, P., Hirayu, H., Magnusson, R. P., Gestautas, J., Portman, L., DeGroot, L. J., and Rapoport, B. Isolation of a complementary cDNA clone for thyroid microsomal antigen. Homology with the gene for thyroid peroxidase. *J. Clin. Invest. 80:*1205–1208, 1987.

66. Smith, T. J., Bahn, R. S., and Gorman, C. A. Hormonal regulation of hyaluronate synthesis in cultured human fibroblasts: Evidence for differences between retroocular and dermal fibroblasts. *J. Clin. Endocrinol. Metab. 69:*1019–1013, 1989.

67. Sunshine, P., Kusumoto, H., Kriss, J. P., Pleshakov, V., and Chien, J. R. Survival time of circulating long-acting thyroid stimulator in neonatal thyrotoxicosis: Implications for diagnosis and therapy of the disorder. *Pediatrics 35:*869, 1965.

68. Stenszky, V., Kozma, L., Balazs, C., Rochlitz, S., Bear, J. C., and Farid, N. R. The genetics of Graves' disease: HLA and disease susceptibility. *J. Clin. Endocrinol. Metab. 61:*735–740, 1985.

69. Topliss, D., How, J., Lewis, M., Row, V., and Volpe, R. Evidence for cell-mediated immunity and specific suppressor T lymphocyte dysfunction in Graves' disease and diabetes mellitus. *J. Clin. Endocrinol. Metab. 57:*700–705, 1983.

70. Weetman, A. P., Cohen, S., Makgoba, M. W., and Borysiewicz, L. K. Expression of an intercellular adhesion molecule, ICAM-1, by human thyroid cells. *J. Endocrinol. 122:*185–191, 1989.

71. Weetman, A. P., Tse, C. K., Randall, W. R., Tsim, K. W., and Barnard, E. A. Acetylcholinesterase antibodies and thyroid autoimmunity. *Clin. Exp. Immunol. 71:*95–99, 1988.

72. Weetman, A. P., Yateman, M. E., Ealey, P. A., Black, C. M., Reimer, C. B., Williams, R. C., Jr.,

Shine, B., and Marshall, N. J. Thyroid stimulating antibody activity between different immunoglobulin G subclasses. *J. Clin. Invest. 86:*723–727, 1990.
73. Zakarija, M. The thyroid-stimulating antibody of Graves' disease: Evidence for restricted heterogeneity. *Horm. Res. 13:*1, 1980.
74. Zanelli, E., Henry, M. Charvet, B., and Malthiery, Y. Evidence for an alternate splicing in the thyroperoxidase messenger from patients with Graves' disease. *Biochem. Biophys. Res. Commun. 170:*735–741, 1990.

Chapter 6

Current Concepts in Follicular Tumors of the Thyroid

VIRGINIA A. LiVOLSI

Follicular nodules are the most common cause of goiter throughout the world—whether in congenital errors of thyroid hormone metabolism, endemic goiter caused by iodine deficiency,[44] or idiopathic nodules. In the United States, it is estimated that about 2–4% of individuals (usually women) harbor clinical nodules, 10% have grossly identifiable nodules in the thyroid, and 40% have microscopic nodules.[3,9,10,29,89,130]

Although pathologists are familiar with the gross and microscopic appearance of nodular goiter, the pathogenesis of the initial events in nodule formation remains elusive.

Despite striking morphologic similarities among all follicular cells, subtle differences must exist, which account for inequality leading to differential growth and responsiveness and hence to nodule formation. Preliminary studies indicate that in at least some nonfunctioning nodules, insulin growth factor receptors are present.[131] Investigators working in nonendemic goiter regions have postulated autoimmune mechanisms for the origin of some nodules.[19,72]

The work of Studer and associates[1,57,95–98,111,120–124] suggests that certain follicular cells or groups thereof are *intrinsically* more rapidly growing than their neighbors. The initial proliferation is a polyclonal one involving one follicle or more likely a group of follicles. These proliferate, while adjacent follicles remain quiescent. Interfollicular stroma and the vessels contained therein participate in the process, and vascular compression leads to focal ischemia, necrosis, and inflammatory and reparative changes. At later times, the same process may affect another group of follicles until large zones of the thyroid are affected. While these changes occur, the hormonal stimuli to the gland continue. However, distortion of vascular supply and follicular dilatation makes the distribution of iodide and thyrotropin uneven. Hence some portion of the gland will "see" excess thyrotropin and focal hyperplasia may occur. The result is alternating areas of hypertrophy and atrophy.

PATHOLOGY

NODULAR GOITER

Grossly nodular goiters range from slightly to massively enlarged glands (weights of 50 to >800 g can be found) with intact capsules and a bumpy external surface. Sectioning will show multiple nodules of varying consistency separated by variable amounts of normal appearing thyroid (in huge goiters, no normal areas may be seen). The nodules are composed chiefly of brown thyroid tissue with variable amounts of hemorrhage, fibrosis, cystic degeneration, calcification, and even ossification. Microscopically, colloid lakes alternate with normal to hyperplastic appearing foci of thyroid, hemorrhage,[118] siderosis, fibrosis, edema, calcification, and bone (Figs. 6.1, 6.2, and 6.3). The appearance of the nodular thyroid is similar whether it occurs in patients in nonendemic or endemic goiter regions; however, in the latter more numerous foci of hyperplasia are seen.[25,86]

FOLLICULAR ADENOMA

A follicular adenoma or solitary adenomatous or adenomatoid nodule is defined as a benign encapsulated mass of follicles, usually showing a uniform pattern throughout the confined nodule.[3,84,86] The features which Meissner[84] used to distinguish histologically between adenoma and adenomatous nodules included: solitary versus multiple nodules; encapsulation versus merely circumscription; uniformity of pattern within the adenoma and divergence from surrounding thyroid; and compression of the surrounding gland by the adenoma and its capsule (Fig. 6.4).

Variants of follicular adenoma include those of variable pattern (microfollicular, trabecular, or solid), variable cytology (oncocytic, with bizarre nuclei) (Fig. 6.5), and unusual patterns such as hyalinizing trabecular adenoma or paraganglioma-like adenoma (Fig. 6.5) and angiomatoid.[18,23,107] Random nuclear atypia (bizarre nuclei) in a thyroid adenoma or nodule do not indicate malignant change; in fact, these probably reflect a degenerative phenomenon similar to that seen in parathyroid adenomas. These nuclei appear large and hyperchromatic (often smudged) and may be rounded or have irregular nuclear contours.

Solitary follicular nodules could be either hyperplasias or true neoplasms. Many pathologists decided to skirt the issue and use the terms "adenomatous" or "adenomatoid" nodule. Hicks *et al.*[55] and Namba *et al.*,[91] using restriction fragment length pleomorphism technology based on the Lyon hypothesis of X chromosome inactivation, proved that most solitary follicular nodules are clonal proliferations and hence neoplastic. The problem with extrapolating these data to all follicular nodules is reflected in the fact that since these studies are based on X chromosome inactivation, they can only be performed on samples from women. Currently only 25% of women are heterozygous for the available gene probes. Hence, postulating that all nodules are clonal may be premature; however, from the studies available this hypothesis appears to hold true. In the future, refinements in DNA technology may allow the study of samples from all women,[133] broadening the experience and answering the question of clonality with larger numbers of cases.

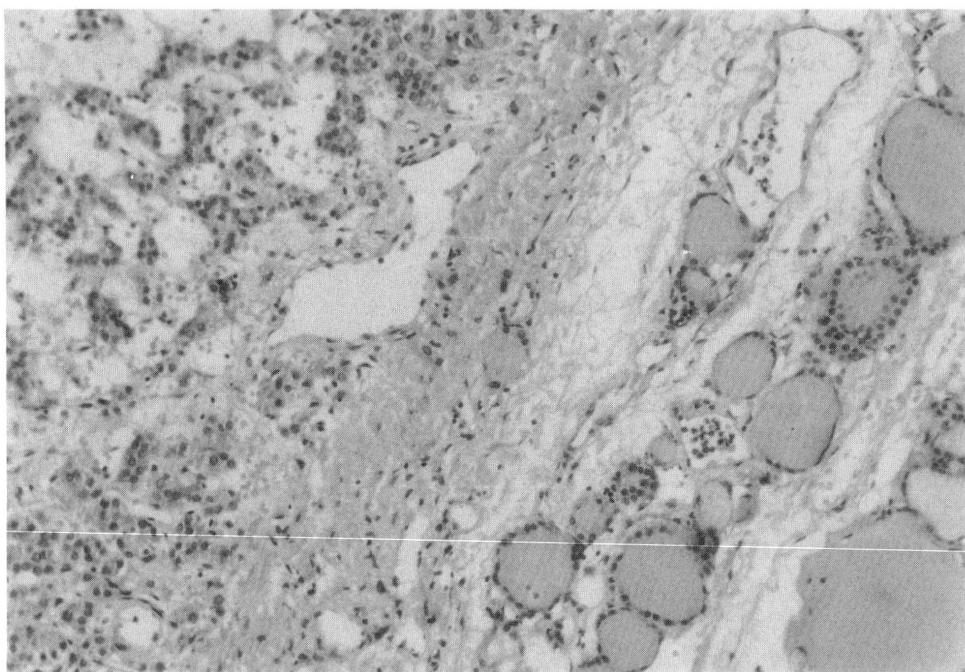

FIG. 6.1. Follicular adenomatous nodule. Not tight nest of follicular epithelium strewn in edematous stroma (*left*); capsule is present in this area.

DNA flow cytometry studies have shown that 27% of follicular adenomas contain aneuploid cell populations[28,56,61,108]; the meaning of these findings with regard to malignant potential is unclear, although some postulate that these represent carcinomas *in situ.*

Studies to detect alterations in *proto-oncogene* sequences in thyroid nodules have shown that nodules in goiters are negative; benign and malignant tumors, however, have shown changes in oncogene expression.[38] One study found that 4 of 36 follicular adenomas contained H-*ras* proto-oncogene mutations.[90,93] In another report, c-*myc* oncogene expression was found in four adenomas but not in normal thyroid.[139] Point mutations of the *gsp* oncogene were identified in 38% of functioning adenomas but in none of the nonfunctional benign or malignant lesions studied by O'Sullivan *et al.*[94]

Studies of gross genetic abnormalities in thyroid adenomas using classic *cytogenetic* techniques have disclosed a number of individual case reports or small series wherein changes have been identified. Antonini *et al.*[6] found clonal and nonclonal chromosomal changes in 4 of 6 adenomas tested; chromosomes 10 and 17 were involved. vanden Berg *et al.*[129] identified a clonal abnormality of chromosome 10 in nodular thyroid tissue that had been radiated as treatment for Hodgkin's disease. vanden Berg *et al.*[128,129] also noted chromosomal anomalies in three follicular adenomas with a clustering that they postulated may be specific for follicular adenomas.

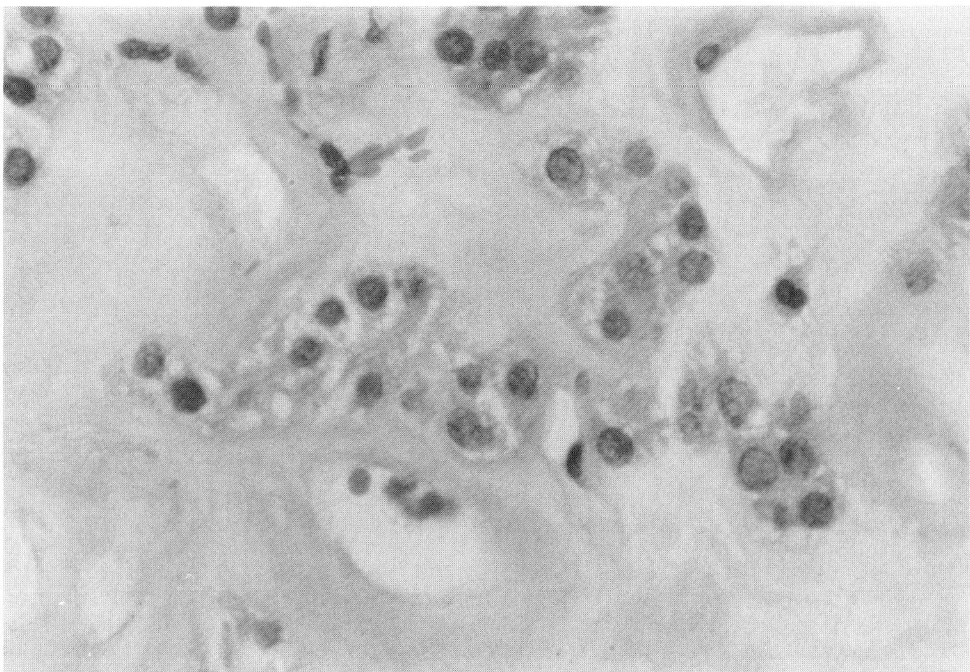

FIG. 6.2. Center of lesion in Figure 6.1. Note hyalinized and edematous stroma between groups of follicular cells.

Are these clonal follicular nodules, especially those with aneuploid cell populations and cytogenetic anomalies,[59,88] to be considered carcinomas *in situ*? Should they all be surgically removed? Since those nodules that have been tested have indeed been excised and since on follow-up all behave in a benign fashion, this question cannot yet be answered. The solitary follicular lesion, which is removed by lobectomy and which when adequately studied histologically shows no evidence of invasion, will neither recur nor metastasize.

ATYPICAL FOLLICULAR ADENOMA

This term proposed by Hazard and Kenyon[51] includes those follicular tumors which for one or more reasons are pathologically disturbing, *but which do not show invasive characteristics*. The features of these tumors that cause concern include the presence of spontaneous necrosis, infarction, numerous mitoses, or unusual cellularity (excluding bizarre cells noted above). Despite these findings, extensive evaluation of the capsule and edges of the tumor fails to disclose invasion.[33,36,51,84] These tumors behave in a benign fashion although the number of patients studied with long-term follow-up is in reality quite small.

FOLLICULAR CARCINOMA OF THE THYROID

Follicular carcinoma comprises about 5% of thyroid cancer in regions where sufficient iodide is present in the diet[27,134,135]; it is a tumor that is more commonly

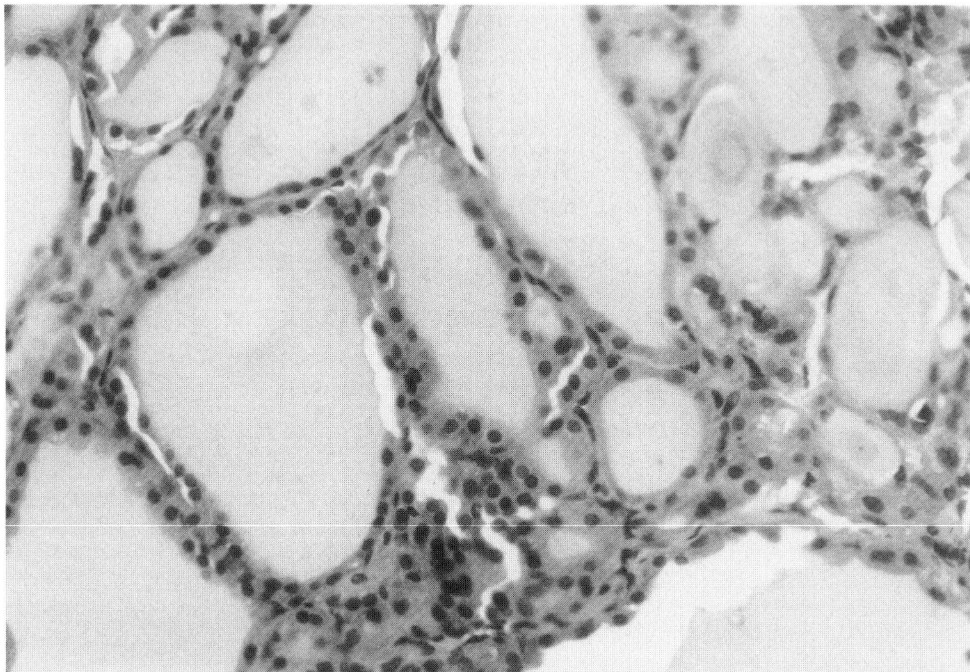

FIG. 6.3.   Nodule in goiter composed of macrofollicles. Oncocytic cells, not classic granular Hürthle cells, line the follicles.

found in endemic goiter areas of the world. The stimulus of thyrotropin (TSH) to the development of follicular carcinoma has been studied in animals and by extrapolation in humans who are iodine-deficient; such patients have excess TSH that may drive the thyroid to undergo neoplastic change.[134] [Confusion exists in the literature as to the incidence of follicular carcinoma among thyroid cancers, since some studies have included as follicular carcinoma the follicular variant of papillary cancer (which has a different biology and clinical course), the insular carcinoma[22] (which probably belongs in a separate group since many of them have papillary areas), and the lesions which many pathologists diagnose as atypical adenoma.] The opinion that perhaps the distinction of papillary from follicular carcinoma is a false one has been put forth[117] since variants of thyroid carcinoma such as the macrofollicular variant[2] and the diffuse follicular variant[117] have been described. It is the current author's opinion that despite these rare variants, there are sufficient clinical and biologic differences between these tumor groups that attempts to subcategorize papillary and follicular carcinoma utilizing established morphologic criteria are still warranted.

Clinically, follicular carcinoma is usually a *solitary mass* in the thyroid with the great majority of such tumors presenting as clinical "lumps." The follicular carcinoma has a marked propensity for vascular invasion (not lymphatics). Follicular carcinoma disseminates hematogenously and characteristically metastasizes to bone, lungs, brain, and liver.[5,26,32,49,64,74–76,104,109,110,115,116,127,136,137,140] Fol-

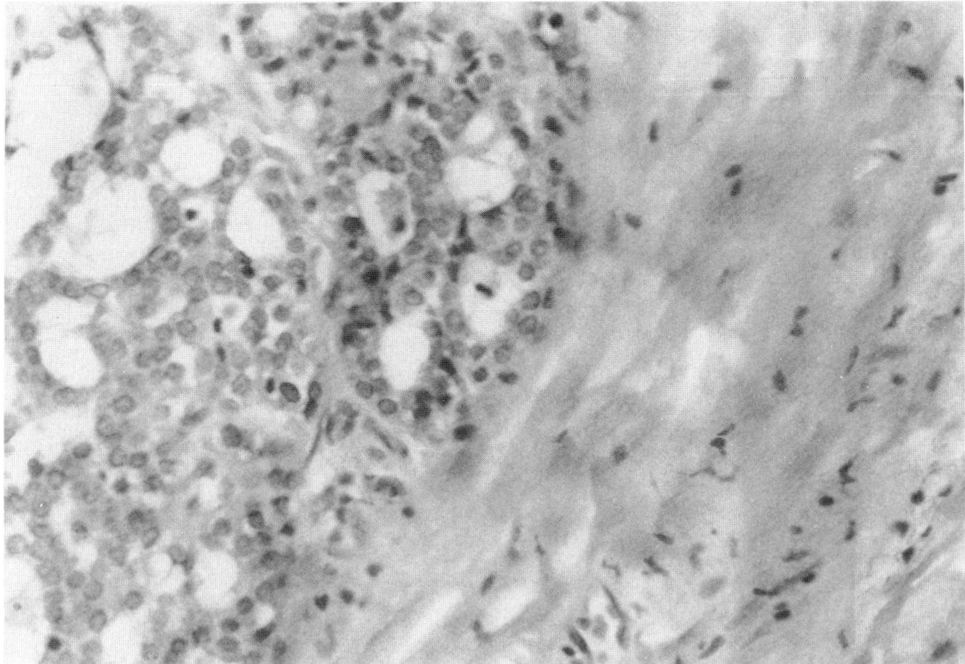

FIG. 6.4. Follicular adenoma. Note thick capsule.

licular cancer metastases may be treatable by radioiodine if there is no normal thyroid tissue present in the neck.[37] For this reason, many surgeons consider total thyroidectomy appropriate therapy for encapsulated follicular cancers. Since it is very difficult, if not impossible, to render a definitive cancer diagnosis from a fine needle aspiration sample or frozen section of such a tumor, delayed completion thyroidectomy may be necessary.

Patients who have follicular carcinoma that is widely invasive fare poorly.[5,26,32,49,74,76,109,110,115,116,127,140] Those individuals with encapsulated follicular tumors confined to the thyroid enjoy a prolonged survival (greater than 80% at 10 years).[74,76,109,115,116,136,137,140] However, if metastases are present at the initial diagnosis [and some patients are referred for a complaint related to a metastasis (*i.e.*, pathologic fracture)[74,76,109,115,140]] or if the patient is elderly, the prognosis is less favorable.[5,14,74,76,109,115,136,137] The major predictive prognostic variables include age over 50 and presence of distant metastasis at diagnosis.[5,14,74,76,109,115,136,140] Size of tumor (greater than 5 cm), extrathyroidal extension, and degree of differentiation are important in some series as well.[5,14,56,109,115,136,140] Immunostaining for thyroglobulin, which becomes less intense as the tumor becomes less well differentiated,[47] may be helpful in some cases. Some authors have found that DNA ploidy studies may also refine the prediction of prognosis with aneuploid tumors having a more aggressive clinical course.[56,62]

Pathologically two main types of follicular carcinoma are recognized: so-called minimally invasive and widely invasive types.

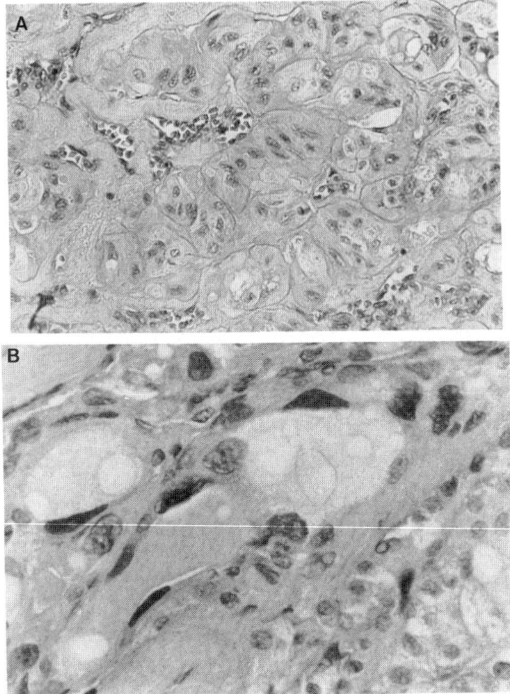

FIG. 6.5. *A*, paraganglioma-like adenoma of the thyroid. This 3-cm lesion was encapsulated and confined to the thyroid. Areas with this morphology can be seen focally in follicular adenomas or nodules and in goiter and thyroiditis. *B*, bizarre nuclei in a follicular adenoma.

The widely invasive follicular carcinoma is a tumor that is clinically and surgically recognized as a cancer; the role of the pathologist in its diagnosis is to confirm that it is of thyroid origin and that it fits into a follicular neoplasm category. Such lesions grossly extend into cervical veins or through the thyroid capsule. Such tumors often are fairly cellular and usually microfollicular and/or focally solid (some pathologists prefer to grade such lesions as "moderately" or "poorly" differentiated[105]; the prognosis is guarded. In the series of Lang *et al.*,[74,76] 80% of the patients with widely invasive cancers developed metastases and about 20% died of tumor. Woolner *et al.*[136,137] found a 50% fatality rate for widely invasive tumors compared with only 3% for those with "minimal invasion." Similar survival statistics are quoted in various series including those of Brennan, Crile, Simpson, and Young.[14,26,115,140]

The minimally invasive follicular carcinoma can be diagnosed only by the pathologist and in the present author's opinion only on the basis of well fixed histologic sections. These lesions are not diagnosable by fine needle aspiration cytology since the diagnosis requires the demonstration of invasion at the edges of the lesion; therefore, sampling of the center as is done in obtaining a cytologic sample cannot be diagnostic. Despite some reports of the value of image analysis for evaluation of nuclear size, contour, and other features in distinguishing follicular cells aspirated from benign and malignant follicular nodules,[7,66] most cytopathologists and histopathologists believe that the diagnosis of follicular carcinoma rests on the examination of tissue sections and especially the tumor capsule.[4,30] Similar problems exist in evaluating such lesions by frozen section.[16,45,70,77,103,113,114] Some authors[71,85] have recommended that intraoperative assessment of such lesions involves the examination of frozen sections from three or four separate areas of the nodule. In the present author's view, this only wastes time and resources and rarely gives useful, *i.e.*, diagnostic, information.

Most authors indicate that the first approach to the diagnosis of a solitary thyroid nodule should be a fine needle aspiration (FNA) biopsy; if surgery is advised on the basis of the FNA results, then frozen section study will yield little definitive diagnostic information. This is especially true for follicular nodules. In our own material,[16] utilizing the experience of one thyroid surgeon, if a follicular nodule was diagnosed as benign by frozen section, it was always benign; if the diagnosis was deferred, the permanent section showed a benign result in 85% of cases. (The only definitely malignant lesions diagnosed by frozen section were follicular variants of papillary cancer.) Other authors have shown that anywhere from 14–31% of the frozen section diagnoses or deferred diagnoses in follicular thyroid lesions are reversed by permanent section. The surgeon should remove the lobe involved by the nodule; since only a small number of these lesions will show evidence of invasion at the time of permanent section, *i.e.*, the majority of them are benign, and since overdiagnosis is more dangerous for the patient than is the delay in making a definitive diagnosis, we discourage frozen section evaluation for these nodules.

Grossly, the minimally invasive follicular carcinoma resembles a follicular adenoma[10,32,36,64]; the lesion is well defined and often encapsulated and on cut section may bulge from the confines of its capsule. The gross appearance may differ slightly in some cases from the benign nodule because of the thickness of the capsule. As Evans[32] has pointed out, the follicular carcinoma tends to be surrounded by a wide thick capsule. The central portion of the lesion is usually homogeneous (except when hemorrhagic foci are present secondary to preoperative biopsy) tan to pink tissue. Although degenerative changes (such as cysts and calcification) may be seen, these are unusual. The central part of the tumor is usually solid.

Microscopically, the minimally invasive follicular carcinoma resembles the benign follicular adenoma (Fig. 6.6); however, it is more likely to demonstrate a microfollicular or trabecular pattern throughout than does a benign adenoma. The follicles are usually regular, small and round. If the lesion shows trabecular areas, these are often irregular.[36,74,75] Significant mitotic activity is often found; this feature is rare in benign adenomas.[36,52,64,74,75,109,110] What are the minimum criteria for making the diagnosis of follicular carcinoma?

"Capsular" invasion is more difficult to define. Some pathologists require vascular invasion to render a diagnosis of follicular carcinoma; others require penetration *through* the capsule of the tumor and still others invasion *into* the capsule.[36,64,74–76,109,110] Kahn and Perzin[64] define capsular invasion as irregular nests or fingers of tumor within the capsule outside the confines of the bulk of the lesion. Evans[32] and Schroder *et al.*[109] agreed that capsular invasion was an

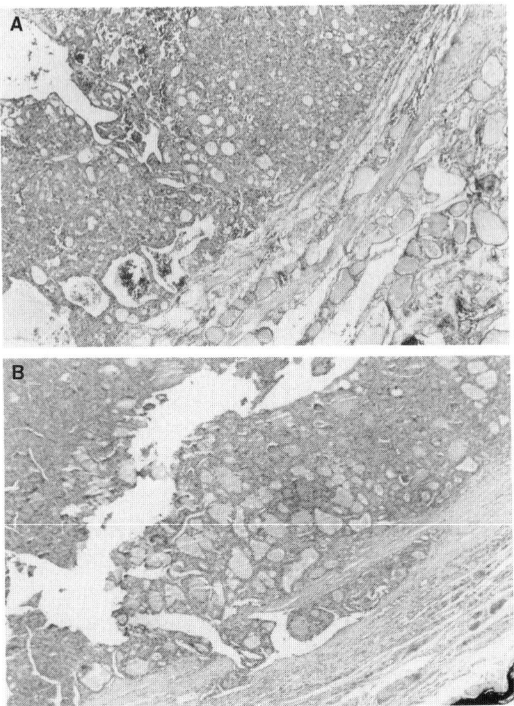

FIG. 6.6.   *A*, follicular neoplasm appears encapsulated in this field. *B*, another area of the tumor-capsule interface shows capsular and probable vascular invasion.

important diagnostic criterion. Hazard and Kenyon[52] noted that smooth, contoured islands of tumor in the capsule may represent vascular invasion. Iida[58] noted that distinguishing capsular invasion from trapping may prove difficult, and he required that the invasive tongues of tumor sever and deflect the collagen fibers in the capsule. Hence, focal herniation into the capsule or the finding of a few follicles in the capsule without apparent reactive fibrosis is insufficient to diagnose cancer in the view of some authors.[74–76,101,109,110] Axiotis *et al.*[8] used immunostaining for laminin and found no diagnostic utility since differences between benign and malignant lesions were minimal.

Schroder *et al.*[109] agree with Franssila *et al.*[36] and Lang *et al.*[76] that prospectively diagnosing follicular carcinoma on the basis of tumor nests in the capsule is dangerous since it is not possible to distinguish between true invasion and trapping in these cases. These three groups of authors therefore, require the complete penetration of the capsule by tumor to prospectively diagnose follicular carcinoma. However, these authors all admit that in a small number of such cases metastases may occur, although usually after many years. Is invasion into the capsule insufficient for the diagnosis of follicular cancer? What follow-up is available in series in which such lesions are diagnosed as cancer? Kahn and Perzin[64] found that 1 in 7 patients with only capsular invasion had metastases (14%). Evans[32] noted that capsular invasion appeared as important as if not more so than venous invasion since 3 of 7 patients with this finding showed metastases. However, in these 3 patients, *metastases were already present* at initial diagnosis.[32,36]

Evans[32] and Kahn and Perzin[64] accept as follicular carcinoma those tumors in which tumor nests are found only within the capsule. I believe that invasion *of* the capsule, invasion *through* the capsule, and/or invasion *into* veins in or beyond the capsule represent the diagnostic criteria for carcinoma in a follicular thyroid neoplasm.

Lang and co-workers[74–76] and Franssila *et al.*[36] consider nests of tumor in the capsule to possibly represent trapping and distortion by fibrosis rather than invasion. These authors require *penetration* of the capsule to diagnose a follicular tumor as carcinoma, preferring not to overdiagnose such lesions.

The criterion for *vascular* invasion applies solely and strictly to vessels in or beyond the capsule, since tumor plugs *within capillaries in the substance of the tumor have no apparent diagnostic and prognostic importance*—this finding alone is not associated with malignant behavior.[36] Kahn and Perzin[64] caution that edema around follicles with a surrounding separation artifact especially in the center of the lesion may mimic tumor in vessels.[36,64]

According to Franssila *et al.*[36] and Kahn and Perzin,[64] the criteria for vascular invasion include invasive tumor forming a plug or polyp in a subendothelial location; the tumor thrombus is covered by endothelium, but the tumor thrombus does not have to be attached to the vessel wall to be acceptable as invasion (Fig. 6.7).

Several studies that attempted to define the vessel wall and endothelium in relationship to the follicular tumor nests near or in them have been published.[36] Staining for elastic tissue in the vein wall is usually futile since the size of the vessels involved is small enough that there is no significant amount of elastic lamina in its wall.[36] Immunostaining for Factor VIII-related antigen, a marker for vascular endothelium is of limited use, since the endothelium of involved, *i.e.*, invaded veins, rarely stains (vascular endothelium of uninvaded or partially invaded vessels does). The reason for this result is unclear, but Harach *et al.*[48] suggested the possibility that the tumor may elaborate some factor that alters the endothelium, allowing for invasion by tumor; this same factor(?s) may interfere with immunostaining and/or expression of Factor VIII-related antigen. Other studies[41,65] have claimed that immunostaining for *Ulex europaeus* lectin, laminin, or basement membrane collagen may prove more successful in defining the relationship of tumor to the endothelial lining of a questionably invaded vein. The present author's experience recapitulates that of Harach *et al.*[48]; only a few veins in a few follicular carcinomas stain for Factor VIII-related antigen. Recent experience with my own material has shown that the endothelial marker CD 34 (hematopoietic marker My10)[119] does decorate endothelial cells of invaded vessels in about two-thirds of the cases studied (three times the number as for Factor VIII).

Hürthle cell nodules are discussed in the context of follicular tumors of the thyroid, since lesions composed entirely or predominantly of these cells should be evaluated using criteria identical to those used for follicular nodules in general.

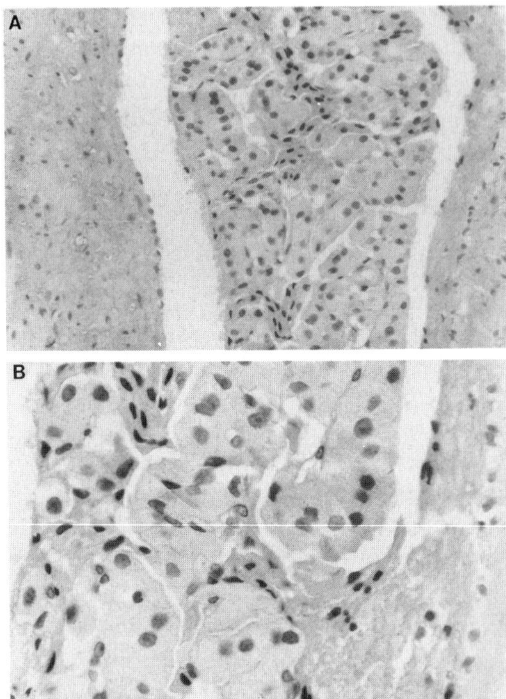

FIG. 6.7.   Vascular invasion is illustrated. *A*, this medium-sized vein outside of the capsule of the tumor shows a tumor plug in its lumen; in this area the tumor does not appear attached to the wall. *B*, this is the same vessel, but in another focus fibrin attaches tumor plug to venous endothelium.

Although one can see oncocytic cytology in adenomatous or nodular goiter, especially in cellular nodules, the eosinophilic change tends to be nongranular and less intensely staining than in true Hürthle cells.[100]

In nodules composed of oncocytes, one can find macrofollicles, microfollicles, or trabecular growth patterns.[17,20] The cells are large with voluminous cytoplasm, which is eosinophilic and granular. The nuclei are large and often irregular; nuclear pleomorphism and even bi- and multinucleation are commonly seen. Such lesions if solitary and encapsulated must be examined for invasion as are similar lesions without oncocytic cytology.[12,13,17,24,31,34,36,39,40,42,43,46,60,83,102,125,126,132] However, our own experience and that reported in the literature indicates that the percentage of Hürthle cell tumors that fulfill criteria for carcinoma is higher than for nononcocytic follicular tumors (average 33% versus <5%).[17] In addition, it has been our experience[17] and that of others[21] that Hürthle cell carcinomas can metastasize to regional nodes unlike follicular non-Hürthle cell cancers.

Because the likelihood of solitary Hürthle cell nodules being malignant is so high, in the absence of clinical or serologic evidence of thyroiditis, the diagnosis of Hürthle cell neoplasm by a FNA requires surgical excision, *i.e.*, thyroid lobectomy. On the other hand, since the great majority of solitary or dominant nodules in the thyroid are follicular, but most have abundant colloid and are adenomatous nodules in goiter, the overwhelming majority of such lesions should be followed clinically with or without medical suppression therapy. Because only about 15% of lesions called follicular neoplasms by FNA (cellular, little colloid, microfollicular pattern) are diagnosed as malignant on histologic evaluation, the urgency for the surgical removal in such cases is less.

THE DIFFERENTIAL DIAGNOSIS OF CAPSULAR INVASION: WHAFFT

In an era when fine needle aspiration represents the initial diagnostic approach to the solitary thyroid nodule,[11,35,45,70,87] the pathologist must exercise extreme caution when attempting to evaluate a follicular lesion. The increasing use of FNA has produced artifactual and/or iatrogenic lesions which mimic capsular invasion[80]; infarction of the nodule may occur, especially in oncocytic lesions.[67,68,80] Distinguishing between these and true capsular invasion may be problematical, but can be aided by historical data, the presence of hemorrhage and hemosiderin, and the focal and geographic pattern of the lesion (Figs. 6.8 and 6.9). We have called these lesions WHAFFT (worrisome histologic alterations following FNA of the thyroid).[80] In the author's consultation practice about 9% of the patients were sent because of WHAFFT effects interfering with interpretation of the nature of the thyroid lesion.

For practical purposes, what should the pathologist do in evaluating a follicular

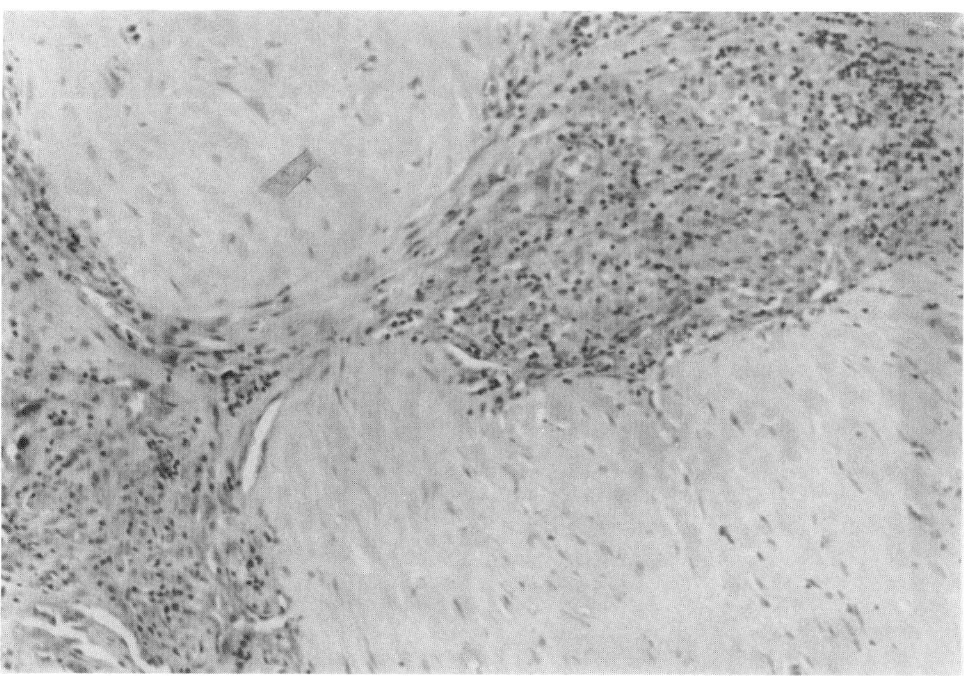

FIG. 6.8. WHAFFT (see text). This geographic streaking of lesional cells through the thick capsule of a follicular adenoma mimics invasion. Note the heavy infiltration of the tumor streak with inflammatory cells.

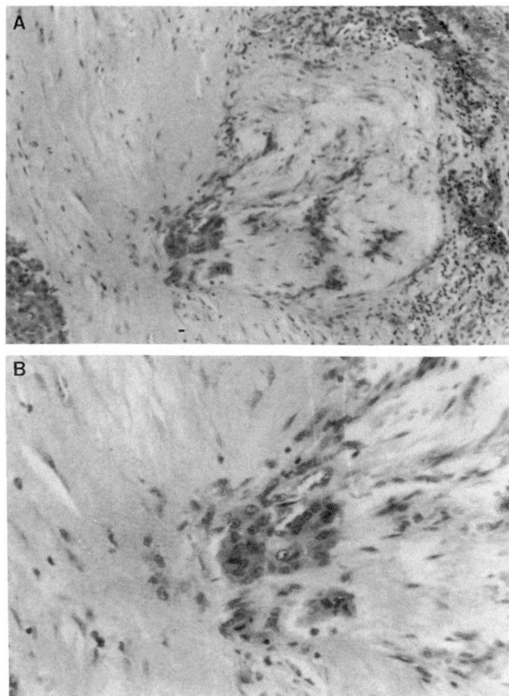

FIG. 6.9.   WHAFFT. *A*, in another case of this phenomenon, there is hemorrhage, granulation tissue, and inflammatory cells with few tumor cells admixed; this area was sole zone of "capsular invasion." *B*, higher power of this focus; note there are only a few follicular cells admixed with the inflammatory reaction.

thyroid nodule histologically? How many sections (blocks) of an encapsulated follicular lesion are needed to prove there is no definite invasion? Lang *et al.*[76] and Franssila *et al.*[36] recommend that 10 blocks be examined. These sections should represent the tumor-capsule-thyroid interface to be considered adequate and representative. For practical purposes, however, the larger the lesion if it is malignant, the more easily invasion will be found, and I believe the recommended 10 blocks of the capsule will probably not miss a significant cancer. Of course, if any of the 10 blocks show irregular tongues of tumor in the capsule or a suspicious area for invasion, further blocks from the lesion should be examined.

None of the modern ancillary techniques assist one in distinguishing benign from malignant follicular tumors. Ultrastructural, morphometric, and flow cytometric analyses have not helped in separating these lesions.[7,15,28,34,39,61,63,73,79,81–83,90,92–94,106,108,112,128,129,139] It may be possible that studies of oncogene expression, TSH receptor biochemistry, or more refined image analysis techniques and/or flow cytometric analysis of multiple parameters may guide us diagnostically in the future.[38,50,53,54,59,69,78,99,138]

REFERENCES

1. Aibi, U., Gerber, H., and Studer, H. Thyroid adenomas: A morphologically and functionally heterogeneous disease. In: *Progress in Thyroid Research*, edited by A. Gordon, J. Gross, and G. Hennemann. Rotterdam, A. A. Balkema Publishers, 1991.

2. Albores-Saavedra, J., Gould, E., Vardaman, C., and Vuitch, F. The macrofollicular variant of papillary thyroid carcinoma: A study of 17 cases. *Lab. Invest. 63:*31A, 1991 (abstract).

3. Al-Moussa, M., and Beck, J. S. Histometry of thyroids containing few and multiple nodules. *J. Clin. Pathol. 39:*483–488, 1986.

4. Altavilla, G., Pascale, M., and Nenci, I. Fine needle aspiration cytology of thyroid gland disease. *Acta Cytol. 34:*251–256, 1990.

5. Andry, G., Chantrain, G., van Glabbeke, M., and Dor, P. Papillary and follicular thyroid carcinoma: Individualization of the treatment according to the prognosis of the disease. *Eur. J. Cancer Clin. Oncol. 24:*1641–1646, 1988.

6. Antonini, P., Venuat, A. M., Linares, G., Caillou, B., Schlumberger, M., Travagli, J. P., Berger, R., and Parmentier, C. Cytogenetic abnormalities in thyroid adenomas. *Cancer Genet. Cytogenet. 52:*157–164, 1991.

7. Arps, H., Sablotny, B., Dietel, M., Niendorf, A., and Schroder, S. DNA cytophotometry in malignant thyroid tumors—Use of different evaluation schemes for prognostic statements. *Virchows Arch. [A] 413:*319–323, 1988.

8. Axiotis, C., Perez, M., Campo, E., Merino, M. J., Charonia, A., and Neumann, R. Laminin in thyroid tumors reflects differentiation and not metastatic potential. *Mod. Pathol. 4:*31A, 1991 (abstract).

9. Beckers, C. Thyroid nodules. *J. Clin. Endocrinol. Metab. 8:*181–192, 1979.

10. Berghout, A., Wiersinga, W. M., Smits, N. J., and Touber, J. L. Interrelationships between age, thyroid volume, thyroid nodularity and thyroid function in patients with sporadic nontoxic goiter. *Am. J. Med. 89:*602–608, 1990.

11. Blum, M. The diagnosis of the thyroid nodule using aspiration biopsy and cytology. *Arch. Intern. Med. 144:*1140–1142, 1984.

12. Bondeson, L., Bondeson, A. G., and Ljungberg, O. Treatment of Hürthle cell neoplasms of the thyroid. *Arch. Surg. 118:*1453, 1983.

13. Bondeson, L., Bondeson, A. G., Ljungberg, O., and Tibblin, S. Oxyphil tumors of the thyroid. Follow-up of 42 surgical cases. *Ann. Surg. 194:*677–680, 1981.

14. Brennan, M. D., Bergstralh, E. J., van Heerden, J. A., and McConahey, W. M. Follicular thyroid cancer treated at the Mayo Clinic 1946 through 1970: Initial manifestations, pathologic findings therapy and outcome. *Mayo Clin. Proc. 66:*11–22, 1991.

15. Bronner, M. P., Clevenger, C. V., Edmonds, P. R., Lowell, D. M., McFarland, M. M., and LiVolsi, V. A. Flow cytometric analysis of DNA content in Hürthle cell adenomas and carcinomas of the thyroid. *Am. J. Clin. Pathol. 89:*764–769, 1988.

16. Bronner, M. P., Hamilton, R., and LiVolsi, V. A. Thyroid follicular nodules: Frozen section experience. *Mod. Pathol. 4:*31A, 1991 (abstract).

17. Bronner, M. P., and LiVolsi, V. A. Oxyphilic (Askanazy/Hürthle cell) tumors of the thyroid: Microscopic features predict biologic behavior. *Surg. Pathol. 1:*137–150, 1988.

18. Bronner, M., LiVolsi, V. A., and Jennings, T. Paraganglioma-like adenomas of the thyroid. *Surg. Pathol. 1:*383–389, 1988.

19. Brown, R. S., Jackson, I. M. D., Pohl, S. L., and Reichlin, S. Do thyroid stimulating immunoglobulins cause nontoxic and toxic multinodular goiter? *Lancet 1:*904–906, 1978.

20. Caplan, R. H., Abellera, M., and Kisken, W. A. Hürthle cell tumors of the thyroid gland: A clinicopathologic review and long-term follow-up. *J.A.M.A. 251:*3114–3117, 1984.

21. Carcangiu, M. L., Bianchi, S., Savino, D., Voynick, I. M., and Rosai, J. Follicular Hürthle cell tumors of the thyroid gland. *Cancer 68:*1944–1953, 1991.

22. Carcangiu, M. L., Zampi, G., and Rosai, J. Poorly differentiated (insular) thyroid carcinoma. *Am. J. Surg. Pathol. 8:*655–668, 1984.

23. Carney, J. A., Ryan, J., and Goellner, J. R. Hyalinizing trabecular adenoma of the thyroid gland. *Am. J. Surg. Pathol. 11:*583–591, 1987.

24. Cooper, D. S., and Schneyer, C. R. Follicular and Hürthle cell carcinoma of the thyroid. *Endocrinol. Metab. Clin. N. Am. 19*:577–591, 1990.

25. Correa, P., and Castro, S. Survey of the pathology of thyroid glands from Cali, Colombia—A goiter area. *Lab. Invest. 10*:39–50, 1961.

26. Crile, G., Pontius, K. I., and Hawk, W. A. Factors influencing the survival of patients with follicular carcinoma of the thyroid gland. *Surg. Gynecol. Obstet. 160*:409–413, 1985.

27. Cuello, C., Correa, P., and Eisenberg, H. Geographic pathology of thyroid carcinoma. *Cancer 23*:230–239, 1969.

28. Cusick E. L., Ewen, S. W. B., Krukowski, Z. H., and Matheson, N. A. DNA aneuploidy in follicular thyroid neoplasia. *Br. J. Surg. 78*:94–98, 1991.

29. DeHaven, J. W., and Sherwin, R. S. The thyroid nodule: Approach to diagnosis and therapy. *Conn. Med. 43*:761–767, 1979.

30. DeJong, S. A., Demeter, J. G., Castelli, M., Jarosz, H., Barbato, A., Brooks, M. H., Braithwaite, S., Emmanuele, M. A., Lawrence, A. M., and Paloyan, E. Follicular cell predominance in the cytologic examination of dominant thyroid nodules indicates a sixty percent incidence of neoplasia. *Surgery 108*:794–800, 1990.

31. El-Naggar, A. K., Batsakis, J. G., Luna, M. A., and Hickey, R. C. Hürthle cell tumors of the thyroid: A flow cytometric DNA analysis. *Arch. Otolaryngol. Head Neck Surg. 114*:520–521, 1988.

32. Evans, H. L. Follicular neoplasms of the thyroid. *Cancer 54*:535–540, 1984.

33. Ferriman, D., Hennebry, T. M., and Tassopoulos, C. N. True thyroid adenoma. *Q. J. Med. 162*:127–139, 1972.

34. Flint, A., Davenport, R. D., Lloyd, R. V., Beckwith, A. L., and Thompson, N. W. Cytophotometric measurements of Hürthle cell tumors of the thyroid gland: Correlation with pathologic features and clinical behavior. *Cancer 61*:110–113, 1988.

35. Frable, W. J. The treatment of thyroid cancer. The role of fine needle aspiration cytology. *Arch. Otolaryngol. Head Neck Surg. 112*:1200–1203, 1986.

36. Franssila, K. O., Ackerman, L. V., Brown, C. L., and Hedinger, C. E. Follicular carcinoma. *Semin. Diagn. Pathol. 2*:101–122, 1985.

37. Frantz, V. K., Quimby, E. H., and Evans, T. C. Radioactive iodine studies of functional thyroid carcinoma. *Radiology 51*:532–552, 1948.

38. Frauman, A. G., and Moses, A. C. Oncogenes and growth factors in thyroid carcinogenesis. *Endocrinol. Metab. Clin. North Am. 19*:479–493, 1990.

39. Galera-Davidson, H., Bibbo, M., Bartels, P. H., Dytch, H. E., Puls, J. H., and Wied, G. L. Correlation between automated DNA ploidy measurements of Hürthle cell tumors and their histopathologic and clinical features. *Anal. Quant. Cytol. Histol. 8*:158–167, 1986.

40. Gonzalez-Campora, R., Herrero-Zapatero, A., Lerma, E., Sanchez, F., and Galera, H. Hürthle cell and mitochondrion-rich cell tumors: A clinicopathologic study. *Cancer 57*:1154–1163, 1986.

41. Gonzalez-Campora, R., Montero, C., Martin-Lacave, I., and Galera, H. Dermonstration of vascular endothelium in thyroid carcinomas using *Ulex europaeus* I agglutinin. *Histopathology 10*:261–266, 1986.

42. Gosain, A. K., and Clark, O. H. Hürthle cell neoplasms: Malignant potential. *Arch. Surg. 119*:515–519, 1984.

43. Gundry, S. R., Burney, R. E., Thompson, N. W., and Lloyd, R. Total thyroidectomy for Hürthle cell neoplasm of the thyroid. *Arch. Surg. 118*:529–532, 1983.

44. Gutenkunst, R., and Scriba, P. C. Goiter and iodine deficiency in Europe. *J. Endocrinol. Invest. 12*:209–220, 1989.

45. Hamburger, J. I., and Hamburger, S. W. Declining role of frozen section in surgical planning for thyroid nodules. *Surgery 98*:307–312, 1985.

46. Har-el, G., Hadar, T., Segal, K., Levy, R., and Sidi, J. Hürthle cell carcinoma of the thyroid gland: A tumor of moderate malignancy. *Cancer 57*:1613–1617, 1986.

47. Harach, H. R., and Franssila, K. O. Thyroglobulin immunostaining in follicular thyroid carcinoma. *Histopathology 13*:43–54, 1988.

48. Harach, H. R., Jasani, B., and Williams, E. D. Factor VIII as a marker of endothelial cells in follicular carcinoma of the thyroid. *J. Clin. Pathol. 36:*1050–1054, 1977.

49. Harness, J. K., Thompson, N. W., McLeod, M. K., Eckhauser, F. E., and Lloyd, R. V. Follicular carcinoma of the thyroid gland: Trends and treatment. *Surgery 96:*972–980, 1984.

50. Hashimoto, T., Matsubara, F., Mizukami, Y., Miyazaki, I., Michigishi, T., and Yanaihara, N. Tumor markers and oncogene expression in thyroid cancer using biochemical and immuno-histochemical studies. *Endocrinol. Jpn. 37:*247–254, 1990.

51. Hazard, J. B., and Kenyon, R. Atypical adenoma of the thyroid. *Arch. Pathol. 58:*554–563, 1954.

52. Hazard, J. B., and Kenyon, R. Encapsulated angioinvasive carcinoma (angioinvasive adenoma) of the thyroid gland. *Am. J. Clin. Pathol. 24:*755–766, 1954.

53. Herriman, M. A., Hay, I. D., Bartlet, D. H., Ritland, S. R., Dahl, R. J., Grant, C. S., and Jenkins, R. B. Cytogenetic and molecular genetic studies of follicular and papillary thyroid cancers. *J. Clin. Invest. 88:*1596–1604, 1991.

54. Herriman, M. A., Talpos, G. B., Mohamed, A. N., Saxe, A., Ratner, S., Lalley, P. A., and Wolman, S. R. Genetic markers in thyroid tumors. *Surgery 110:*941–948, 1991.

55. Hicks, D. G., LiVolsi, V. A., Neidich, J. A., Puck, J. M., and Kant, J. A. Clonal analysis of solitary follicular nodules of the thyroid. *Am. J. Pathol. 137:*553–562, 1990.

56. Hruban, R. H., Huvos, A. G., Traganos, F., Reuter, V., Lieberman, P. H., and Melamed, M. R. Follicular neoplasms of the thyroid in men older than 50 years of age. *Am. J. Clin. Pathol. 94:*527–532, 1990.

57. Huber, G., Derwah, I. M., Kaempf, J., Peter, H. J., Gerber, H., and Studer, H. Generation of intercellular heterogeneity of growth and function in cloned rat thyroid cells (FRTL-5). *J. Clin. Endocrinol. Metab. 126:*1639–1645, 1990.

58. Iida, F. The fate and surgical significance of adenoma of the thyroid gland. *Surg. Gynecol. Obstet. 136:*536–540, 1973.

59. Jenkins, R. B., Hay, I. D., Herath, J. F., Schultz, C. G., Spurbeck, J. L., Grant, C. S., Goellner, J. R., and DeWald, G. W. Frequent occurrence of cytogenetic abnormalities in sporadic nonmedullary thyroid carcinoma. *Cancer 66:*1213–1220, 1990.

60. Johnson, T. L., Lloyd, R. V., Burney, R. E., and Thompson, N. W. Hürthle cell thyroid tumors: An immunohistochemical study. *Cancer 59:*107–112, 1987.

61. Joensuu, H., Klemi, P., and Eerola, E. DNA aneuploidy in follicular adenomas of the thyroid gland. *Am. J. Pathol. 124:*373–376, 1987.

62. Joensuu, H., Klemi, P., Eerola, E., and Tuominen, J. Influence of cellular DNA content on survival in differentiated thyroid cancer. *Cancer 58:*2462–2467, 1986.

63. Johannessen, J. V., Sobrinho-Simoes, M., Lindmo, T., and Tangen, K. O. The diagnostic value of flow cytometric DNA measurements in selected disorders of the human thyroid. *Am. J. Clin. Pathol. 77:*20–25, 1982.

64. Kahn, N., and Perzin, K. H. Follicular carcinoma of the thyroid: An evaluation of the histologic criteria used for diagnosis. *Pathol. Annu. 18:*221–253, 1983.

65. Kendall, C. H., Sanderson, P. R., Cope, J., and Talbot, L. C. Follicular thyroid tumours: A study of laminin and type IV collagen in basement membrane and endothelium. *J. Clin. Pathol. 38:*1100–1105, 1985.

66. Kini, S. R. *Guides to Clinical Aspiration Biopsy: Thyroid.* New York, Igaku-Shoin, 1987.

67. Kini, S. R., Miller, J. M., and Hamburger, J. I. Cytopathology of Hürthle cell lesions of the thyroid gland by fine needle aspiration. *Acta Cytol. 25:*647–652, 1981.

68. Kini, S. R., Miller, J. M., Abrash, M. P., Gaba, A., and Johnson, T. Pose fine needle aspiration biopsy infarction in thyroid nodules. *Mod. Pathol. 1:*48A, 1988 (abstract).

69. Knyazev, P. G., Nikiforova, I. F., Serova, O. M., and Pluzhnkiova, G. F. Distribution and rearrangements of alleles of c-Ha-ras-1 protooncogene and their correlation with the development of lung, ovarian, and thyroid cancers. *Neoplasma 37:*647–655, 1990.

70. Kopald, K. H., Layfield, L. J., Mohrmann, R., Foshag, L. J., and Giuliano, A. E. Clarifying the role of fine needle aspiration cytologic evaluation and frozen section examination in the operative management of thyroid cancer. *Arch. Surg. 124:*1201–1205, 1989.

71. Kraemer, B. B. Frozen section and the thyroid. *Semin. Diagn. Pathol. 4:*169–189, 1987.

72. Kraiem, Z., Glaser, B., Yigla, M., Pauker, J., Sadeh, O., and Sheinfeld, M. Toxic multinodular goiter: A variant of autoimmune hyperthyroidism. *J. Clin. Endocrinol. Metab.* 65:659–664, 1987.

73. Kumar, A., Shah, D. H., and Thakare, U. R. Biochemical characterization of serum thyroglobulin from patients with bone metastases from follicular carcinoma of the thyroid. *Indian J. Biochem. Biophys.* 28:198–202, 1991.

74. Lang, W., Choritz, H., and Hundeshagen, H. Risk factors in follicular thyroid carcinomas. A retrospective follow-up study covering a 14 year period with emphasis on morphological findings. *Am. J. Surg. Pathol.* 10:246–255, 1986.

75. Lang, W., and Georgii, G. Minimal invasive cancer in the thyroid. *Clin. Oncol.* 1:527–537, 1982.

76. Lang, W., Georgii, G., Stauch, G., and Kienzie, E. The differentiation of atypical adenomas and encapsulated follicular carcinomas in the thyroid gland. *Virchows Arch [A] 385:*125–141, 1980.

77. Layfield, L. J., Mohrmann, R. L., Kopald, K. H., and Giuliamo, A. E. Use of aspiration cytology and frozen section examination for management of benign and malignant thyroid nodules. *Cancer 68:*130–134, 1991.

78. Lemoine, N. R., Staddon, S., Bond, J., Wyllie, F. S., Shaw, J. J., and Wynford-Thomas, D. Partial transformation of human thyroid epithelial cells by mutant HA-ras oncogene. *Oncogene 5:*1833–1837, 1990.

79. Lemoine, N. R., Wyllie, F. S., Lillehaug, J. R., Staddon, S. L., Hughes, C. M., Aasland, R., Shaw, J., Varhaug, J. E., Brown, C. L., Gullick, W. J., and Wynford-Thomas, D. Absence of abnormalities of the c-erbB-1 and c-erbB-2 protooncogenes in human thyroid neoplasia. *Eur. J. Cancer 26:*777–779, 1990.

80. LiVolsi, V. A., and Merino, M. J. Worrisome histologic alterations following fine needle aspiration of the thyroid. *Lab. Invest.* 62:59A, 1990 (abstract).

81. Luck, J. B., Mumaw, V. R., and Frable, W. J. Fine needle aspiration biopsy of the thyroid: Differential diagnosis by videoplan image analysis. *Acta Cytol.* 26:793–796, 1982.

82. Lukacs, G. L., Balazs, G., and Zs-Nagy, I. Cytofluorimetric measurements on the DNA contents of tumor cells in human thyroid gland. *J. Cancer Res. Clin. Oncol.* 95:265–271, 1979.

83. McLeod, M. K., Thompson, N. W., Hudson, J. L., Gaglio, J. A., Lloyd, R. V., Harness, J. K., Nishiyama, R., and Cheung, P. S. Y. Flow cytometric measurements of nuclear DNA and ploidy analysis in Hürthle cell neoplasms of the thyroid. *Arch. Surg.* 123:849–854, 1988.

84. Meissner, W. A. Surgical pathology. In: *Surgery of the Thyroid Gland*, edited by C. E. Sedgwick. Philadelphia, W.B. Saunders Co., 1974, pp. 24–40.

85. Meissner, W. A. Follicular carcinoma of the thyroid; frozen section diagnosis. *Am. J. Surg. Pathol.* 1:171–175, 1977.

86. Meissner, W. A., and Warren, S. *Tumors of the Thyroid Gland,* Fascicle 4, second series. Washington, DC, Armed Forces Institute of Pathology, 1969.

87. Miller, J. M. Evaluation of thyroid nodules: Accent on needle biopsy. *Med. Clin. North. Am.* 69:1063–1077, 1985.

88. Montironi, R., Scarpelli, M., Sisti, S., Mariuzzi, G. M., Collan, Y., and Pesonen, E. Sources and nature of variation in DNA analysis of follicular thyroid adenoma. *Pathol. Res. Pract.* 185:579–583, 1989.

89. Mortensen, J. D., Woolner, L. B., and Bennett, W. A. Gross and microscopic findings in clinically normal thyroid glands. *J. Clin. Endocrinol. Metab.* 15:1270–1280, 1955.

90. Namba, H., Gutman, R. A., Matsuo, K., Alvarez, A., and Fagin, J. A. H-*ras* protooncogene mutations in human thyroid neoplasms. *J. Clin. Endocrinol. Metab.* 71:223–229, 1990.

91. Namba, H., Matsuo, K., and Fagin, J. A. Clonal composition of benign and malignant human thyroid tumors. *J. Clin. Invest.* 86:120–125, 1990.

92. Namba, H., Ross, J. L., Goodman, D., and Fagin, J. A. Solitary polyclonal autonomous thyroid nodule: A rare cause of childhood hyperthyroidism. *J. Clin. Invest.* 72:1108–1112, 1991.

93. Namba, H., Rubin, S. A. and Fagin, J. A. Point mutations of *ras* oncogene are an early event in thyroid tumorigenesis. *Mol. Endocrinol.* 4:1474–1479, 1990.

94. O'Sullivan, C., Barton, C. M., Staddon, S. L., Brown, C. L., and Lemoine, N. R. Activating point mutations of the *gsp* oncogene in human thyroid adenomas. *Mol. Carcinog.* 4:345–349, 1991.

95. Peter, H. J., Gerber, H., Studer, H., and Smeds, S. Pathogenesis of heterogeneity in human multinodular goiter. *J. Clin. Invest. 76:*1992–2002, 1985.

96. Peter, H. J., Studer, H., Forster, R., and Gerber, H. The pathogenesis of "hot" and "cold" follicles in multinodular goiters. *J. Clin. Endocrinol. Metab. 55:*941–946, 1982.

97. Peter, H. J., Studer, H., and Groscurth, P. Autonomous growth, but not autonomous function in embryonic human thyroids: A clue to understanding autonomous goiter growth? *J. Clin. Endocrinol. Metab. 66:*968–973, 1988.

98. Ramelli, F., Studer, H., and Bruggisser, D. Pathogenesis of thyroid nodules in multinodular goiter. *Am. J. Pathol. 109:*215–223, 1982.

99. Reuse, S., Maenhaut, C., and Dumont, J. E. Regulation of protooncogenes c-*fos* and c-*myc* expressions by protein tyrosine kinase, protein kinase C and cyclic AMP mitogenic pathways in dog primary thyrocytes: A positive and negative control by cyclic AMP on c-*myc* expression. *Exp. Cell Res. 189:*33–40, 1990.

100. Roediger, W. E. W. The oxyphil and C cells of the human thyroid gland. *Cancer 36:*1758–1770, 1975.

101. Rosai, J., and Carcangiu, M. L. Pathology of thyroid tumors: Some recent and old questions. *Hum. Pathol. 15:*1008–1012, 1984.

102. Rosen, I. B., Luk, S., and Katz, I. Hürthle cell tumor behavior: Dilemma and resolution. *Surgery 98:*777–783, 1985.

103. Rosen, Y., Rosenblatt, P., and Saltzman, E. Intraoperative pathologic diagnosis of thyroid neoplasms. *Cancer 66:*2001–2006, 1990.

104. Ruegemer, J. J., Hay, I. D., Bergstralh, E. J., Ryan, J. J., Offord, K. P., and Gorman, C. A. Distant metastases in differentiated thyroid carcinoma: A multivariate analysis of prognostic variables. *J. Clin. Endocrinol. Metab. 67:*501–508, 1988.

105. Sakamoto, A., Kasai, N., and Sugano, H. Poorly differentiated carcinoma of the thyroid. A clinicopathologic entity for a high risk group of papillary and follicular carcinomas. *Cancer 52:*1849–1855, 1983.

106. Salmon, I., Kiss, R., Franc, B., Gasperin, P., Heimann, R., Pasteels, J. L., and Verhest, A. Comparison of morphonuclear features in normal, benign and neoplastic thyroid tissue by digital cell image analysis. *Anal. Quant. Cytol. Histol. 14:*47–54, 1992.

107. Sambade, C., Franssila, K., Cameselle-Teijeiro, J., Nesland, J., and Sobrinho-Simoes, M. Hyalinizing trabecular adenoma: A misnomer for a peculiar tumor of the thyroid gland. *Endocr. Pathol. 2:*83–91, 1991.

108. Schelfhout, L. J. D. M., Corneliese, C. J., Goslings, B. M., Hamming, J. F., Kuipers-Dukshoorn, N. J., vandeVelde, C. J. H., and Fleuren, G. J. Frequency and degree of aneuploidy in benign and malignant thyroid neoplasms. *Int. J. Cancer 45:*16–20, 1990.

109. Schroder, S., Baisch, H., Rehpenning, W., Muller-Gartner, H. W., Schulz-Bischof, K., Sablotny, B., Meiners, I., Bocker, W., and Schreiber, H. W. Morphologie und Prognose des folliculären Schilddrusencarcinoms—Eine klinisch-pathologische und DNA-cytometrische Untersuchung an 95 Tumoren. *Langenbecks Arch. Chir. 370:*3–24, 1987.

110. Schroder, S., Pfannschmidt, N., Draile, H., Arps, H., and Bocker, W. The encapsulated follicular carcinoma of the thyroid. *Virchows Arch. [A] 402:*259–273, 1984.

111. Schurch, M., Peter, H. J., Gerber, H., and Studer, H. Cold follicles in a multinodular human goiter arise partly from a falling iodide pump and partly from deficient iodine organification. *J. Clin. Endocrinol. Metab. 71:*1224–1229, 1990.

112. Schurmann, G., Mattfeldt, T., Feichter, G., Koretz, K., Moller, P., and Buhr, H. Stereology, flow cytometry and immunohistochemistry of follicular neoplasms of the thyroid gland. *Hum. Pathol. 22:*179–184, 1991.

113. Shaha, A., DiMaio, T., Webber, C., and Jaffe, B. M. Intraoperative decision making during thyroid surgery based on the results of preoperative needle biopsy and frozen section. *Surgery 108:*964–971, 1990.

114. Shaha, A., Gleich, L., DiMaio, T., and Jaffe, B. M. Accuracy and pitfalls of frozen section during thyroid surgery. *J. Surg. Oncol. 44:*84–92, 1990.

115. Simpson, W. J., McKinney, S. E., Carruthers, J. S., Gospodarowicz, M. K., Sutcliffe, S. B., and

Panzarella, T. Papillary and follicular thyroid cancer: Prognostic factors in 1578 patients. *Am. J. Med. 83*:479–488, 1987.

116. Simpson, W. J., Panzarella, T., Carruthers, J. S., Gospodarowicz, M. K., and Sutcliffe, S. B. Papillary and follicular thyroid cancer: Impact of therapy in 1578 patients. *Int. J. Radiol. Oncol. Biol. Phys. 14*:1063–1075, 1988.

117. Sobrinho-Simões, M., Soares, J., Carniero, F., and Limbert, E. Diffuse follicular variant of papillary carcinoma of the thyroid: Report of eight cases of a distinct aggressive type of thyroid tumor. *Surg. Pathol. 3*:189–203, 1990.

118. Soderstrom, N., Lindgren, J., and Tibblin, S. Hemorrhagic thyroid cysts in nodular goitre. *Lancet 23*:531–532, 1974.

119. Strauss, L. C., Rowley, S. K., Loken, M. R., Stuart, R. K., and Civin, C. I. Primitive normal lymphohematopoietic progenitor cells express the MY-10 antigen: Further characterization. *Blood 64*:117A, 1984 (abstract).

120. Studer, H. Growth control and follicular cell neoplasia. In: *Frontiers in Thyroidology*, edited by G. Medeiros-Neto and E. Gaitan. New York, Plenum Medical Books, 1987, Vol. 1, pp. 131–137.

121. Studer, H., Hunziker, H. R., and Ruchti, C. Morphologic and functional substrate of thyrotoxicosis caused by nodular goiters. *Am. J. Med. 65*:227–234, 1978.

122. Studer, H., Peter, H. J., and Gerber, H. Morphologic and functional changes in developing goiters. In: *Thyroid Disorders Associated with Iodine Deficiency and Excess,* edited by R. Hall and J. Kobberling. New York, Raven Press, 1985, pp. 229–241.

123. Studer, H., Peter, H. J., and Gerber, H. Natural heterogeneity of thyroid cells: The basis for understanding thyroid function and nodular goiter growth. *Endocr. Rev. 10*:125–135, 1989.

124. Studer, H., and Ramelli, F. Simple goiter and its variants: Euthyroid and hyperthyroid. *Endocr. Rev. 3*:40–61, 1982.

125. Thompson, N. W., Dunn, E. L., Batsakis, J. G., and Nishiyama, R. H. Hürthle cell lesions of the thyroid gland. *Surg. Gynecol. Obstet. 139*:555–560, 1974.

126. Tollefson, H. R., Shah, J. P., and Huvos, A. G. Hürthle cell carcinoma of the thyroid. *Am. J. Surg. 130*:390–394, 1975.

127. Tubiana, M., Schlumberger, M., Rougier, P., LaPlanche, A., Benhamori, E., Gardet, P., Caillou, B., Travagli, J. P., and Parmentier, C. Long-term results and prognostic factors in patients with well differentiated thyroid carcinoma. *Cancer 55*:794–804, 1985.

128. vanden Berg, E., Oosterhuis, J. W., deJong, B., Buist, J., Vos, A. M., Dam, A., and Vermeij, B. Cytogenetics of thyroid follicular adenomas. *Cancer Genet. Cytogenet. 44*:217–222, 1990.

129. vanden Berg, E., vanDoormaal, J. J., Oosterhuis, J. W., deJong, B., Buist, J., Vos, A. M., Dam, A., and Vermeij, B. Cytogenetic study of a nodular hyperplasia of the thyroid after irradiation for Hodgkin's disease. *Cancer Genet. Cytogenet. 53*:15–21, 1991.

130. Vander, J. B., Gaston, E. A., and Dawber, T. R. The significance of nontoxic thyroid nodules. *Ann. Intern. Med. 69*:537–540, 1968.

131. Vannelli, G. B., Barni, T., Modigliani, U., Paulin, I., Serio, M., Maggi, M., Fiorelli, G., and Balboni, G. C. Insulin-like growth factor I receptors in nonfunctioning thyroid nodules. *J. Clin. Endocrinol. Metab. 71*:1175–1182, 1990.

132. Watson, R. G., Brennan, M. D., Goellner, J. R., vanHeerden, J. A., McConahey, W. M., and Taylor, W. F. Invasive Hürthle cell carcinoma of the thyroid: Natural history and management. *Mayo Clin. Proc. 59*:851–855, 1984.

133. Weber, J. L., and May, P. E. Abundant class of human DNA polymorphisms which can be typed using the polymerase chain reaction. *Am. J. Hum. Genet. 44*:388–396, 1989.

134. Williams, E. D. TSH and thyroid cancer. In: *Proceedings of the International Symposium: Physiological Regulation and Biological Function of Thyreotropin,* edited by E. F. Pfeiffer and G. M. Reaven. Hormone and Metabolic Research Suppl. Series Vol. 23, 1989, pp. 72–75.

135. Williams, E. D., Doniach, I., Bjarnson, O., and Michie, W. Thyroid cancer in an iodide rich area. *Cancer 39*:215–222, 1977.

136. Woolner, L. B. Thyroid carcinoma: Pathologic consideration with data on prognosis. *Semin. Nucl. Med. 1*:481–502, 1971.

137. Woolner, L. B., Beahrs, O. H., Black, B. M., McConahey, W. M., and Keating, F. R. Classification and diagnosis of thyroid carcinoma. *Am. J. Surg. 102:*354–387, 1961.
138. Wynford-Thomas, D., Bond, J. A., Wyllie, F. S., Burns, J. S., Williams, E. D., Jones, T., Sheer, D., and Lemoine, N. R. Conditional immortalization of human thyroid epithelial cells: A tool for analysis of oncogene action. *Mol. Cell. Biol. 10:*5365–5377, 1990.
139. Yamashita, S., Ong, J., Fagin, J. A., and Melmed, S. Expression of the *myc* cellular protooncogene in human thyroid tissue. *J. Clin. Endocrinol. Metab. 63:*1170–1173, 1986.
140. Young, R. L., Mazzaferri, E. L., Rahe, A. J., and Dorfman, S. G. Pure follicular carcinoma: Impact of therapy in 214 patients. *J. Nucl. Med. 21:*733–737, 1980.

Chapter 7

Papillary Carcinoma

JUAN ROSAI

Papillary carcinoma is a malignant epithelial tumor showing evidence of follicular cell differentiation and characterized by the formation of papillae and/ or a set of distinctive nuclear changes.

GENERAL FEATURES

Papillary carcinoma constitutes 65–80% of all thyroid cancers in the United States.[87] Apparently, its relative incidence as compared to that of follicular carcinoma is even greater in areas of high iodine intake.[69,142]

There is a proven association between radiation exposure to the neck and subsequent development of papillary and related thyroid carcinomas.[8,66,122] In most instances, the radiation had been administered during childhood, and the average interval until the development of malignancy had been approximately 20 years[5]; however, cases have also been reported of papillary thyroid carcinoma developing shortly following the administration of high-dose radiation to the neck for malignant tumors.[13,62,98] In two large series of thyroid papillary carcinoma, the numbers of patients who gave a history of previous irradiation to the neck were 6.0% and 6.6%, respectively.[21,94]

It has been claimed that there is an increased incidence of papillary carcinoma in Graves' disease, but this has not been conclusively proven.[42,46,107,113] It has been postulated that in those patients with Graves' disease who develop thyroid carcinoma, the thyroid-stimulating antibodies that are responsible for the former may play a role in the tumor development.[47]

Papillary carcinoma seems to be more common in glands affected by autoimmune thyroiditis,[30,109] but a definite statistical relationship still needs to be proven. Hyperplastic nodules or adenomas are present in about 40% of the glands harboring papillary carcinomas, but these probably represent coincidental events.[21]

Cases of papillary carcinoma have been reported in families,[90] in patients with ataxia-telangiectasia,[104] in individuals with multiple endocrine neoplasia syndrome,[68] and in association with parathyroid tumors,[65] carotid body tumors,[3] and a variety of colorectal abnormalities. The latter include sporadic adenocarcinoma, polyposis coli, Gardner syndrome, and Cowden syndrome.[112]

138

CLINICAL FEATURES

Papillary carcinoma is more common in women. The female/male ratio in most series ranges between 2:1 and 3:1,[49,61,94] but is substantially higher in Japan (9:1 to 13:1). The mean age at the time of diagnosis has ranged from 31 to 49 years. Several authors have noted a shift to a younger range in recent years, and have attributed this to earlier diagnosis.[18,36] Papillary carcinoma constitutes 90% or more of all cases of thyroid carcinoma in childhood.

GROSS FEATURES

The typical carcinoma appears grossly as an invasive neoplasm of ill-defined margins, firm consistency, whitish color, and a granular cut surface. Calcifications are common. The size is extremely variable, the mean diameter being between 2 and 3 cm.

Some notable variations in the gross appearance are related to the variants described below. This applies to the well-circumscribed and fleshy appearance resembling adenoma that can be seen in the follicular variant, and the partial or complete cystic change that is characteristic of the encapsulated type.

Fresh tumor necrosis is exceptional in papillary carcinoma. Its presence should suggest an alternative diagnosis or the development within of a more aggressive component of either poorly differentiated or undifferentiated nature.

MICROSCOPIC FEATURES

The two cardinal morphologic features of papillary carcinoma are the papillae and the nuclear changes.

PAPILLAE

These structures are formed by a central fibrovascular stalk covered by neoplastic epithelium (Fig. 7.1). The better developed papillae are long, with a complex arborizing pattern; some are straight and slender, others are short and stubby. Yet another configuration, perhaps secondary to fusion of individual papillae, is a cribriform pattern reminiscent of that seen in intraductal carcinoma of the breast.[24,26]

The amount and composition of the papillary stalk are variable. In most instances, it is made up of loose connective tissue and variously sized vessels. In some cases, it is swollen by edema fluid or occupied by an abundant hyaline material. Sometimes it is infiltrated by lymphocytes or clusters of macrophages, some of which may be foamy or hemosiderin-laden. Psammoma bodies and other calcific concretions may be present. Exceptionally, it may contain mature adipose tissue.[137] It is not rare to find follicles within the papillary stalks.

It is often stressed that for papillae to qualify as such, they should contain a central fibrovascular stalk, in contrast to the infolding epithelium of benign lesions. However, exceptions to this rule are plentiful. Some of the "abortive" papillae of papillary carcinoma are devoid of this stalk, whereas in some benign conditions such as diffuse hyperplasia, nodular hyperplasia, or adenoma with

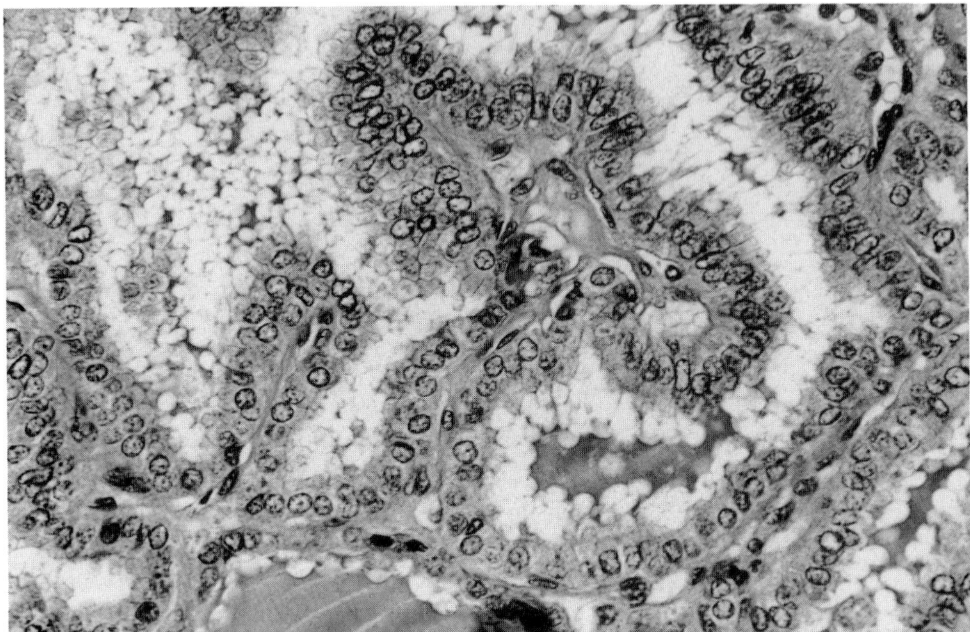

FIG. 7.1. Typical microscopic appearance of papillary carcinoma. The lining is made up of one layer of cuboidal to low columnar cells having irregularly distributed vesicular nuclei. The colloid shows prominently scalloped edges.

papillary hyperplasia, the papillary structures within them may contain well-developed fibrovascular stalks.

In its most typical form, papillary carcinoma shows a predominance of papillary structures throughout the tumor. Yet, it is rare for it to be composed exclusively of papillae. In most instances, the papillae are admixed with neoplastic follicles having similar nuclear features, the proportion between the two structures varying greatly from case to case. This can be indicated in the report by the expressions "with papillary predominance" or "with follicular predominance," depending on the case. The term "mixed carcinoma" should not be used for these tumors. As long as the cells in the neoplastic follicles share the nuclear features seen in the papillae, the natural history of the tumor will be that of a papillary carcinoma. When the follicular predominance over the papillae is complete, the tumor should be placed into the follicular variant of papillary carcinoma.

NUCLEAR FEATURES

The nuclei of the papillary carcinoma cells have in most instances a distinctive appearance, which has now acquired a diagnostic significance just as important as that of the papillae themselves (Fig. 7.2).

These nuclei are usually round or slightly oval. The contours may appear superficially smooth, but close inspection of thinner preparations will reveal subtle irregularities in the form of indentations, crenellations, and folds. These nuclear irregularities may manifest in the form of pseudoinclusions or grooves.

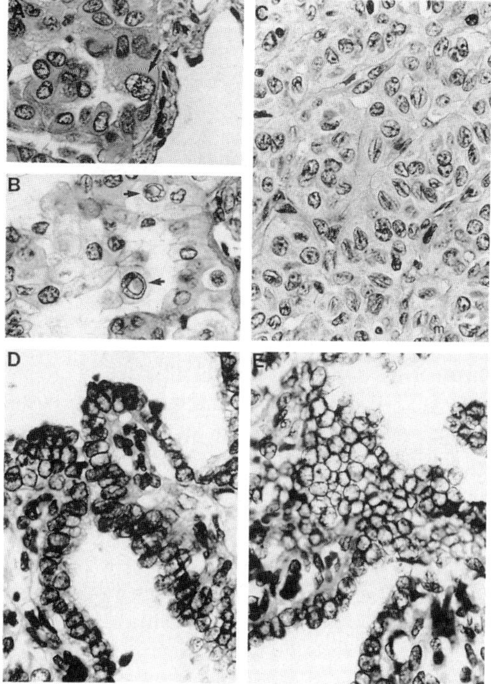

FIG. 7.2. Typical nuclear features of papillary carcinoma cells. *A*, the large nucleus located in the center of the photograph has a finely irregular ("serrated") appearance (*arrow*). *B*, two large nuclear pseudoinclusions are evident (*arrows*). *C*, many of the nuclei show prominent longitudinal grooves. *D*, typical ground glass nuclei showing marked overlapping. *E*, "egg basket" appearance resulting from tangential sectioning of ground glass nuclei.

The former arise from deep cytoplasmic invaginations and result in nuclear acidophilic inclusion-like round structures.[2,75] The nuclear grooves are more common in oval-shaped nuclei and are usually parallel to their long axis.[27]

Another peculiar and rather constant feature of the nucleus of papillary carcinoma cells is represented by an "empty" appearance of the nucleoplasm, accompanied by an irregular thickening of the nuclear membrane. The nucleolus, which may be prominent, is often located against the nuclear membrane. These nuclei have been variously described as pale, clear, optically clear, watery, empty, ground glass, and Orphan Annie's eyes. This appearance is well seen in fixed paraffin-embedded material (regardless of the fixative used), but is inconspicuous or altogether absent in frozen sections or smears from the same cases.[22,139] This had led to the conclusion that it represents an artifact of fixation and/or embedding, although it probably reflects some intrinsic physicochemical alteration of the chromatin structure or associated nuclear proteins.

Mitotic figures are exceptional or absent in papillary carcinoma; their presence in more than an occasional number should suggest the presence of a poorly differentiated neoplasm.[85]

The cytoplasm of papillary carcinoma cells is rather nondescript. In most instances, it is modest in amount, slightly to moderately eosinophilic to ampho-philic, and cuboidal. Variations include pale cells, cells with a finely granular cytoplasm (due to richness of mitochondria), and cells with a diffusely acidophilic cytoplasm (due to cytoplasmic filaments).

OTHER MORPHOLOGIC FEATURES

In addition to the papillary and follicular patterns, papillary carcinoma can grow in solid or trabecular formations. There is usually a focal change, but it may involve most or all of the neoplasm. It should not be taken as evidence that the tumor has become undifferentiated or even poorly differentiated, as long as the typical nuclear features of papillary carcinoma persist in it. Squamous metaplasia is also common. It can be focal or extensive; in its most characteristic form, it presents as concentric whorls of keratinized cells surrounded by papillary foci. Squamous metaplasia is most common in the areas of tumor surrounded by abundant stromal reaction.

Another structure typically associated with papillary carcinoma is the psammoma body. This is a round calcific concretion exhibiting concentric lamination. It is found in roughly half of the cases and is particularly common in those tumors featuring a predominantly papillary pattern of growth. The mechanism of formation is controversial, but there is good evidence that the nidus is represented by a single necrotic tumor cell, with successive layers of calcium salt deposit.[76] Psammoma bodies are not entirely specific for papillary carcinoma; however, they are so rare in benign thyroid diseases that their presence should immediately suggest the presence of a papillary carcinoma.[83] When found in an area of inflammation and dense fibrosis, they usually are indicative of a papillary cancer that has regressed at that site. When found in an otherwise normal thyroid, the chances are high that a papillary carcinoma is present nearby. If present in an otherwise normal cervical lymph node, there is a high probability that the node is involved by a metastatic papillary carcinoma which is not apparent at that particular level.

Psammoma bodies have also been described in cases of follicular carcinoma, but most of these would probably be classified at present as the follicular variant of papillary carcinoma. Psammoma bodies can also occur in medullary carcinoma and have even been described in metastatic carcinoma to the thyroid.[119]

An abundant fibrous stroma is common in papillary carcinoma. In most instances, it presents in the form of wide hyaline bands. The fibrosing tendencies of this tumor are particularly evident at the advancing edge. Some of this stromal reaction has a very cellular ("desmoplastic") appearance; rarely, it acquires a nodular fasciitis-like or fibromatosis-like quality and is so abundant as to obscure the neoplastic component.[25] In other cases, a prominent myxoid change may be encountered.[108]

Approximately one-third of papillary carcinomas show a moderate to marked lymphocytic infiltration; this change tends to be more pronounced at the tumor periphery and within the fibrovascular papillary stalks. It may represent a host reaction to the tumor or the expression of a pre-existing autoimmune thyroiditis.[80,127] The stroma of papillary carcinoma may also contain aggregates of S-100 protein-positive cells, which have been interpreted as of Langerhans/reticulum cell type.[126]

Secondary cystic changes are common, particularly in the very papillary tumors. Most of these cysts are lined by papillary formation, but others are covered by an attenuated single-layered, flat epithelium having a deceptively benign appearance.

Blood vessel invasion is not as common as in follicular carcinoma, but it occurs.[21] Invasion of lymph vessels is a much more common phenomenon; when very extensive, the possibility of the tumor belonging to the diffuse sclerosing variant should be considered.

ULTRASTRUCTURAL FEATURES

The characteristic nuclei of papillary carcinoma cells exhibit a finely dispersed chromatin, a highly folded nuclear membrane, and an apparent paucity of nuclear pores[10,75,77] (Fig. 7.3). The nuclear folds may result in large invaginations within the nucleus that correspond to the inclusion-like formations seen with the light microscope. The cytoplasm is rich in mitochondria, lysosomes, and filaments. The latter are particularly numerous in foci of squamous metaplasia, in which

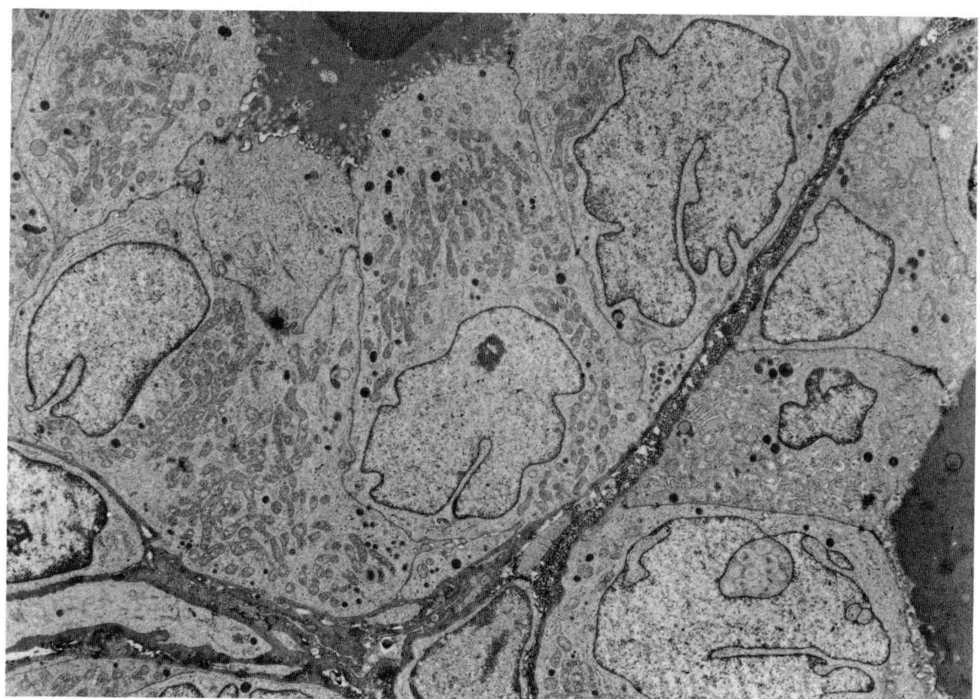

FIG. 7.3.   Ultrastructural appearance of papillary carcinoma. The cells covering the papillae are tall cuboidal. The cytoplasm contains a relatively large number of mitochondria and scattered lysosomes. The nucleus is characteristically indented; this corresponding to the grooves seen in light microscopic preparations (original magnification, ×8,400). (Photo courtesy of Dr. Robert Erlandson, Memorial Sloan-Kettering Cancer Center, New York, NY.)

they may be accompanied by keratohyaline granules. The apical surface exhibits microvillous differentiation.

IMMUNOHISTOCHEMICAL FEATURES

Papillary carcinoma cells are consistently positive for thyroglobulin, although the intensity of the reaction tends to be less pronounced than in follicular neoplasms.[111,133] The tumor cells are also immunoreactive for keratin and vimentin, the two markers often being expressed in the same cell.[138,143] The keratins found are not only of the low molecular weight type present in the normal thyroid, but also of high molecular weight. Since the latter are usually not encountered in the normal thyroid gland or in follicular neoplasms, it has been suggested that they may be useful in the differential diagnosis.[120] One should keep in mind, though, that the abnormal follicular epithelium of Hashimoto's thyroiditis also expresses high molecular weight keratins.[67]

OTHER SPECIAL TECHNIQUES

Biochemical studies of the thyroglobulin (TGB) secreted by papillary (as well as follicular) carcinomas suggest that, at least in some cases, there are structural differences with the TGB secreted by the normal gland. These include a lesser degree of iodination, a lesser degree of binding to some monoclonal antibodies, a lesser degree of absorption in affinity chromatography on a concanavalin A-Sepharose column, a decrease in high-mannose-type oligosaccharides with a corresponding increase of other neutral oligosaccharides, and replacement of sialylated oligosaccharides for phosphorylated oligosaccharides.[133] A set of monoclonal antibodies raised against the thyroglobulin of a papillary carcinoma and thought to recognize iodine-related (hormonogenic) epitopes was found to stain preferentially the colloid but not the cytoplasm in normal or hyperplastic glands, and to exhibit an inverse pattern in papillary carcinoma, in which the intraluminal colloid was negative whereas the cytoplasm was strongly stained (usually apically but sometimes also basolaterally).[133]

Estrogen receptor protein has been detected immunohistochemically in the nuclei of papillary carcinoma cells in a high proportion of cases, independently of the hormonal status of the patients.[40]

DNA analysis, performed either by static or flow cytometric techniques, has shown that about 80% of papillary carcinomas are diploid. One chromosomal analysis study showed that most papillary carcinomas were characterized by normal stemlines.[15] In another study, clonal karyotypical abnormalities were detected in 4 of 7 cases, all of them involving 10q[73]; in yet another, a 7:10 (q35:q21) was documented.[6]

In several reported series, most of the tumors causing death belonged to the aneuploid group.[7,35,74,129] It should be noted that nearly all of these patients would have already been identifiable as being in the high-risk group in view of their age and sex.

Several types of oncogene alterations have been described in papillary carcinoma.[50] An increase in the expression of the oncogene *ras* product (p21 antigen) was detected immunohistochemically by Mizukami *et al.*[101] in the apical surface of papillary carcinoma cells, when compared with those of normal, inflamed, hyperplastic, or benign neoplastic glands, but the significance of this finding is not known. Johnson *et al.*[78] showed that p21 antigen was more strongly expressed in papillary carcinoma and other thyroid diseases than in the normal gland; however, no significant differences were found between neoplastic and nonneoplastic conditions, or between benign and malignant tumors.

Wright *et al.*[145] found by transfection techniques an incidence of *ras* point mutation of 17% for papillary carcinoma and of 53% for follicular carcinoma; they speculated that this statistically significant difference was probably related to the known differences in epidemiology, pathology, and clinical behavior between the two tumors.

A group of Italian investigators has studied 16 papillary carcinomas for transforming activity and detected it in 10 (62%).[17,53] This was found to be due to activation of three different oncogenes, identified in four cases as *PTC* (rearrangement), *TRK* (rearrangement), and N-*ras* (point mutation). The *PTC* oncogene (short for papillary thyroid carcinoma) is thought to represent a rearranged form of the *ret* proto-oncogene and has been assigned to chromosome 10 q11-q12.[41,56] Since both *PTC* and *TRK* display a tyrosine protein kinase activity, the authors proposed that the activation of this class of oncogenes is specifically involved in the pathogenesis of papillary carcinoma.[17]

Wyllie *et al.*[146] failed to detect evidence of rearrangement or amplification of c-*myc* or of any other member of the "nuclear" oncogene family in papillary carcinoma or any of the other thyroid neoplasms they studied. Mizukami *et al.*[102] were also unable to find differences in c-*myc* expression between benign and malignant thyroid tumors. They found instead a possibly higher expression of epidermal growth factor among the papillary carcinomas that recurred when compared with those that did not.

CYTOLOGIC FEATURES

Cytologic specimens from papillary carcinoma tend to be very cellular, with scanty or absent colloid. When the latter is present, it often exhibits a peculiar streaking and smearing effect, sometimes referred to as a "bubble gum" appearance.

Papillary formations may be found, admixed with flat monolayers of cells. These may be combined with syncytium-like formations and follicles, as discussed in Chapter 8.

The individual tumor cells may be low columnar or cuboidal. The nuclei have a fine ("powdery" or "dusty") chromatin pattern and an irregular contour, with frequent creases and grooves. Intranuclear pseudoinclusions representing cytoplasmic invaginations are common and represent one of the most important diagnostic features of papillary carcinoma.[31,86] The ground glass appearance constantly seen in histologic sections is inconspicuous in cytologic preparations. Multiple small or large nucleoli are usually identified. The cytoplasm is variable in amount and tinctorial qualities; it may appear pale, foamy, vacuolated, or dense. Psammoma bodies may be identified.[81]

A difficult problem is created by the papillary carcinomas with cystic degeneration, since the aspirate may show lymphocytes, foamy macrophages, and few or no tumor cells.[55]

SPREAD AND METASTASES

One of the most striking properties of papillary carcinoma is its tendency for multicentric involvement of the gland. Controversy exists as to whether this is the result of intrathyroidal lymph vessel spread or of true multicentric transformation of the follicular epithelium.

In most reported series, the incidence of multicentricity has ranged from 18 to 22%.[21] The outstanding exception is the figure of 87.5% reported by Russell *et al.*[115] in a whole-mount study of 80 well-differentiated thyroid carcinomas, most of which were of the papillary type.

Extrathyroid extension into the soft tissues of the neck has been reported in 10–34% of the cases.[19,33,135,144] The growth may take place along fascial planes, perineural spaces, and within skeletal muscle; in advanced stages, direct extension into larynx, trachea, esophagus, or skin can be encountered.[136]

Papillary carcinoma has a great tendency to metastasize to cervical lymph nodes. One-third of the patients have clinically evident lymphadenopathy at the time of presentation.[21] Even in cases thought to be negative on palpation, microscopic examination will reveal metastatic tumor in approximately one-half.[51] The deposits are usually on the same side as the tumor, but bilateral involvement occurs in about one-tenth of the cases.[105] Spread to mediastinal nodes is usually secondary to extensive cervical disease.

Nodal metastases of papillary carcinoma have a tendency to undergo cystic degeneration and/or to grow in an obvious papillary pattern, even when these features are not well developed in the primary tumor. The cystic change can be so pronounced as to result in a misdiagnosis of branchial cleft cyst on microscopic examination. The presence of papillae, nuclear abnormalities, and/or psammoma bodies provides the clues for the diagnosis, which can be easily confirmed with an immunohistochemical stain for thyroglobulin.

Blood-borne metastasis also occurs, although less commonly than with most other thyroid malignancies. The incidence ranges from 4 to 14% in the various series.[21,60,70,144] The lung is by far the most common site, and deposits can occur in the absence of cervical nodal involvement.[116] Other sites include the skeletal system, liver, and central nervous system.

TREATMENT

The treatment of papillary carcinoma remains controversial. In the past, the standard approach was the performance of a total thyroidectomy together with a radical lymph node dissection on the side of the tumor, the rationale for this aggressive approach being the high frequency of intraglandular spread/multicentricity and of regional lymph node metastases. The performance of a formal cervical lymphadenectomy has been largely abandoned, in part because of the demonstration that it fails to remove a good number of the first-station lymph nodes, but mainly because no detectable improvements in prognosis have been documented as a result of this operation.[57,72,106] Currently, the approach toward these nodes is to leave them undisturbed if they appear grossly normal and to perform a modified lymph node dissection (with preservation of the sternomastoid muscle) is they appear involved.

As far as the thyroid gland itself is concerned, some groups strongly advocate the performance of a total thyroidectomy and follow this procedure with the administration of radioactive iodine in an attempt to ablate any possible metastatic sites.[32,59,91,94,95] Other groups regard this approach as unnecessarily radical and maintain that similarly good results can be obtained with a lesser operation followed by suppression of thyroid-stimulating hormone secretion, without the addition of radioactive iodine postoperatively.[34,37,123] Our own experience[21] and the evaluation of two recent large series on the subject[141,150] suggest that the latter, more conservative approach is just as effective and perhaps preferable for the majority of the cases, *i.e.*, those papillary carcinomas appearing clinically and scintigraphically localized to one lobe, not belonging to one of the microscopically unfavorable variants (such as diffuse sclerosing or tall/columnar), and occurring in low-risk group patients (women under the age of 50 or men under the age of 40). The specific type of operation, *i.e.*, whether lobectomy, lobectomy with isthmusectomy, or subtotal thyroidectomy, seems to be of no great significance.

PROGNOSIS

The overall probability of long-term survival for patients with papillary carcinoma is excellent, to the point that in some series the figures are not significantly different from those of a normal population of similar age.[36,96]

Factors shown to be associated with a worsened prognosis are the following:

1. Age. This is of great importance. In most series, no deaths from papillary carcinoma are seen below the age of 40 years, the probability of a fatal outcome increasing markedly with each decade.[19,21,38,88,121]

2. Sex. In most series, women have fared better than men, but the difference has not been as significant as for age.[92,121,128] Cady *et al.*[19] proposed dividing patients with well-differentiated (including papillary) carcinomas into two groups on the basis of the two factors listed above: a low-risk group (comprising men 40 years of age or younger and women 50 years of age or younger), and a high-risk group (older patients); almost all deaths from papillary carcinoma will occur in the latter.

3. Tumor size. The probability of tumor recurrence increases when the tumor size exceeds 5 cm. The best prognosis is associated with papillary carcinomas measuring 1.5 cm in diameter or less.[96]

4. Multicentricity. We have found that tumors in which this feature is easily detectable are associated with increased chances of nodal and pulmonary metastases and a corresponding decrease in disease-free survival rates.[21]

5. Blood vessel invasion. According to most authors, this feature is of only modest prognostic importance, barely significant at the statistical level.[18,21,61]

6. Extrathyroid extension. This constitutes one of the worst morphologic prognostic signs in papillary carcinoma. It is associated with an over 6-fold increase in the number of tumor deaths.[21]

7. Distant metastases. The occurrence of lung metastases is associated with a moderate but obvious deleterious effect on prognosis, whereas the development of bone metastases carries an ominous prognostic significance, even when they concentrate ^{131}I.[21,70,97]

8. Aneuploidy. See above under "Other Special Techniques."

9. High microscopic grade. This rare event, which is related to the following item, is associated with a more aggressive clinical course.[96]

10. Progression to a poorly differentiated (including "insular") or undifferentiated (anaplastic) pattern (Figs. 7.4 and 7.5). Both of these types of dedifferentiation carry a decidedly adverse prognostic significance. This is particularly true of the latter.

Features associated with an improved prognosis include total encapsulation, pushing margins of growth, and cystic changes[21]; these three features often coexist.

Features not bearing statistically prognostic significance include history of head and neck irradiation in childhood, relative numbers of papillae and follicles, presence and type of fibrosis, presence of trabecular and/or solid areas (as long as the typical nuclear features of papillary carcinoma are retained), presence and amount of squamous metaplasia, presence and number of psammoma bodies, and

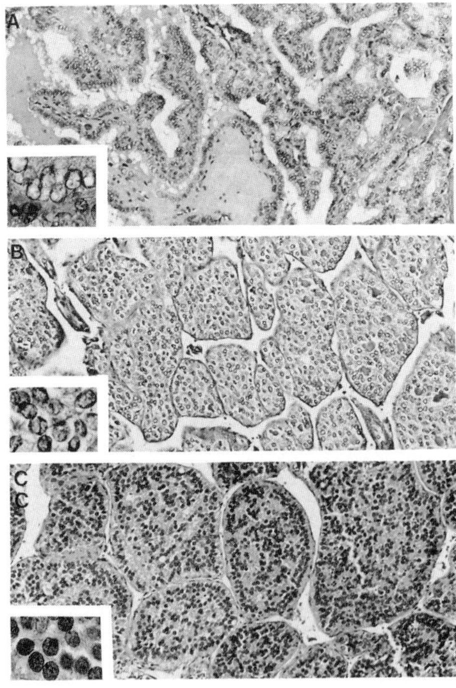

FIG. 7.4.   Progressive transformation of papillary carcinoma into poorly differentiated ("insular") carcinoma. *A,* typical papillary carcinoma as seen in the original excision, performed in 1975. *B,* in the local recurrence in 1984, the papillary pattern has been replaced by an insular pattern. *C,* in another local recurrence from 1987, the insular pattern is fully developed. These architectural changes were paralleled by similarly notable changes in the nuclear appearance, as seen in the *insets.* (Courtesy of Dr. Aidan Carney, Mayo Clinic, Rochester, MN.)

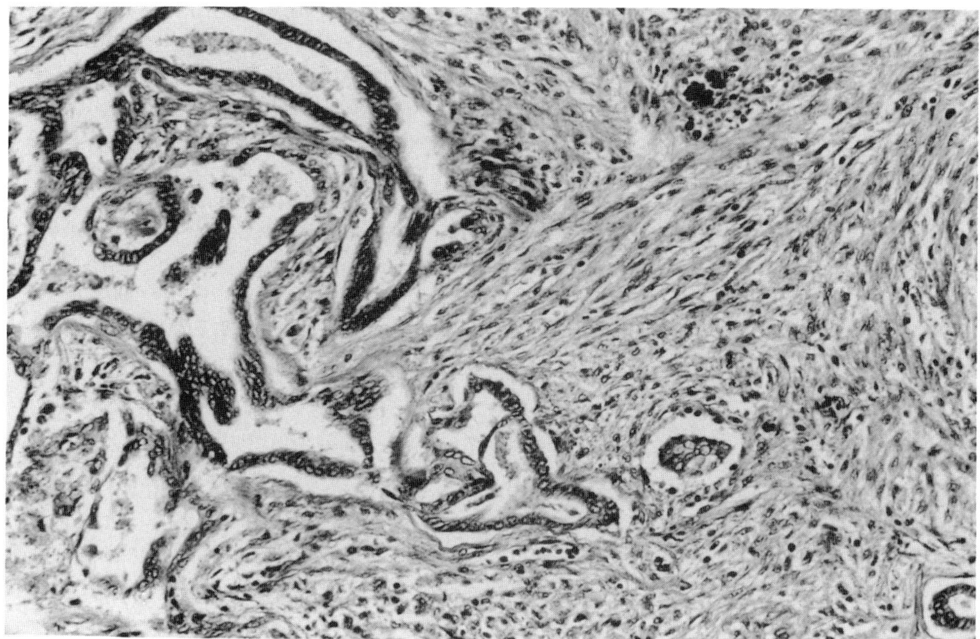

FIG. 7.5.   Undifferentiated carcinoma of spindle cell type with residual papillary carcinoma. There is a sharp segregation of the two components.

presence or absence of cervical lymph node metastases.[117] Another parameter that does not carry prognosis significance in most series is the type of therapy carried out, as already mentioned.[34,36,37,139]

PAPILLARY CARCINOMA VARIANTS

PAPILLARY MICROCARCINOMA

The WHO Committee[64] defines this variant as a papillary carcinoma measuring 1.0 cm or less in diameter. This roughly corresponds to the entity traditionally designated as occult sclerosing carcinoma,[82] also known as nonencapsulated sclerosing tumor[63] and occult papillary carcinoma.[71] It is a common finding in population-based autopsy studies and (as an incidental finding) in carefully examined thyroidectomy specimens.[14,16,58,84,118,148,149] The reported incidence in autopsy material has ranged in most series from 4 to 20%, the highest figure being 35.6% in the series of Harach *et al.*[58]

In one surgical series of papillary carcinomas, the number of microcarcinomas was 6.4%, most having been found either incidentally or because of the development of cervical lymph node metastases.[21] Because of their small size, these lesions are likely to be missed grossly unless a careful and systematic search for them is carried out.

Microscopically, the typical lesion has an irregular, scar-like configuration. The neoplastic elements predominate at the periphery of the fibrotic area, but others are seen entrapped in the center. The features of papillary carcinoma are present in them, including typical nuclear changes, psammoma bodies, and occasionally even well-formed papillae. In most areas, however, the tumor cells display a follicular or solid architecture.

Some papillary microcarcinomas are accompanied by little or no fibrosis (Fig. 7.6). Conversely, others are totally surrounded by an extremely thick fibrous capsule, which may be focally calcified.

That these lesions are malignant has been proven by the repeated demonstration that they can metastasize to regional nodes.[54] However, the overall prognosis is remarkably good: in one series, 93% of the patients were free of disease on follow-up, and there was not even a single instance of distant metastases.[21] Nevertheless, exceptional examples of these tumors metastasizing through the bloodstream and resulting in death are on record.[5,110,134]

ENCAPSULATED VARIANT

One of the most distinctive features of papillary carcinoma is its capacity to invade the surrounding gland. There exists, however, a type of papillary carcinoma that is totally surrounded by a fibrous capsule which may be intact or focally infiltrated by tumor growth. This type, designated as the encapsulated variant of papillary carcinoma, comprises about 10% of all cases of papillary carcinoma.[21,61,125] In the past, tumors with these features were sometimes designated papillary adenomas.[99] The fact that they have been found associated with cervical lymph node metastases in over one-quarter of the cases is clear-cut

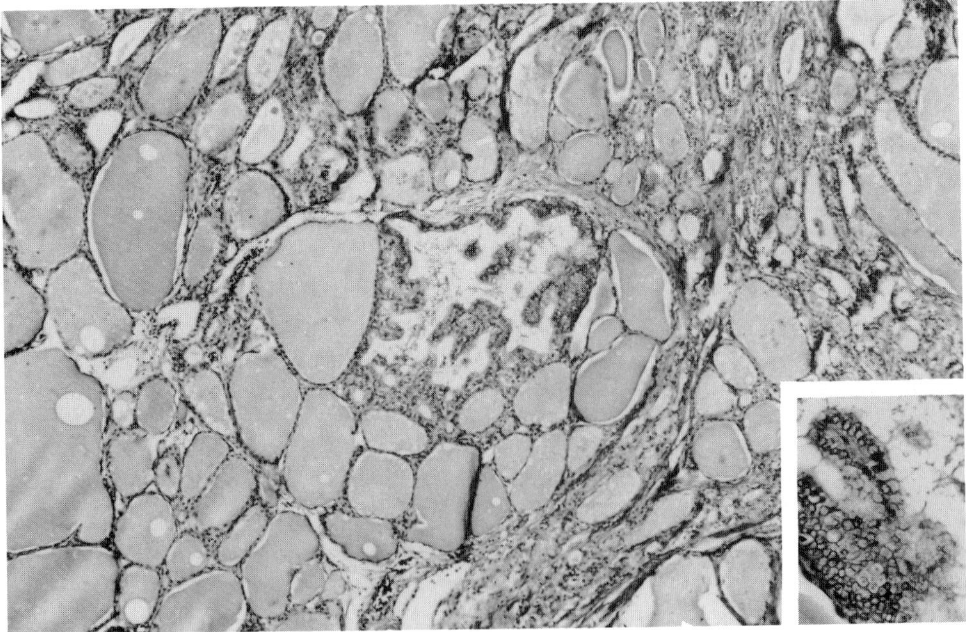

FIG. 7.6.   Papillary microcarcinoma with scanty fibrosis. The architectural and cytologic features are typical of the papillary family of neoplasms, the latter being particularly well appreciated in the *inset.*

evidence that these lesions should be regarded as malignant.[21,125] The main differential diagnosis is follicular adenoma with papillary hyperplasia. The important point to remember is that for a lesion to qualify as encapsulated papillary carcinoma, it should have the typical architecture as well as the nuclear changes of this tumor type. When thus defined, encapsulated papillary carcinoma will be found to be associated with an excellent prognosis; regional nodal metastases may be present, but blood-borne metastases are exceptional and the survival rate is nearly 100%.[43,125]

FOLLICULAR VARIANT

This designation is given to papillary carcinomas with an exclusively or almost exclusively follicular pattern of growth.[21,29,88,114] This variant shares many features with conventional papillary carcinoma: capsule formation is usually absent or incomplete, fibrous septa are common and sometimes extensive, and scattered psammoma bodies may be found in the interfollicular stroma. The follicles themselves offer many clues—some are markedly elongated, resembling tubular glands, whereas others exhibit irregularities of their lining epithelium with formations of folds, ridges, buds, and other intraluminal protrusions which probably represent rudimentary attempts at making papillae. On occasion, the neoplastic follicles are very large, the appearance thus simulating that of nodular hyperplasia; this has been referred to as the "macrofollicular variant" of papillary carcinoma.[4] Regardless of follicle size, the nuclei of the lining cells have features analogous to those of conventional papillary carcinoma and different from those of follicular carcinoma[45] (Fig. 7.7). The colloid within the lumina of the neoplastic follicle often has a strong and homogeneous eosinophilic quality and a scalloped configuration, the latter being similar to that seen in markedly hyperplastic glands.

Careful search for papillae will usually demonstrate some; however, it is important to remember that identification of papillae is not a requisite for the diagnosis of this variant; as a matter of fact, if papillae are easily found, the tumor should not be classified as the follicular variant.

Support for the interpretation that this tumor belongs to the papillary family of thyroid neoplasms derives from the facts that some of these tumors have multicentric foci within the thyroid having a conventional papillary appearance,[114] that the natural history of these tumors conforms in practically all regards to that of conventional papillary carcinoma, that the nodal metastases often have a papillary configuration, and that the types of keratin expressed by the tumor cells match those of papillary rather than follicular carcinoma.[100,147]

ENCAPSULATED FOLLICULAR VARIANT AND RELATED LESIONS

There exists a form of papillary carcinoma, the encapsulated follicular type, which combines features of two variants. As the name indicates, this is a totally encapsulated neoplasm (with or without capsular and/or blood vessel invasion) having the cytoarchitectural features of the follicular variant of papillary carcinoma. In order for this diagnosis to be made, those features need to be displayed prominently throughout the neoplasm. Sometimes, an encapsulated nodule with

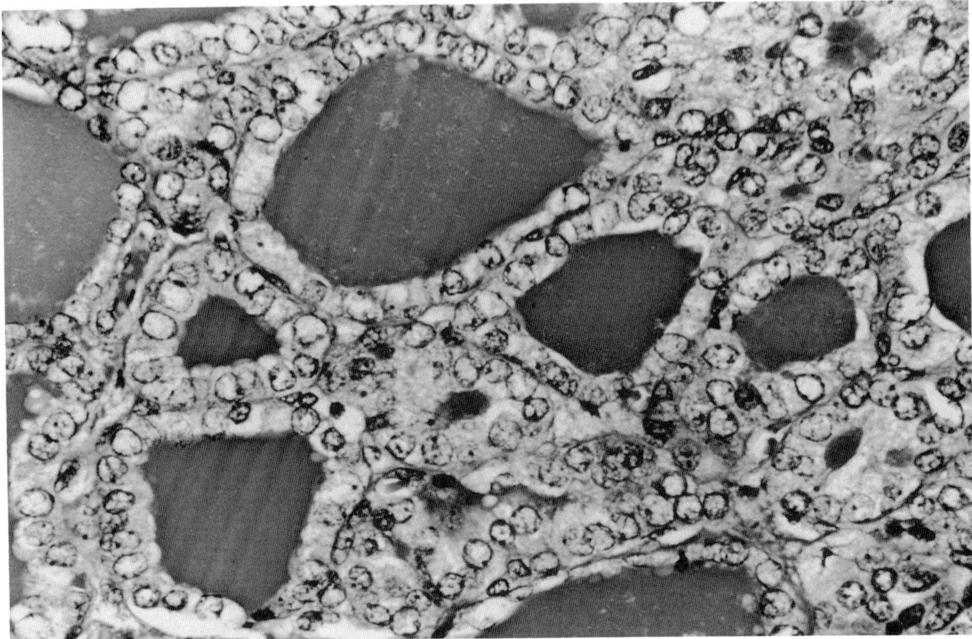

FIG. 7.7. Follicular variant of papillary carcinoma. The nuclei have the characteristic ground glass overlapping quality. The cytoplasm is clear, and the intraluminal colloid has a homogeneous acidophilic staining quality.

a follicular pattern of growth exhibiting capsular and/or vascular invasion (and therefore clearly malignant) will have some features suggestive of papillary carcinoma (such as vesicular nuclei or darkly staining colloid) but will lack others. In such instances, assignment to a follicular versus papillary carcinoma category becomes extremely subjective and probably unwarranted. We prefer to designate such tumors as *well-differentiated carcinoma, not otherwise specified,* instead of pushing them artificially into one category or another.

A related and equally difficult diagnostic dilemma arises when some of the cytologic and/or architectural features of papillary carcinoma are found *focally* with a lesion having otherwise the appearance of a benign follicular lesion, *i.e.,* a hyperplastic (adenomatoid) nodule or a follicular adenoma. Closer examination of the process may allow it to be placed into one of the following three categories:

1. A focus of typical papillary carcinoma (usually of the follicular variant rather than the conventional type) merging with areas having a great resemblance to an adenomatoid nodule, but in which high-power examination reveals numerous foci of transition, as well as the presence in some of the benign-looking follicles of nuclear features similar to the ones in the more typical foci. We interpret this as an extreme variation of the follicular variant of papillary carcinoma, in which the tumor resembles more an adenomatoid nodule (because of the large size of some follicles) than an adenoma.[4,93]

2. A focus of typical papillary carcinoma (usually of the conventional but

sometimes of the follicular variant type) within a lesion which appears otherwise perfectly benign, with no areas of transition between them. This very rare phenomenon could be interpreted as a papillary carcinoma arising in either an adenomatoid nodule or a follicular adenoma.[93]

3. A lesion having the features of an adenomatoid nodule or an adenoma in which occasional follicles are lined by follicular cells having vesicular nuclei, some of which may approach a ground glass appearance. If no supporting morphologic features for papillary carcinoma exist (such as tubular follicles, abortive papillae, or darkly staining colloid), we do not regard these nuclear changes as sufficient for a diagnosis of malignancy.

Needless to say, the distinction between these three situations (admitting that they are indeed pathogenetically distinct, which may not necessarily be the case) is not always possible. Table 7.1 is an attempt to guide the reader through this bewildering list of possibilities involving encapsulated well-differentiated thyroid lesions having a predominant or exclusively follicular pattern of growth. Fortunately, the practical implications of the differential diagnosis in this field are relatively minor, in view of the fact that the outcome is likely to be favorable regardless. This being the case, a conservative diagnostic attitude and—even more important—a conservative therapeutic approach are warranted.

SOLID/TRABECULAR VARIANT

It is not unusual for papillary carcinoma to exhibit foci of solid and/or trabecular growth. The phenomenon seems to be more common in children. The term "solid/trabecular" variant should be used when all or nearly all of a tumor not belonging to any of the other variants has a solid and/or trabecular appearance. This variant is rare, but it is important to be aware of its existence in order not to overdiagnose it as poorly differentiated or undifferentiated. Diagnostic clues include the presence of irregular fibrous trabeculae within the tumor, an occasional psammoma body, and clusters of lymphocytes in or around the tumor. An important requirement is that the typical nuclear features of papillary carcinoma must be retained. When this is the case, the tumor behavior will not be significantly different from that of the conventional type of papillary carcinoma.

DIFFUSE SCLEROSING VARIANT

This variant, originally proposed by Vickery *et al.*[140] is characterized by the following features: 1) diffuse involvement of one or, more commonly, both lobes; 2) numerous small papillary formations located within intrathyroidal cleft-like spaces, probably representing lymph vessels; 3) extensive squamous metaplasia; 4) large numbers of psammoma bodies; 5) marked lymphocytic infiltration, and 6) prominent fibrosis. Of all these features, the widespread lymphatic permeation is the most important, since it is probably responsible for the other morphologic findings and the tumor behavior (Fig. 7.8).

When compared with conventional papillary carcinoma, this variant exhibits the following characteristics: 1) similar predilection for the female sex; 2) greater

TABLE 7.1. DIFFERENTIAL DIAGNOSIS OF ENCAPSULATED THYROID LESIONS WITH A PREDOMINANTLY OR EXCLUSIVELY FOLLICULAR PATTERN OF GROWTH

Capsular and/or Vascular Invasion	Cytoarchitectural Features of Papillary Carcinoma, Follicular Variant		Terminology
Present	Absent		Well-differentiated carcinoma, follicular type
	Imperfectly developed		Well-differentiated carcinoma, not otherwise specified
	Well-developed, widespread		Well-differentiated carcinoma, papillary type (encapsulated follicular variant)
Absent	Absent		Follicular adenoma
	Imperfectly developed		Follicular adenoma
	Well developed, widespread		Well-differentiated carcinoma, papillary type (encapsulated follicular variant)
	Well developed, focal	Rest of nodule showing similar nuclear features on closer inspection	Well-differentiated carcinoma, papillary type (encapsulated follicular variant)
		Rest of nodule perfectly benign	Follicular adenoma with focal well differentiated carcinoma, papillary type (follicular variant)*

* This type is exceptionally rare. A somewhat more common situation is that in which the focal carcinoma in the benign follicular nodule has a typical papillary configuration.

incidence of cervical lymph node involvement; 3) greater incidence of pulmonary metastases; and 4) lesser probability of disease-free survival on follow-up.

An interesting clinical observation is the fact that there is a greater delay in diagnosis, explainable by the fact that the diffuse glandular enlargement simulates thyroiditis clinically and on thyroid scan.[20] Despite the high incidence of pulmonary metastases, the death rate is very low[20,28,52,103,124,130]; perhaps the young age of most patients with this variant counterbalances the adverse clinical significance of the other findings.

In one series, a "dominant" tumor nodule was found in over half of the cases,[20] suggesting that this variant (like its conventional counterpart) starts as a single tumor mass and that its subsequent appearance is the result of an early widespread permeation of intrathyroid lymph vessels, as originally proposed by Lindsay.[88]

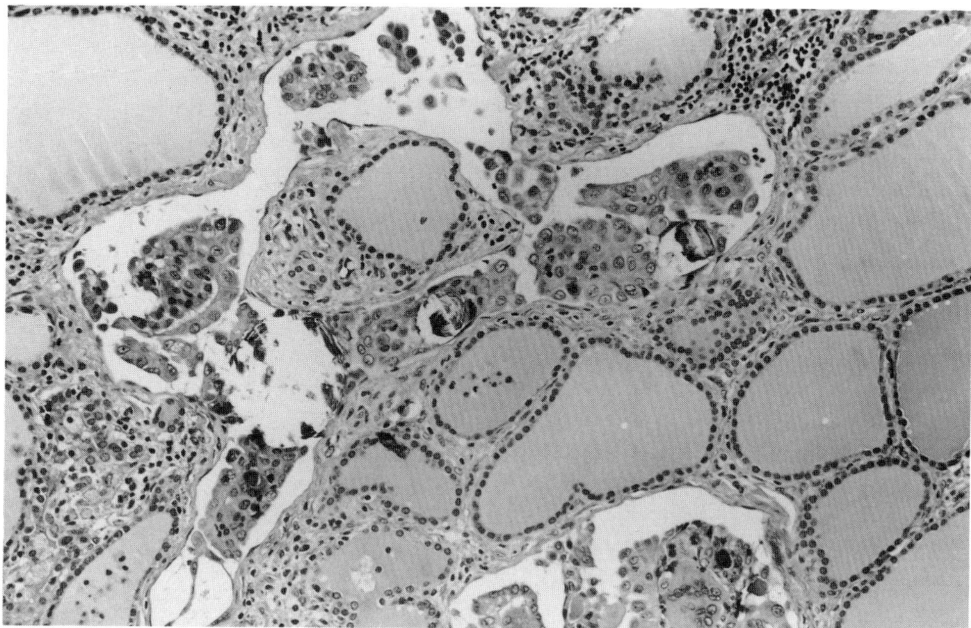

FIG. 7.8. Diffuse sclerosing variant of papillary carcinoma. The tumor is growing within endothelial-lined spaces and is associated with psammoma body formation and fibrosis.

TALL AND COLUMNAR CELL VARIANTS

Hawk and Hazard[61] first proposed the existence of the tall cell variant of papillary carcinoma. They stated that it tends to occur in older patients and to be of large size (usually over 5 cm). Extrathyroid extension is frequent, and there is a greater incidence of blood vessel invasion. The papillae are well formed and are covered by cells that are twice as tall as they are wide.[135] These cells often have a rather abundant acidophilic ("pink") cytoplasm. Mitotic figures can be found easily (in striking contrast with conventional papillary carcinoma), and the nuclei are normo- or hyperchromatic.[140] Flint *et al.*[48] found no difference in DNA content, chromatin texture, or nuclear size or shape between tall cell variant and conventional papillary carcinomas. The behavior of the tall cell variant of papillary carcinoma is more aggressive than that of the conventional form, the mortality rate being 25% in the series of Hawk and Hazard.[61]

Columnar cell carcinoma differs from both the conventional and the tall cell forms of papillary carcinoma because of the presence of prominent nuclear stratification (Fig. 7.9). In addition, the nuclei may lack the typical features of papillary carcinoma.[44,132] LiVolsi[89] commented on the fact that the cytoplasm tends to be very clear, to the point of exhibiting subnuclear vacuolization reminiscent of that seen in secretory endometrium. The few reported cases have run a very aggressive clinical course. It is not clear what the relationship is between the tall and the columnar variants. It is of interest, though, that a case combining features of both types has been reported,[1] and we have seen similar examples.

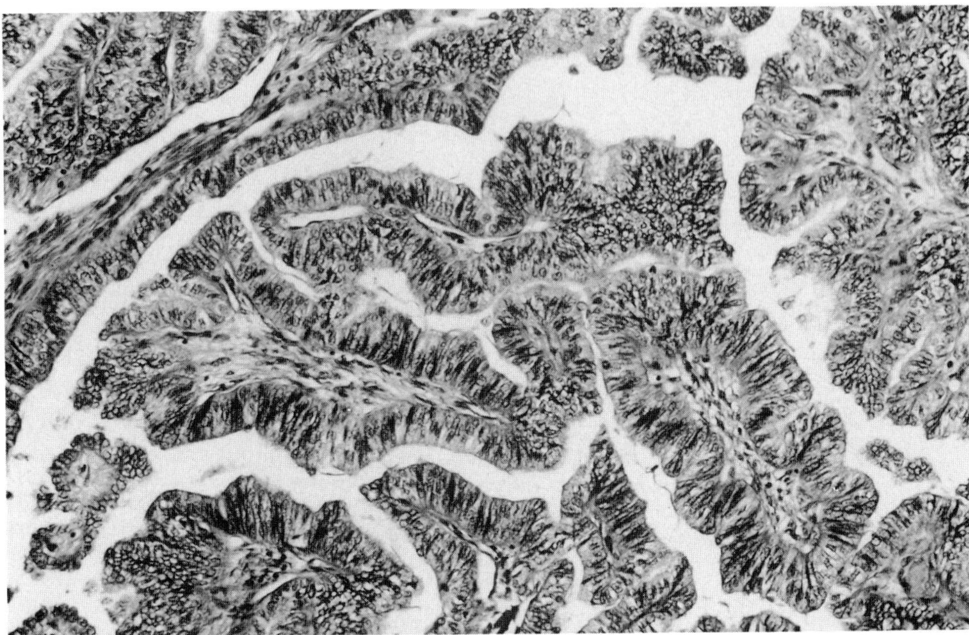

FIG. 7.9. Columnar cell variant of papillary carcinoma. The tumor cells have a columnar shape and there is marked stratification of nuclei.

DIFFERENTIAL DIAGNOSIS

The differential diagnosis of papillary thyroid carcinoma includes several benign and malignant conditions.

NODULAR HYPERPLASIA AND FOLLICULAR ADENOMA

On occasion, one or more of the nodules of nodular hyperplasia (adenomatoid goiter) may feature well-developed papillary structures. This may also be the case, although much less commonly, with follicular adenoma. The latter has been referred to as adenoma with papillary hyperplasia and hyperplastic papillary adenoma, the former term being preferable. The features of these benign papillary structures are similar regardless of whether they occur in one condition or the other. They are characteristically short and blunt, and they face the lumina of cystically dilated follicles. A central fibrovascular core is usually poorly developed or absent; instead, the stroma is likely to be edematous and to enclose numerous follicles. However, on occasion they are complex and branching (Fig. 7.10). More importantly, the follicular cells having these formations are tall cuboidal or columnar, with basally located nuclei which tend to be perfectly round and normo/hyperchromatic, *i.e.*, substantially different from those typically seen in papillary carcinoma (Fig. 7.11). Immunohistochemically, staining for keratin in formalin-fixed, paraffin-embedded material is usually patchy and limited to the low molecular weight forms of this marker, in contrast to the diffuse and intense staining usually seen in papillary carcinoma.[12] Furthermore, it has been shown

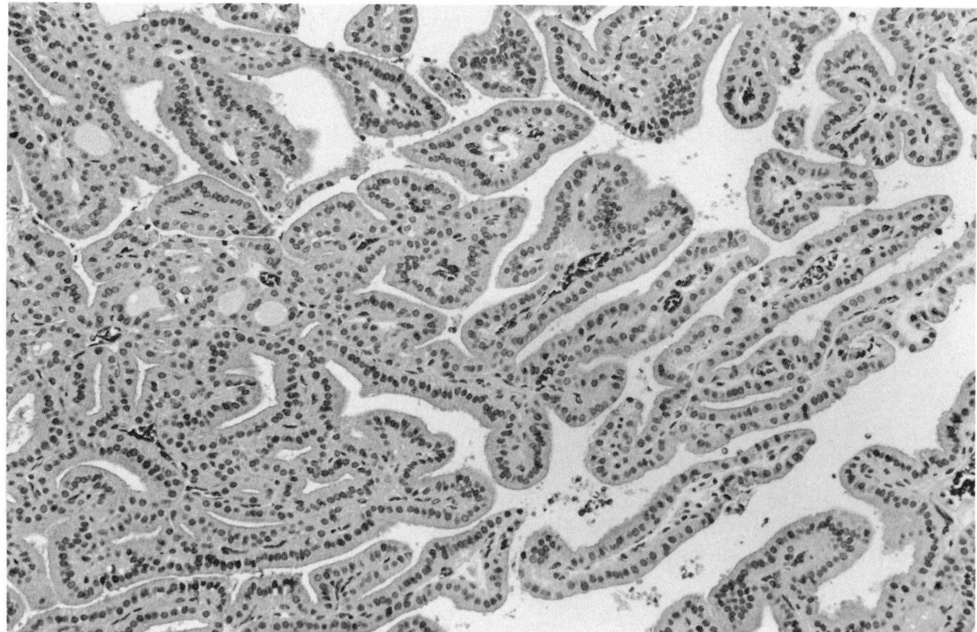

Fig. 7.10. Hyperplastic thyroid nodule featuring well developed papillae.

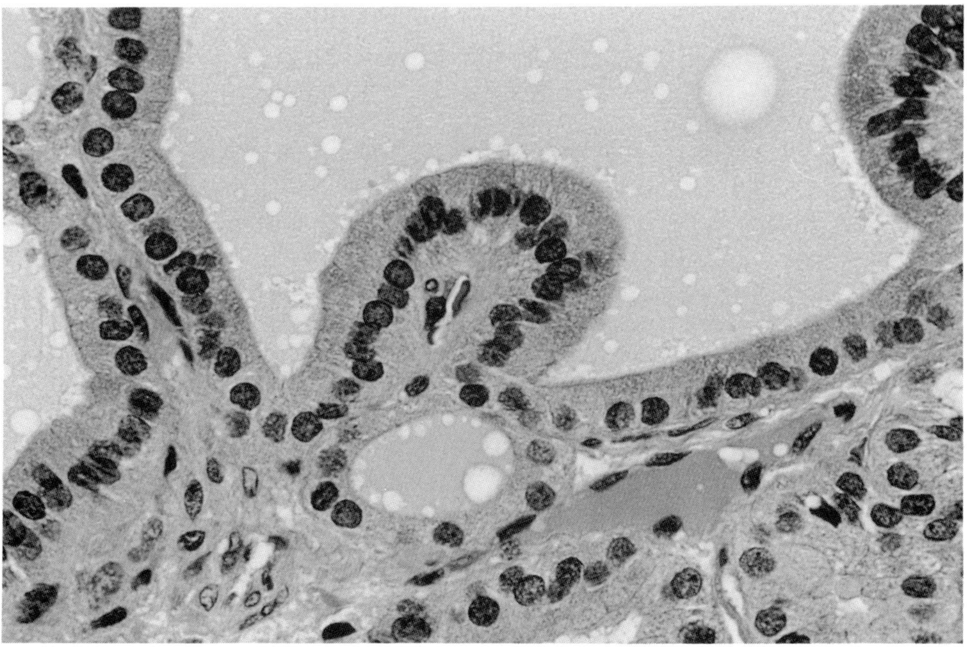

Fig. 7.11. High-power view of the same case. The follicular cells covering the papillae are tall columnar. The nuclei are basally located, small, and hyperchromatic.

that the apical surface of benign papillae stain slightly or not at all with Alcian blue or epithelial membrane antigen, whereas that in the papillae of papillary carcinoma usually reacts strongly.[39]

Hyalinizing Trabecular Adenoma

This entity resembles papillary carcinoma by virtue of the nuclear features (some exhibiting grooves and pseudoinclusions) and the occasional occurrence of psammoma body-like formations.[23] It is distinguished from papillary carcinoma by the prominence of hyalinization and the fact that the tumor cells are arranged in trabeculae and compact clusters.

Papillary Oncocytic Neoplasms

The large majority of oncocytic thyroid neoplasms exhibit follicular, trabecular, and/or solid patterns of growth. It is for this reason that they are regarded by most as a subtype of follicular neoplasms. In some oncocytic tumors, particularly those with a macrofollicular pattern of growth, the septa separating the follicles are very thin, so that when cut tangentially they may simulate papillae. There are, however, rare oncocytic neoplasms that exhibit a papillary configuration throughout (Fig. 7.12). These papillae are covered by a single layer of oncocytic cells of either cuboidal or columnar shape. The nuclei, although vesicular, usually lack a well-developed ground glass appearance. Some of these tumors are invasive and seem to behave similarly to conventional papillary carcinoma, *i.e.*, they have a tendency for regional lymph node involvement. Their long-term behavior is said to be comparable to that of their nononcocytic counterparts,[11] but our own

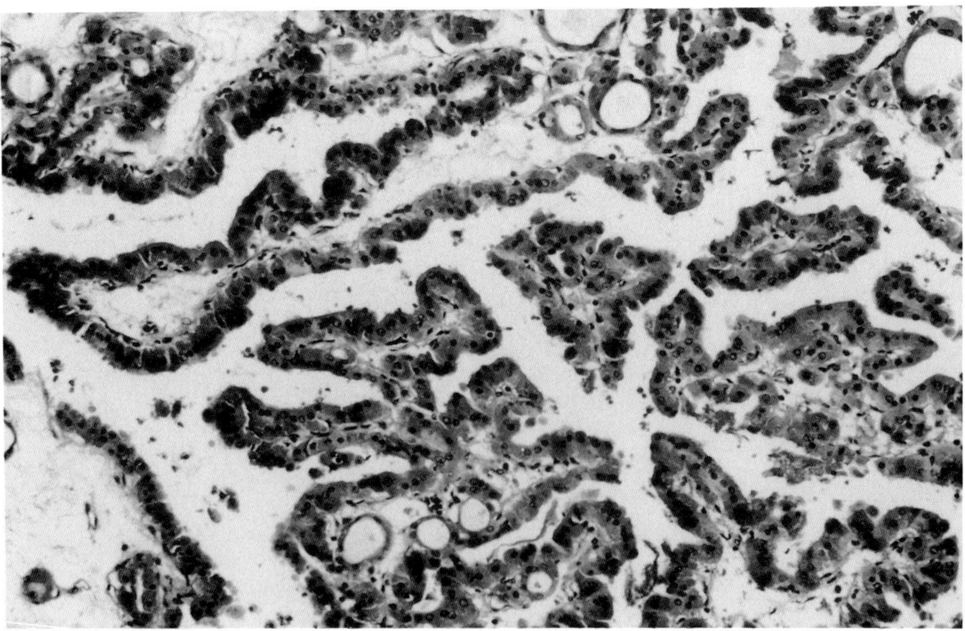

FIG. 7.12.   Oncocytic neoplasm with a well-developed papillary pattern of growth.

experience suggests that they might behave more aggressively.[9] In the reported series of papillary carcinoma, the incidence of the oncocytic type has ranged from 1.1 to 11.3%.[131] For these invasive papillary neoplasms exhibiting true oncocytic features, we prefer the designation of *oncocytic papillary carcinoma.*

Other oncocytic papillary neoplasms are totally encapsulated and exhibit no signs of either capsular or blood vessel invasion.[9] The position of these lesions in the classification scheme of thyroid neoplasia remains controversial. The dilemma is whether to regard them as encapsulated papillary carcinomas of oncocytic type or as oncocytic adenomas with papillary hyperplasia. We favor the latter interpretation, in view of the fact that we have found no documentation of metastases in our series or in those of others.[9,11] However, since the issue is not settled, we recommend that these tumors be designated for the time being with the noncommittal term of *encapsulated papillary oncocytic neoplasms.* A conservative surgical approach seems justified.

Papillary Variant of Medullary Carcinoma

Medullary carcinomas rarely may exhibit a true papillary pattern of growth, in which the constituent tumor cells are aligned along fibrovascular stalks. In the cases described by Kakudo *et al.*[79] the tumors also contained solid foci characteristic of typical medullary carcinomas. The presence of calcitonin/immunoreactivity and the negativity for thyroglobulin should allow for an easy distinction.

More common than the true papillary variant of medullary carcinoma is the so-called "pseudopapillary" variant, which results from artifactual separation of groups of tumor cells.

Hashimoto's Thyroiditis

Some cases of Hashimoto's disease simulate papillary thyroid carcinoma because the nuclei of the oncocytic follicular cells may be vesicular and slightly overlapping, their appearance thus approaching that of the ground glass nuclei of papillary carcinoma. Furthermore, papillary formations may appear in Hashimoto's thyroiditis when the disease is associated with the changes of diffuse hyperplasia ("hashitoxicosis") or nodular hyperplasia ("nodular Hashimoto's thyroiditis"). The criteria for distinguishing them from the papillae of papillary carcinoma are similar to those listed under "Nodular Hyperplasia and Follicular Adenoma."

REFERENCES

1. Akslen, L. A., and Varhaug, J. E. Thyroid carcinoma with mixed tall-cell and columnar-cell features. *Am. J. Clin. Pathol. 94:*442–445, 1990.
2. Albores-Saavedra, J., Altamirano-Dimas, M., Alcorta-Anguizola, B., and Smith, M. Fine structure of human papillary thyroid carcinoma. *Cancer 28:*763–774, 1971.
3. Albores-Saavedra, J., and Duran, M. E. Association of thyroid carcinoma and chemodectoma. *Am. J. Surg. 116:*887–890, 1968.
4. Albores-Saavedra, J., Gould, E., Vardaman, C., and Vuitch, F. The macrofollicular variant of papillary thyroid carcinoma. A study of 17 cases. *Hum. Pathol. 22:*1195–1205, 1991.

5. Allo, M. D., Christianson, W., and Koivunen, D. Not all "occult papillary" carcinomas are "minimal." *Surgery 104:*971–976, 1988.
6. Antonini, P., Venuat, A. M., Linares, G., *et al.* Translocation (7;10)(q35:q21) in a differentiated papillary carcinoma of the thyroid. *Cancer Genet. Cytogenet. 41:*139–144, 1989.
7. Bäckdahl, M. Nuclear DNA Content and Prognosis in Papillary, Follicular and Medullary Carcinomas of the Thyroid, Dissertation. Stockholm, Karolinska Medical Institute, 1985.
8. Bakri, K., Shimaoka, K., Rao, U., and Tsukada, Y. Adenosquamous carcinoma of the thyroid after radiotherapy for Hodgkin's disease. A case report and review. *Cancer 52:*465–470, 1983.
9. Barbuto, D., Carcangiu, M. L., and Rosai, J. Papillary Hürthle cell neoplasms of the thyroid gland. A study of 20 cases. *Mod. Pathol. 3:*7A, 1990 (abstract).
10. Beaumont, A., Ben Othman, S., and Fragu, P. The fine structure of papillary carcinoma of the thyroid. *Histopathology 5:*377–388, 1981.
11. Beckner, M., and Oertel, J. Papillary carcinomas of the oxyphil cell subtype. *Lab. Invest. 56:*5A, 1987 (abstract).
12. Bennett, W. P., Bhan, A. K., and Vickery, A. L. Keratin expression as a diagnostic adjunct in thyroid tumors with papillary architecture. *Lab. Invest. 58:*9A, 1988 (abstract).
13. Block, M. A., Miller, M. J., and Horn, R. Carcinoma of the thyroid after external radiation to the neck in adults. *Am. J. Surg. 118:*764–768, 1969.
14. Bocker, W., Schroder, S., and Dralle, H. Minimal thyroid neoplasia. *Recent Results Cancer Res. 106:*131–138, 1988.
15. Bondeson, I., Bengtsson, A., Bondeson, A. G., *et al.* Chromosome studies in thyroid neoplasia. *Cancer 64:*680–685, 1989.
16. Bondeson, I., and Ljungberg, L. Occult papillary thyroid carcinoma in the young and the aged. *Cancer 53:*1790–1791, 1984.
17. Borganzone, I., Pierotti, M. A., Monzini, N., *et al.* High frequency of activation of tyrosine kinase oncogenes in human papillary thyroid carcinoma. *Oncogene 4:*1457–1462, 1989.
18. Cady, B., Sedgwick, C. E., Meissner, W. A., *et al.* Changing clinical, pathologic, therapeutic, and survival patterns in differentiated thyroid carcinoma. *Ann. Surg. 184:*541–553, 1976.
19. Cady, B., Sedgwick, C. E., Meissner, W. A., *et al.* Risk factor analysis in differentiated thyroid cancer. *Cancer 43:*810–820, 1979.
20. Carcangiu, M. L., and Bianchi, S. Diffuse sclerosing variant of papillary thyroid carcinoma. Clinicopathologic study of 15 cases. *Am. J. Surg. Pathol. 13:*1041–1049, 1989.
21. Carcangiu, M. L., Zampi, G., Pupi, A., *et al.* Papillary carcinoma of the thyroid. A clinicopathologic study of 241 cases treated at the University of Florence, Italy. *Cancer 55:*805–828, 1985.
22. Carcangiu, M. L., Zampi, G., and Rosai, J. Papillary thyroid carcinoma. A study of its many morphologic expressions and clinical correlates. *Pathol. Annu. 20 (Part 1):*1–44, 1985.
23. Carney, J. A., Ryan, J., and Goellner, J. R. Hyalinizing trabecular adenoma of the thyroid gland. *Am. J. Surg. Pathol. 11:*583–591, 1987.
24. Chan, J. K. C. Papillary carcinoma of thyroid: Classical and variants. *Histol. Histopathol. 5:*241–257, 1990.
25. Chan, J. K. C., Carcangiu, M. L., and Rosai, J. Papillary carcinoma of thyroid with exuberant nodular fasciitis-like stroma. Report of three cases. *Am. J. Clin Pathol. 95:*309–314, 1991.
26. Chan, J. K. C., and Loo, K. T. Cribriform variant of papillary thyroid carcinoma. *Arch. Pathol. Lab. Med. 114:*622–624, 1990.
27. Chan, J. K. C., and Saw, D. The grooved nucleus. A useful diagnostic criterion of papillary carcinoma of the thyroid. *Am. J. Surg. Pathol. 10:*672–679, 1986.
28. Chan, J. C. K., Tsui, M. S., and Tse, C. H. Diffuse sclerosing variant of papillary carcinoma of the thyroid. A histological and immunohistochemical study of three cases. *Histopathology 11:*191–201, 1987.
29. Chen, K. T. K., and Rosai, J. Follicular variant of thyroid papillary carcinoma. A clinicopathologic study of six cases. *Am. J. Surg. Pathol. 1:*123–130, 1977.
30. Chesky, V. E., Hellwig, C. A., and Welch, J. W. Cancer of the thyroid associated with Hashimoto's disease: An analysis of 48 cases. *Am. Surg. 28:*678–685, 1962.
31. Christ, M. L., and Haja, J. Intranuclear cytoplasmic inclusions (invaginations) in thyroid aspirations: Frequency and specificity. Acta Cytol. 23:327–331, 1979.

32. Clark, O. H. Total thyroidectomy. The treatment of choice for patients with differentiated thyroid cancer. *Ann. Surg. 196:*361–370, 1981.
33. Cody, H. S., and Shah, J. P. Locally invasive, well-differentiated thyroid cancer. *Am. J. Surg. 142:*480–483, 1981.
34. Cohn, K. H., Bäckdahl, M., Forsslund, G., *et al.* Biologic considerations and operative strategy in papillary thyroid carcinoma. Arguments against the routine performance of total thyroidectomy. *Surgery 96:*957–971, 1984.
35. Cohn, K. H., Bäckdahl, M., Forsslund, G., *et al.* Prognostic value of nuclear DNA content in papillary thyroid carcinoma. *World J. Surg. 8:*474–480, 1984.
36. Crile, G. Changing end results in patients with papillary carcinoma of the thyroid. *Surg. Gynecol. Obstet. 131:*460–468, 1971.
37. Crile, G., Antunez, A. R., Esselstyne, C. B., *et al.* The advantages of subtotal thyroidectomy and suppression of TSH in the primary treatment of papillary carcinoma of the thyroid. *Cancer 55:*2691–2697, 1985.
38. Crile, G., and Hazard, J. B. Relationship of the age of the patient to the natural history and prognosis of carcinoma of the thyroid. *Ann. Surg. 138:*33–38, 1953.
39. Damiani, S., Fratamico, F., Lapertosa, G., *et al.* Alcian blue and epithelial membrane antigen are useful markers in differentiating benign from malignant papillae in thyroid. *Virchows Arch. [A] 419:*131–135, 1991.
40. Diaz, N. M., Wick, M. R., and Mazoujian, G. Estrogen receptor protein (ERP) in papillary thyroid carcinoma: An immunohistochemical analysis of 30 cases. *Lab. Invest. 64:*32A, 1991 (abstract).
41. Donghi, R., Sozzi, G., Pierotti, M. A., *et al.* The oncogene associated with human papillary thyroid carcinoma (PTC) is assigned to chromosome 10 q11-q12 in the same region as multiple endocrine neoplasia type 2A (MEN2A). *Oncogene 4:*521–523, 1989.
42. Doniach, I. Aetiologic consideration of thyroid carcinoma. In: *Tumours of the Thyroid Gland,* edited by D. Smithers. Edinburgh, E&S Livingstone, 1970, pp. 66–67.
43. Evans, H. L. Encapsulated papillary neoplasms of the thyroid. A study of 14 cases followed for a minimum of 10 years. *Am. J. Surg. Pathol. 11:*592–597, 1987.
44. Evans, H. L. Columnar-cell carcinoma of the thyroid. A report of two cases of an aggressive variant of thyroid carcinoma. *Am. J. Clin. Pathol. 85:*77–80, 1986.
45. Evans, H. L. Follicular neoplasms of the thyroid: A study of 44 cases followed for a minimum of 10 years, with emphasis of differential diagnosis. *Cancer 54:*535–540, 1984.
46. Farbota, L. M., Calandra, D. B., Lawrence, A. M., and Paloyan, E. Thyroid carcinoma in Graves' disease. *Surgery 98:*1148–1152, 1985.
47. Filetti, S., Belfiore, A., Amir, S. M., *et al.* The role of thyroid-stimulating antibodies of Graves' disease in differentiated thyroid cancer. *N. Engl. J. Med. 318:*753–759, 1988.
48. Flint, A., Davenport, R. D., and Lloyd, R. V. The tall cell variant of papillary carcinoma of the thyroid gland. Comparison with the common form of papillary carcinoma by DNA and morphometric analysis. *Arch. Pathol. Lab. Med. 115:*169–171, 1991.
49. Fransilla, K. O. Is the differentiation between papillary and follicular thyroid carcinoma valid? *Cancer 32:*853–864, 1973.
50. Frauman, A. G., and Moses, A. C. Oncogenes and growth factors in thyroid carcinogenesis. *Endocrinol. Metab. Clin. North Am. 19:*479–494, 1990.
51. Frazell, E. L., and Foote, F. W. Papillary thyroid carcinoma. Pathological findings in cases with and without clinical evidence of cervical node involvement. *Cancer 8:*1165–1166, 1955.
52. Fujimoto, Y., Obara, T., Ito, Y., *et al.* Diffuse sclerosing variant of papillary carcinoma of the thyroid. Clinical importance, surgical treatment, and follow-up study. *Cancer 66:*2306–2312, 1990.
53. Fusco, A., Grieco, M., Santoro, M., *et al.* A new oncogene in human thyroid papillary carcinomas and their lymphnodal metastases. *Nature 328:*170–172, 1987.
54. Gikas, P. W., Labow, S. S., DiGiulio, W., and Finger, J. Occult metastasis from occult papillary carcinoma of the thyroid. *Cancer 20:*2100–2104, 1967.
55. Goellner, J. R., and Johnson, D. A. Cytology of cystic papillary carcinoma of the thyroid. *Acta Cytol. 26:*797–799, 1982.

56. Grieco, M., Santoro, M., Berlingieri, M. T., *et al.* PTC is a novel rearranged form of the *ret* proto-oncogene and is frequently detected *in vivo* in human thyroid papillary carcinomas. *Cell 60*:557–563, 1990.
57. Hamming, J. F., van de Velde, C. J., Goslings, B. M., *et al.* Preoperative diagnosis and treatment of metastases to the regional lymph nodes in papillary carcinoma of the thyroid. *Surg. Gynecol. Obstet. 169*:107–114, 1989.
58. Harach, H. R., Franssila, K. O., and Wasenius, V. M. Occult papillary carcinoma of the thyroid: A "normal" finding in Finland. A systematic autopsy study. *Cancer 56*:531–538, 1985.
59. Harness, J. K., Thompson, H. W., McLeod, M. K., *et al.* Follicular carcinoma of the thyroid gland. Trends and treatment. *Surgery 96*:972–980, 1984.
60. Harness, J. K., Thompson, H. W., Sisson, J. C., and Beierwaltes, W. H. Differentiated thyroid carcinomas: Treatment of distant metastases. *Arch. Surg. 108*:410–419, 1974.
61. Hawk, W. A., and Hazard, J. B. The many appearances of papillary carcinoma of the thyroid. *Cleve. Clin. Q. 43*:207–216, 1976.
62. Hawkins, M. M., and Kingston, J. E. Malignant thyroid tumours following childhood cancer. *Lancet 2*:804, 1988.
63. Hazard, J. B. Small papillary carcinoma of the thyroid. A study with special reference to so-called nonencapsulated sclerosing tumor. *Lab. Invest. 9*:86–97, 1960.
64. Hedinger, C. *Histological Typing of Thyroid Tumors.* Berlin, Springer Verlag, 1988.
65. Hedman, I., and Tisell, L. E. Associated hyperparathyroidism and nonmedullary thyroid carcinoma. The etiologic role of radiation. *Surgery 95*:392–397, 1984.
66. Hempelmann, I. H., Hall, W. J., Phillips, M., *et al.* Neoplasms in persons treated with x-rays in infancy. Fourth survey in 20 years. *J. Natl. Cancer. Inst. 55*:519–530, 1975.
67. Henzen-Logmans, S. C., Mullink, H., Ramaekers, F. C., *et al.* Expression of cytokeratins and vimentin in epithelial cells of normal and pathologic thyroid tissue. *Virchows Arch. [A] 410*:347–354, 1987.
68. Hernandez, O. L., Saavedra, J. A., Benavides, G., *et al.* Multiple endocrine neoplasia. *Am. J. Clin. Pathol. 78*:527–532, 1982.
69. Hofstädter, F. Frequency and morphology of malignant tumors of the thyroid before and after the introduction of iodine-prophylaxis. *Virchows Arch [A] 385*:263–270, 1980.
70. Hoie, J., Stenwig, A. E., Kullmann, G., and Lindegaard, M. Distant metastases in papillary thyroid cancer. A review of 91 patients. *Cancer 61*:1–6, 1988.
71. Hubert, J. P., Kiernan, P. D., Beahrs, O. H., *et al.* Occult papillary carcinoma of the thyroid. *Arch. Surg. 115*:394–398, 1980.
72. Hutter, R. V. P., Frazell, E. L., and Foote, F. W. Elective radical neck dissection. An assessment of its use in the management of papillary thyroid cancer. *CA 20*:87–93, 1970.
73. Jenkins, R. B., Hay, I. D., Herath, J. F., *et al.* Frequent occurrence of cytogenetic abnormalities in sporadic nonmedullary thyroid carcinoma. *Cancer 66*:1213–1220, 1990.
74. Joensuu, H., Klemi, P., Eerola, E., and Tuominen, J. Influence of cellular DNA content on survival in differentiated thyroid cancer. *Cancer 58*:2462–2467, 1986.
75. Johannessen, J. V., Gould, V. E., and Jao, W. The fine structure of human thyroid cancer. *Hum. Pathol. 9*:385–400, 1978.
76. Johannessen, J. V., and Sobrinho-Simões, M. The origin and significance of thyroid psammoma bodies. *Lab. Invest. 43*:287–296, 1980.
77. Johannessen, J. V., Sobrinho-Simões, M., Finseth, I., and Pilström, L. Papillary carcinomas of the thyroid have pore-deficinet nuclei. *Int. J. Cancer 30*:409–411, 1982.
78. Johnson, T. L., Lloyd, R. V., and Thor, A. Expression of *ras* oncogene p21 antigen in normal and proliferative thyroid tissues. *Am. J. Pathol. 127*:60–65, 1987.
79. Kakudo, K., Miyanchyi, A., Yakai, S. I., *et al.* C-cell carcinoma of the thyroid, papillary type. *Acta Pathol. Jpn. 29*:633–659, 1979.
80. Kamma, H., Fujii, K., and Ogata, T. Lymphocytic infiltration in juvenile thyroid carcinoma. *Cancer 62*:1988–1993, 1988.
81. Kini, S. R. Guides to clinical aspiration biopsy. *Thyroid.* New York, Igaku-Shoin, 1987, pp. 121–187.

82. Klinck, G. H., and Winship, T. Occult sclerosing carcinoma of the thyroid. *Cancer 8:*701–706, 1955.
83. Klinck, G. H., and Winship, T. Psammoma bodies and thyroid cancer. *Cancer 12:*656–662, 1959.
84. Lang, W., Borrusch, H., and Bauer, L. Occult carcinomas of the thyroid. Evaluation of 1,020 sequential autopsies. *Am. J. Clin. Pathol. 90:*72–76, 1988.
85. Lee, T. K., Myers, R. T., Marshall, R. B., *et al.* The significance of mitotic rate. A retrospective study of 127 thyroid carcinomas. *Hum. Pathol. 16:*1042–1046, 1985.
86. Lew, W., Orell, S., and Henderson, D. W. Intranuclear vacuoles in nonpapillary carcinoma of the thyroid. A report of 3 cases. *Acta Cytol. 28:*581–586, 1984.
87. Lieberman, P. H., Fotte, F. W., and Schottenfeld, D. A study of the pathology of thyroid cancer, 1930–1960. *Clin. Bull. 2:*7–12, 1972.
88. Lindsay, S. *Carcinoma of the Thyroid Gland. A Clinical and Pathologic Study of 293 Patients at the University of California Hospital.* Springfield, IL, Charles C, Thomas, 1960.
89. LiVolsi, V. A. Surgical pathology of the thyroid. In: *Major Problems in Pathology,* edited by J. L. Bennington. Philadelphia, W. B. Saunders, 1990, vol. 22.
90. Lote, K., Andersen, K., Nordal, E., and Brennhovd, I. O. Familial occurrence of papillary thyroid carcinoma. *Cancer 46:*1291–1297, 1980.
91. Maheshwari, Y. K., Hill, C. S., Haynie, T. P., *et al.* I-131 therapy in differentiated thyroid carcinoma. M. D. Anderson Hospital experience. *Cancer 47:*664–681, 1981.
92. Mazzaferri, E. L. Papillary thyroid carcinoma: Factors influencing prognosis and current therapy. *Semin. Oncol. 14:*315–332, 1987.
93. Mazzaferri, E. L,, and Oertel, J. E. The pathology and prognosis of thyroid cancer. In: *Surgery of the Thyroid and Parathyroid Glands,* vol. 6 of *Clinical Surgery International,* edited by E. L. Kaplan. Edinburgh, Churchill Livingstone, 1983, pp. 22–23.
94. Mazzaferri, E. L., and Young, R. L. Papillary thyroid carcinoma. A 10 year follow-up report of the impact of therapy in 576 patients. *Am. J. Med. 70:*511–518, 1981.
95. Mazzaferri, E. L., Young, R. L., Oertel, J. E., *et al.* Papillary thyroid carcinoma: The impact of therapy in 576 patients. *Medicine (Baltimore) 56:*171–196, 1977.
96. McConahey, W. M., Hay, I. D., Woolner, L. B., *et al.* Papillary thyroid cancer treated at the Mayo Clinic, 1946 through 1970. Initial manifestations, pathologic findings, therapy, and outcome. *Mayo Clin. Proc. 61:*978–996, 1986.
97. McCormack, K. R. Bone metastases from thyroid carcinoma. *Cancer 19:*181–184, 1966.
98. McDougall, I. R., Coleman, C. N., Burke, J. S., *et al.* Thyroid carcinoma after high dose external radiotherapy for Hodgkin's disease. Report of three cases. *Cancer 45:*2056–2060, 1980.
99. Meissner, W. A., and Warren, S. Tumors of the thyroid gland. *Atlas of Tumor Pathology,* 2nd Series, Fascicle 4. Washington, DC, Armed Forces Institute of Pathology, 1969, pp. 50–52.
100. Miettinen, M., Franssila, K., Lehto, V. P., *et al.* Expression of intermediate filament proteins in thyroid gland and thyroid tumors. *Lab. Invest. 50:*262–269, 1984.
101. Mizukami, Y., Nonomura, A., Hashimoto, T., *et al.* Immunohistochemical demonstration of *ras* p21 oncogene product in normal, benign, and malignant human thyroid disease. *Cancer 61:*873–880, 1988.
102. Mizukami, Y., Nonomura, A., Hashimoto, T., *et al.* Immunohistochemical demonstration of epidermal growth fact and c-*myc* oncogene product in normal, benign, and malignant thyroid tissues. *Histopathology 18:*11–18, 1991.
103. Mizukami, Y., Nonomura, A., Michigishi, T., *et al.* Diffuse sclerosing variant of papillary carcinoma of the thyroid: Report of three cases. *Acta Pathol. Jpn. 40:*676–682, 1990.
104. Narita, T., and Takagi, K. Ataxia-telangiectasia with dysgerminoma of right ovary, papillary carcinoma of thyroid, and adenocarcinoma of pancreas. *Cancer 54:*1113–1116, 1984.
105. Noguchi, M., Kumaki, T., Taniya, T., and Miyazaki, I. Bilateral cervical lymph node metastases in well-differentiated thyroid cancer. *Arch. Surg. 125:*804–806, 1990.
106. Noguchi, S., and Murakami, N. The value of lymph-node dissection in patients with differentiated thyroid cancer. *Surg. Clin. North Am. 67:*251–261, 1987.
107. Olen, E., Klinck, G. H. Thyroid carcinoma occurring in Graves' disease. *Arch. Intern. Med. 117:*432–435, 1966.

108. Ostrowski, M. A., Asa, S. L., Chamberlain, D., *et al.* Myxomatous change in papillary carcinoma of the thyroid. *Surg. Pathol. 2:*249–256, 1989.
109. Ott, R. A., Calandra, D. B., McCall, A., *et al.* The incidence of thyroid carcinoma in patients with Hashimoto's thyroiditis and solitary cold nodules. *Surgery 98:*1202–1206, 1985.
110. Patchefsky, A. S., Keller, I. B., and Mansfield, C. M. Solitary vertebral column metastasis from occult sclerosing carcinoma of the thyroid gland. *Am. J. Clin. Pathol. 53:*596–601, 1970.
111. Permanetter, W., Nathrath, W. B., and Lohrs, U. Immunohistochemical analysis of thyroglobulin and keratin in benign and malignant thyroid tumours. *Virchows Arch. [A] 398:*221–228, 1982.
112. Plail, R. O., Bussey, H. J., Glazer, G., and Thomson, J. P. Adenomatous polyposis. An association with carcinoma of the thyroid. *Br. J. Surg. 74:*377–380, 1987.
113. Rieger, R., Pimpl, W., Money, S., *et al.* Hyperthyroidism and concurrent thyroid malignancies. *Surgery 106:*6–10, 1989.
114. Rosai, J., Zampi, G., and Carcangiu, M. L. Papillary carcinoma of the thyroid. A discussion of its several morphologic expressions, with particular emphasis on the follicular variant. *Am. J. Surg. Pathol. 76:*809–817, 1983.
115. Russell, W. O., Ibanez, M. L., Clark, R. L., and White, E. C. Thyroid carcinoma. Classification, intraglandular dissemination, and clinicopathological study based upon whole organ sections of 80 glands. *Cancer 16:*1425–1460, 1963.
116. Samaan, N. A., Schultz, P. N., Haynie, T. P., and Ordonez, N. G. Pulmonary metastasis of differentiated thyroid carcinoma: treatment results in 101 patients. *J. Clin. Endocrinol. Metab. 65:*376–380, 1985.
117. Samaan, N. A., Schultz, P. N., Ordonez, N. G., *et al.* A comparison of thyroid carcinoma in those who have and have not had head and neck irradiation in childhood. *J. Clin. Endocrinol. Metab. 64:*219–223, 1987.
118. Sampson, R. J., Oka, H., Key, C. R., *et al.* Metastases from occult thyroid carcinoma: An autopsy study from Hiroshima and Nagasaki, Japan. *Cancer 25:*803–811, 1970.
119. Satoh, Y., Sakamoto, A., Yamada, K., and Kasai, N. Psammoma bodies in metastatic carcinoma to the thyroid. *Mod. Pathol. 3:*267–270, 1990.
120. Schelfhout, L. J., van Muijen, G. N., and Fleuren, G. J. Expression of keratin 19 distinguishes papillary thyroid carcinoma from follicular carcinoma and follicular thyroid adenoma. *Am. J. Clin. Pathol. 92:*654–658, 1989.
121. Schindler, A. M., van Melle, G., Evequoz, B., and Scazziga, B. Prognostic factors in papillary carcinoma of the thyroid. *Cancer 68:*324–330, 1991.
122. Schneider, A. B., Pinsky, S., Bekerman, C., and Ryo, U. Y. Characteristics of 108 thyroid cancers detected by screening in a population with a history of head and neck irradiation. *Cancer 46:*1218–1227, 1980.
123. Schroder, D. M., Chambors, A., and France, C. J. Operative strategy for thyroid cancer. Is total thyroidectomy worth the price? *Cancer 58:*2320–2328, 1986.
124. Schröder, S., Bay, V., Dunke, K., *et al.* Diffuse sclerosing variant of papillary thyroid carcinoma. S-100 protein immunocytochemistry and prognosis. *Virchows Arch. [A] 416:*367–371, 1990.
125. Schröder, S., Bocker, W., Dralle, H., *et al.* The encapsulated papillary carcinoma of the thyroid. A morphologic subtype of the papillary thyroid carcinoma. *Cancer 54:*90–93, 1984.
126. Schröder, S., Schwarz, W., Rehpenning, W., *et al.* Dendritic/Langerhans cells and prognosis in patients with papillary thyroid carcinomas. *Am. J. Clin. Pathol. 89:*295–300, 1989.
127. Selzer, G., Kahn, L. B., and Albertyn, L. Primary malignant tumors of the thyroid gland. A clinicopathologic study of 254 cases. *Cancer 40:*1501–1510, 1977.
128. Simpson, W. J., McKinney, S. E., Carruthers, J. S., *et al.* Papillary and follicular thyroid cancer. Prognostic factors in 1,578 patients. *Am. J. Med. 83:*479–488, 1987.
129. Smith, S. A., Hay, I. D., Goellner, *et al.* Mortality from papillary thyroid carcinoma. A case-control study of 56 lethal cases. *Cancer 62:*1381–1388, 1988.
130. Soares, J., Limbert, E., and Sobrinho-Simões, M. Diffuse sclerosing variant of papillary thyroid carcinoma. A clinocopathologic study of 10 cases. *Pathol. Res. Pract. 185:*200–206, 1989.
131. Sobrinho-Simões, M., Nesland, J. M., Holm, R., *et al.* Hürthle cell and mitochondrion-rich

papillary carcinomas of the thyroid gland. An ultrastructural and immunocytochemical study. *Ultrastruct. Pathol. 8:*131–142, 1985.

132. Sobrinho-Simões, M., Nesland, J. M., and Johannessen, J. V. Columnar-cell carcinoma. Another variant of poorly differentiated carcinoma of the thyroid. *Am. J. Clin. Pathol. 89:*264–267, 1988.

133. Stanta, G., Carcangiu, M. L., and Rosai, J. The biochemical and immunohistochemical profile of thyroid neoplasia. *Pathol Annu. 23* (Part 1):129–157, 1988.

134. Strate, S. M., Lee, E. L., and Childres, J. H. Occult papillary carcinoma of the thyroid with distant metastases. *Cancer 54:*1093–1100, 1984.

135. Tscholl-Ducommun, J., and Hedinger, C. E. Papillary thyroid carcinomas. Morphology and prognosis. *Virchows Arch. [A] 396:*19–39, 1982.

136. Tsumori, T., Nakao, K., Miyata, M., *et al.* Clinicopathologic study of thyroid carcinoma infiltrating the trachea. *Cancer 56:*2843–2848, 1985.

137. Vestfrid, M. A. Papillary carcinoma of the thyroid gland with lipomatous stroma: Report of a peculiar histological type of thyroid tumour. *Histopathology 10:*97–100, 1986.

138. Viale, G., Dell'Orto, P., Coggi, G., and Gambacorta, M. Coexpression of cytokeratins and vimentin in normal and diseased thyroid glands. Lack of diagnostic utility of vimentin immunostaining. *Am. J. Surg. Pathol. 13:*1034–1040, 1989.

139. Vickery, A. L. Thyroid papillary carcinoma. Pathological and philosophical controversies. *Am. J. Surg. Pathol. 7:*797–807, 1983.

140. Vickery, A. L., Carcangiu, M. L., Johannessen, J. V., and Sobrinho-Simoes, M. Papillary carcinoma. *Semin. Diagn. Pathol. 2:*90–100, 1985.

141. Vickery, A. L., Wang, C. A., and Walker, A. M. Treatment of intrathyroidal papillary carcinoma of the thyroid. *Cancer 60:*2587–2595, 1987.

142. Williams, E. D., Doniach, I., Bjarnason, O., and Michie, W. Thyroid cancer in an iodine-rich area. A histopathologic study. *Cancer 39:*215–222, 1977.

143. Wilson, N. W., Pambakian, H., Richardson, T. C., *et al.* Epithelial markers in thyroid carcinoma. An immunoperoxidase study. *Histopathology 10:*815–819, 1986.

144. Woolner, A. L. B., Beahrs, O. H., Black, B. M., *et al.* Classification and prognosis of thyroid carcinoma: A study of 885 cases observed in a thirty-year period. *Am. J. Surg. 102:*354–387, 1981.

145. Wright, P. A., Lemoine, N. R., Mayall, E. S., *et al.* Papillary and follicular thyroid carcinomas show a different pattern of *ras* oncogene mutation. *Br. J. Cancer 60:*576–577, 1989.

146. Wyllie, F. S., Lemoine, N. R., Williams, E. D., and Wynford-Thomas, D. Structure and expression of nuclear oncogenes in multistage thyroid tumorigenesis. *Br. J. Cancer 60:*561–565, 1989.

147. Yagi, Y., Yagi, S., and Saku, T. The localization of cytoskeletal proteins and thyroglobulin in thyroid microcarcinoma in comparison with clinically manifested thyroid carcinoma. *Cancer 56:*1967–1971, 1985.

148. Yamamoto, Y., Maeda, T., Izumi, K., and Otsuka, H. Occult papillary carcinoma of the thyroid. A study of 408 autopsy cases. *Cancer 65:*1173–1179, 1990.

149. Yamashita, H., Nakayama, I., Noguchi, S., *et al.* Minute carcinoma of the thyroid and its development to advanced carcinoma. *Acta Pathol. Jpn. 35:*781–788, 1985.

150. Zimmerman, D., Hay, I. D., Gough, I. R., *et al.* Papillary thyroid carcinoma in children and adults: Long-term follow-up of 1,039 patients conservatively treated at one institution during three decades. *Surgery 104:*1157–1166, 1988.

ity (%) Chapter 8

Fine Needle Aspiration of the Thyroid

BARBARA F. ATKINSON

Thyroid aspiration is now generally accepted as the first step in the evaluation of a thyroid nodule. Other indications for aspiration include evaluation of diffuse goiter, follow-up radiation-exposed individuals, screening for familial medullary carcinoma, and cyst drainage.[12] Since thyroid nodules are present in 4–7% of adults, it is important to find a technique that can separate those nodules which are probably benign and can be followed clinically from those which need to be resected.

Aspiration is a cost-effective and reliable method for selecting thyroid nodules for observation or excision.[48] Fine needle aspiration (FNA) can be performed at the time of a patient's first visit to the endocrinologist so that the cytologic interpretation is available at the same time as thyroid function and/or antibody studies.

Recent studies have shown that aspiration cytology has better sensitivity, specificity, and positive predictive value than pertechnetate scanning and ultrasound imaging in such predictions[1,59] (Table 8.1). In another study high-resolution ultrasonography was found to be useful in demonstrating a typical malignant pattern in 64.3% of carcinomas, but FNA was even better, demonstrating abnormal findings in 92.4% of carcinomas.[101]

The thyroid aspirate diagnosis should be used to support the clinical impression. Either clinical impression or aspiration diagnosis may ultimately dictate surgical removal of a nodule but the findings of both should be considered. The clinician needs to assess the level of clinical suspicion. Cytopathologic diagnosis should clearly categorize the lesion as probably benign so that the patient can be followed, versus suspicious or malignant, in which case excision is indicated. Either a specific diagnosis or the differential diagnosis of the lesion should also be given.

TABLE 8.1. COMPARISON OF DIAGNOSTIC MODALITIES FOR EVALUATION OF THYROID NODULES[a]

	Thyroid FNA	Pertechnetate Scan	Ultrasound Imaging
Sensitivity (%)	92	82	73
Specificity (%)	85	34	58
Positive predictive value (%)	41	11	19

[a] Modified from Jones, *et al.*[59]

If there is a reasonable chance that a malignant tumor may be present, the diagnosis should include a phrase such as "suspicious for . . ., suggest surgical excision if clinically indicated." With this type of diagnostic approach there is the potential for surgical biopsy of some lesions that are found to be benign including nodular goiter, Hashimoto's thyroiditis, and follicular adenoma, but the risk of missing a malignant tumor is minimized.

When a diagnosis of a benign lesion such as nodular goiter or Hashimoto's thyroiditis is made, the clinician can feel comfortable following the patient if the clinical impression was also benign. If the diagnosis unequivocally shows a malignant tumor, then surgical treatment can be planned. The most difficult cases are those in which there is some epithelial atypia present, but not enough for a definite diagnosis of suspicious or malignant. In this instance the clinical judgments of both the cytopathologist and the endocrinologist must be combined in order to arrive at an appropriate management decision based on the complete clinical picture and the cytologic information. As in other cytologic specimen types, it is essential to have clinical information available during interpretation of the specimen. A good rapport with the endocrinologist is essential so that he/she fully understands the diagnosis and implications.

ACCURACY AND USE

Numerous studies have analyzed the diagnostic accuracy of FNA. In the last few years most have found that the results are excellent,[22,33,47,61,74] but at least one study[24] found that FNA was less reliable than expected. It is difficult to compare studies and to arrive at a generally accepted rate for sensitivity and specificity of thyroid FNA. Patient selection is different and investigators handle categories such as indeterminate, uncertain, suspicious, or follicular neoplasia in different ways for purposes of calculating statistics. For example, in one study which found a 27.8% discrepancy between FNA and surgical excision those cases with inadequate material for diagnosis were classified as discrepant.[47]

In the series by LaRosa *et al.*[74] of 5608 aspirates, false-negative results were 2.3%, and false-positive findings were only 1.1%. The risk of a nodule being malignant in this series was 4.46%. Cytologic categories of malignant, probably malignant, probably benign, and benign were used for calculation of statistics. The overall sensitivity was 97.8%, specificity was 97.7%, and accuracy was 97.7%. These results are excellent; most cytopathologists and clinicians would accept an even lower specificity in order to be sure not to miss tumors.

Hamming *et al.*[51] separated patients into three categories on the basis of high, moderate, and low clinical suspicion. The criteria for the high suspicion group were medullary carcinoma/multiple endocrine neoplasia 2 in patient's family, rapid growth of tumor, very firm nodule, fixation to adjacent structures, vocal cord paralysis, enlarged regional lymph nodes, or distant metastases. Criteria for moderate suspicion were age under 20 or over 60, history of neck irradiation, male sex with solitary nodule, dubious fixation, or a nodule with a diameter over 4 cm which was partially cystic. Low suspicion included everything else.

The overall rate of cancer found by these authors was 23%. In this study sensitivity was 92%, specificity was 71%, and accuracy was 75%. With the categories of high, moderate and low clinical suspicion, the rate of cancer detection by FNA was 71, 14, and 11%, respectively; sensitivity was 95, 89, and 88%. Diagnostic specificity was 88, 72, and 67%, and accuracy was 93, 75, and 69% for categories of high, moderate, and low clinical suspicion, respectively. Their conclusion was that all patients with high clinical suspicion should have a surgical excision regardless of the aspirate diagnosis. A surgical excision is also indicated in patients with low clinical suspicion but a malignant or uncertain diagnosis by FNA.

The management decision is whether to recommend a surgical resection or to prescribe a trial of thyroid hormone treatment to suppress further growth. Patients with nodular goiter or Hashimoto's thyroiditis treated with thyroid hormone often show regression of the nodule or at least no further increase in size of the nodule. Even when a nodule is diagnosed as benign by aspirate but clinical suspicion is high or the lesion increases in size during hormone suppression, a biopsy should be performed, since the aspiration may have missed the critical area.

Hall *et al.*[47] reviewed sources of diagnostic error that affected their diagnostic yield. Discrepant diagnoses were found in 20 cases (27.8% of cases with subsequent surgical biopsy). Six of these discrepant cases were due to insufficient material for diagnosis, and 2 were due to sampling errors (a papillary carcinoma and a follicular adenoma not present on the aspirate specimen). The remaining 12 cases were classified as cytodiagnostic errors, all of which were related to the diagnosis of follicular lesions. Seven that were diagnosed as follicular or Hürthle cell neoplasm proved to be nodular goiter. One follicular tumor and one Hürthle cell tumor were found to be papillary carcinoma. Lastly, three aspirates diagnosed as papillary carcinoma proved to be follicular or Hürthle cell adenomas. Because of the difficulties in cytologic diagnosis of follicular lesions, these patients are the most likely to be found to have only nodular goiter after surgery.

If FNA is used to screen patients, then the number of patients referred for surgery is lower than if only scan, ultrasound, and clinical suspicion are used. Several studies have recently examined whether the rate of surgery has been decreased by the addition of FNA in patient management and the value of FNA has been confirmed.[17,60,90] Ng *et al.*[90] found that the percentage of resections decreased from 90 to 60%, while the proportion of patients in whom cancer was found increased from 18.4 to 26.2%. Kendall[61] reviewed 3 years' experience and found that resections for nodular goiter were reduced from 40 to 3% while the yield of neoplastic lesions increased from 16 to 69%.

Julian *et al.*[60] found that when FNA was used for screening, surgery was avoided and not just delayed. The mean follow-up period was 4.7 years. With this time, none of their patients developed new indications for surgery, and of the patients who had subsequent surgery, no cancer cases were found.

An important question in patient management is whether a diagnosis of negative means that the patient does not have neoplastic disease. Grant *et al.*[42] from the Mayo Clinic studied patients who had a diagnosis of a benign lesion by FNA and who were followed without surgery for a mean of 6.1 years. In that time they uncovered only 3 false-negative results out of 39 patients, a rate of 7.7%. Although this rate may increase with longer follow-up times, if the patient has multiple screenings over time, no significant lesion should be missed. For instance, a papillary carcinoma could be quite small and its course indolent, but with multiple screenings it is not likely to be missed.

Other issues in surgical management of thyroid disease are still being debated, including the need for total thyroidectomy and the place of frozen section in diagnosis of thyroid lesions.[49] Some surgeons recommend total or subtotal thyroidectomy[14,28] for treatment of lesions diagnosed as malignant or indeterminate by FNA. Many others think lobectomy is adequate when the diagnosis is suspicious or indeterminate. It may be difficult on a frozen section to determine if a tumor is an adenoma or carcinoma, the same difficulty that is encountered in FNA diagnosis. Frozen section has been compared to FNA in several recent studies.[72,99,102] All demonstrate successful diagnosis by FNA and suggest that it is at least as accurate as frozen section diagnosis. The combination of preoperative FNA and gross examination of the specimen by a pathologist during surgery may eliminate the need for frozen section in most cases. Hamburger and Husain[49] conclude that "reduction or elimination of useless or redundant frozen section procedures reduces costs as well as anesthesia duration."

TECHNIQUE

The technique for performing a FNA of the thyroid is the same as that for aspiration of other superficial lesions. It has been described in more detail in several texts and journals.[35,63] Aspiration may be done with the patient either sitting or lying down. The neck should be fully extended. All slides and material should be laid out ready for use prior to the aspiration. A 21- or 23-gauge needle is commonly used, but in some practices 18- or 19-gauge needles are preferred.

When the needle is inserted, it should be aimed at the periphery of the lesion. Suction should be maintained as the needle is moved within the lesion. This takes advantage of the cutting action of the needle bore to obtain mini-biopsy type pieces of tissue. Suction is relaxed prior to removal of the needle. Direct smear slides are made as the sample is expressed from the syringe into liquid fixative.

Several aspirates are usually taken from each lesion. If possible, the aspirates should be taken from the peripheral areas of the whole nodule. If a cyst is encountered, the contents are drained and sent to the laboratory. It should be emphasized that additional samples from thyroid adjacent to the cyst should be taken in order to rule out the presence of a cystic papillary carcinoma.[89]

In many practices the pathologist personally performs the fine needle aspirations. There are several advantages to this approach: excellent correlation of aspirate findings and clinical information, the degree of clinical suspicion of the nodule can be personally assessed, and slides will be perfectly smeared and fixed. Hall *et al.*[47] document that pathologists are better at obtaining an adequate sample than either community- or hospital-based clinicians. On the other hand if a clinician gives the laboratory the appropriate clinical information and if they learn how to correctly perform, smear, and fix specimens, then excellent results are obtained.

Use of Saccomano's carbowax fixation method allows the clinician to provide the laboratory with a perfectly fixed specimen. After the aspirate is completed, the needle is flushed directly into a liquid fixative such as Saccomano's carbowax solution.[5] This minimizes the difficulty of smearing and fixing the specimen since the slides are prepared by the laboratory. The fixative is distributed in plastic centrifuge tubes, which can be stored until used. The specimen tube can then be sent or mailed to the laboratory. Cytospin preparations and cell blocks are prepared.

Carbowax is an ideal fixative for bloody thyroid aspirates, which are usually found. This method of fixation lyses the red blood cells to produce a proteinaceous background which allows a cell block to be made even in the most sparsely cellular specimen.

If the direct smear technique is used, additional material can be obtained by flushing the material that remains in the needle bore into liquid fixative. A cell block with fragments of tissue often gives the cytopathologist an added measure of confidence in the diagnosis. A specimen prepared in this way involves additional cost for the laboratory because of the materials and the time involved, but the advantage of excellent fixation, recovery of all of the material and the cell block makes the added effort worthwhile.

DIAGNOSTIC CRITERIA

Many studies have examined the value of thyroid FNA.[1,70,91,104] There have also been several book chapters which discuss and illustrate diagnostic criteria,[6,12,35,53,80] as well as excellent books on thyroid surgical pathology[81] and FNA diagnosis[63] which may be helpful as additional resources.

The most important step in diagnosis of thyroid aspirates is to have a mind's eye picture of normal follicular epithelium to use as an internal comparison. The size of the nuclei, the delicacy of the cytoplasm, the variety of follicle sizes, and the organization of cells in the follicle are all particularly important. Follicular cells are small and have a high nuclear to cytoplasmic ratio and delicate, inconspicuous cytoplasm. Cell size is small with nuclei about the size of an activated lymphocyte. Chromatin is relatively hyperchromatic and nucleoli are usually absent or small.

Follicular cells are best recognized as follicle groups and sheets (Fig. 8.1). In a benign specimen it is rare to be able to identify single follicular cells. Variability in size of follicles (both in amount of colloid and the number of cells in each group) is an important "benign" sign. There is regular spacing of the nuclei within the follicle group, although allowance must be made for piling and overlap related to placement of the follicle on the slide. Molding of nuclei is unusual. Presence of colloid in the background of the smear is another important benign sign.

It is essential to ensure that there are adequate numbers of follicular groups present. Many cytopathologists require that at least six benign follicular groups be present on each of several aspirates.[48,50] The usual benign specimen of nodule goiter is sparsely cellular; however, these minimum requirements must be

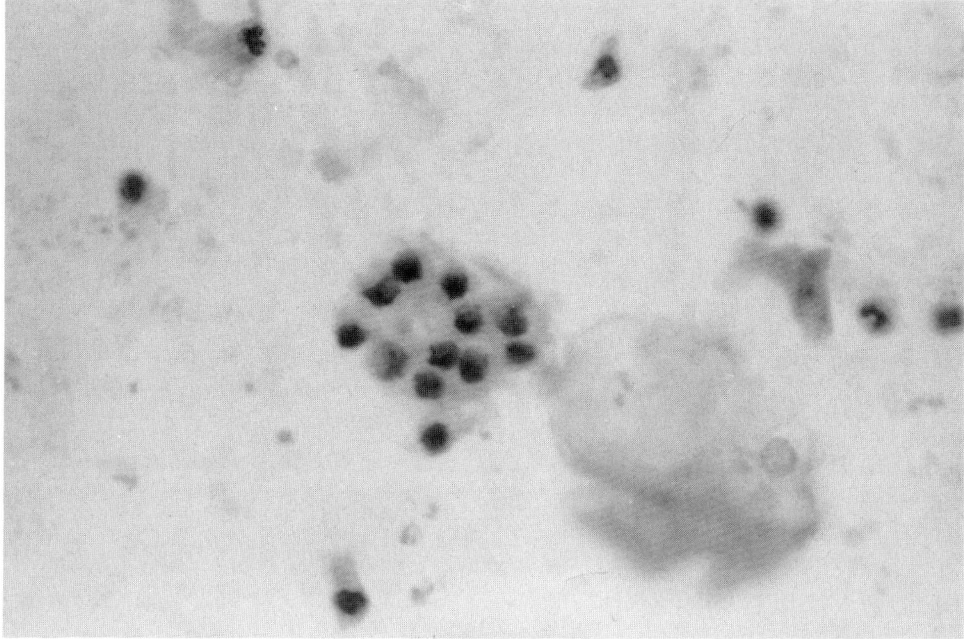

FIG. 8.1. Nodular goiter. Normal follicular cells and colloid are seen. Notice that the cells in this follicular group are small when seen in comparison to the inflammatory cells in the background. The chromatin pattern is slightly hyperchromatic and the chromatin is relatively even. Small micronucleoli may be present. The cytoplasm is relatively scant, and the nuclei are evenly spaced within the follicle group. Cytoplasmic borders of follicular cells are generally not well documented. The colloid is formed into a follicle-shaped aggregate. The size of this colloid aggregate indicates the size of the follicle from which it came from (Papanicolaou stain, ×250).

achieved. In general, high cellularity is one of the best indicators of a follicular tumor, but if abundant cellularity is present, it is important to consider whether this is usual for specimens received from a particular aspirator.

If the specimen is adequate but cellularity is marginal, it is appropriate to make a diagnosis of scant specimen and suggest clinical follow-up with re-aspiration at the time of the next visit. If there are not enough follicles for a diagnosis then immediate re-aspiration is necessary.

Often when the lesion is a cyst, a large quantity of fluid is obtained by aspiration. Such a specimen usually has macrophages, some colloid, rare inflammatory cells, and no follicular epithelium (Figure 8.2). It is appropriate in such a case to make the diagnosis of "suggestive of a cyst, but no follicular epithelium present." However, given this scenario, some would make a diagnosis of "unsatisfactory." The cystic material is quite characteristic (pigmented macrophages, debris and often colloid), and the lesion usually disappears after aspiration.

The differential diagnosis of most nodular lesions of the thyroid is quite straightforward. Some lesions, however, pose particularly difficult diagnostic problems, including Hashimoto's thyroiditis and follicular lesions. Graves' disease

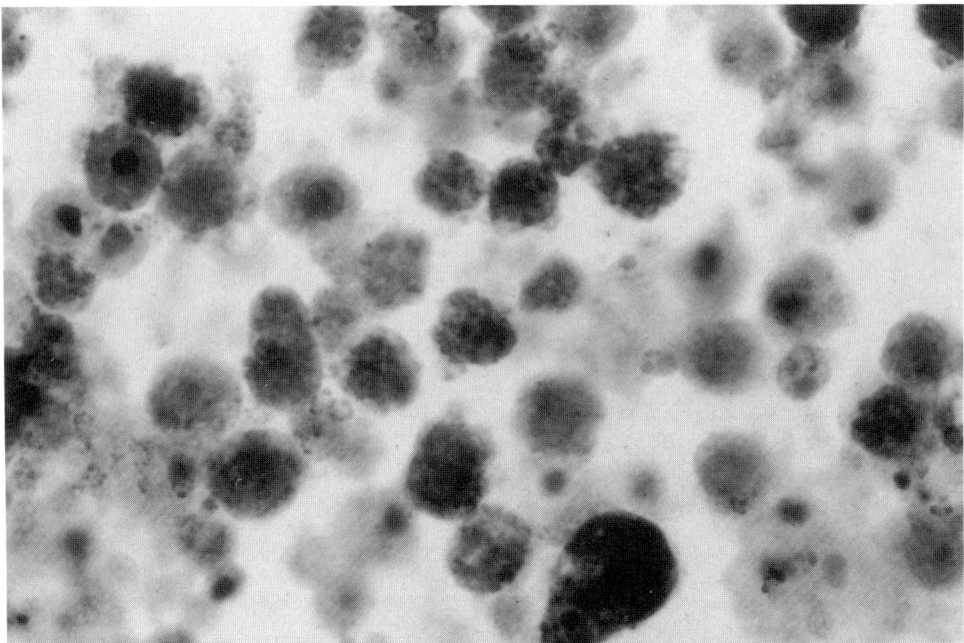

FIG. 8.2.　Cyst in nodular goiter. The presence of macrophages filled with cystic, colloid debris such as seen here is typical of nodular goiter with cyst formation. Most cells do not have visible nuclei, and many cells are quite degenerate (Papanicolaou stain, ×400).

TABLE 8.2.　DIFFERENTIAL DIAGNOSIS OF THYROID NODULES

1. Nodular goiter
2. Hashimoto's thyroiditis
3. Papillary carcinoma
4. Follicular neoplasia
5. Medullary carcinoma
6. Malignant lymphoma
7. Anaplastic carcinoma
8. Metastatic carcinoma and other tumors

is very difficult and sometimes impossible to evaluate by FNA because the degree of nuclear abnormality of the follicular cells is greater than that usually seen in many malignant tumors. These findings have been discussed by Jayaram *et al.*[58] In general FNA is not recommended in patients with active Graves' disease. Atypical findings associated with carbamizole treatment have also been described.[105] Evaluation of hot nodules is discussed by Liel *et al.*[79] Particular care must be taken in evaluation by FNA of a nodule in a pregnant patient because follicular cells may be very active. Nucleoli are present and vacuolated cytoplasm may be seen.[10]

The differential diagnosis of thyroid nodular disease is summarized in Table 8.2. A discussion of the major cytologic features or each of these entities will follow.

Nodular Goiter

Most aspirates are obtained from cases of nodular goiter since this is such a common disease. In such aspirates the nuclei of the follicular cells are normal-sized, colloid clumps of varying sizes are present, and macrophages are common (Figs 8.1 and 8.3). The best diagnostic criteria are the presence of variable-sized follicles and colloid. Cellularity is usually scant. The epithelial cells have variable amounts of cytoplasm. This often indicates that some Hürthle cell change is present, another characteristic finding of nodular goiter.

Cell blocks are particularly useful for determining growth patterns and structure (Fig. 8.4). Variably sized follicles and colloid are usually quite prominent in nodular goiter. Hyperplastic papillae and fragments of dilated follicles are the two most specific features for distinguishing nodular goiter from follicular neoplasm in a cell block.[73] The presence of nuclear atypia and non-honeycomb patterns may indicate follicular tumor.

Hürthle cells are identified by their abundant, dense cytoplasm (Fig. 8.5). Nuclei of these cells are variable and often they are normal. They may also show large, active-appearing nuclei having either a vesicular chromatin pattern with a nucleolus or a large, hyperchromatic nucleus having an irregular shape. It is

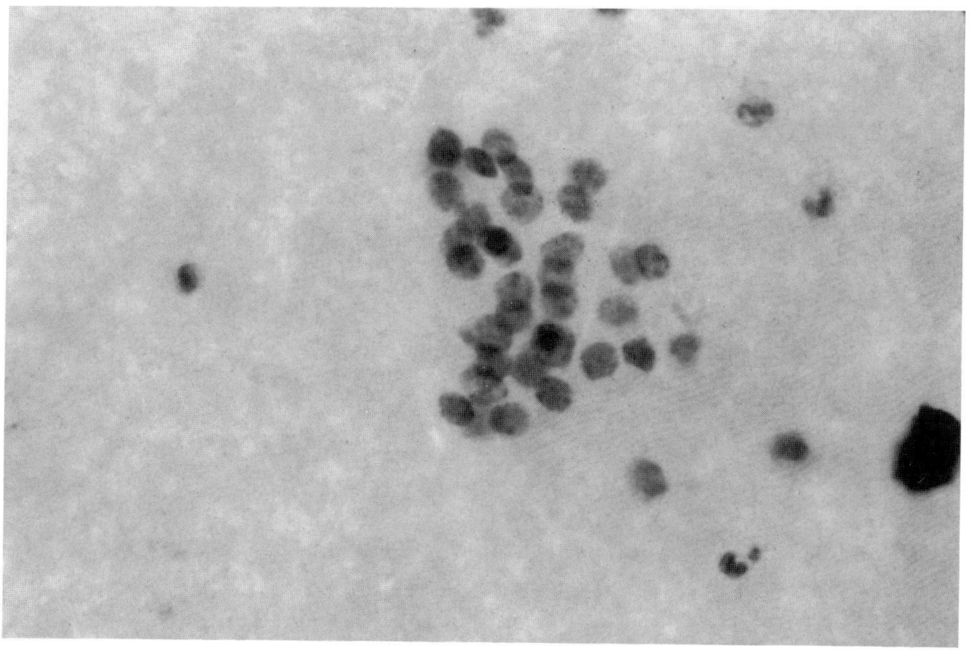

FIG. 8.3. Nodular goiter. Normal follicular epithelium is seen in this cytospin preparation. The lysed bloody background is commonly seen when Saccomano's carbowax fixation is used. The nuclei stand out clearly against the lysed blood, but the cytoplasm of the cells is indistinct and the cytoplasmic borders are not apparent. The follicle structure can be identified here. Notice the small size of the nuclei, only slightly bigger than normal lymphocytes, and the relatively hyperchromatic appearance of the chromatin. The cells are uniformly spaced within the follicle structure (Papanicolaou stain, ×400).

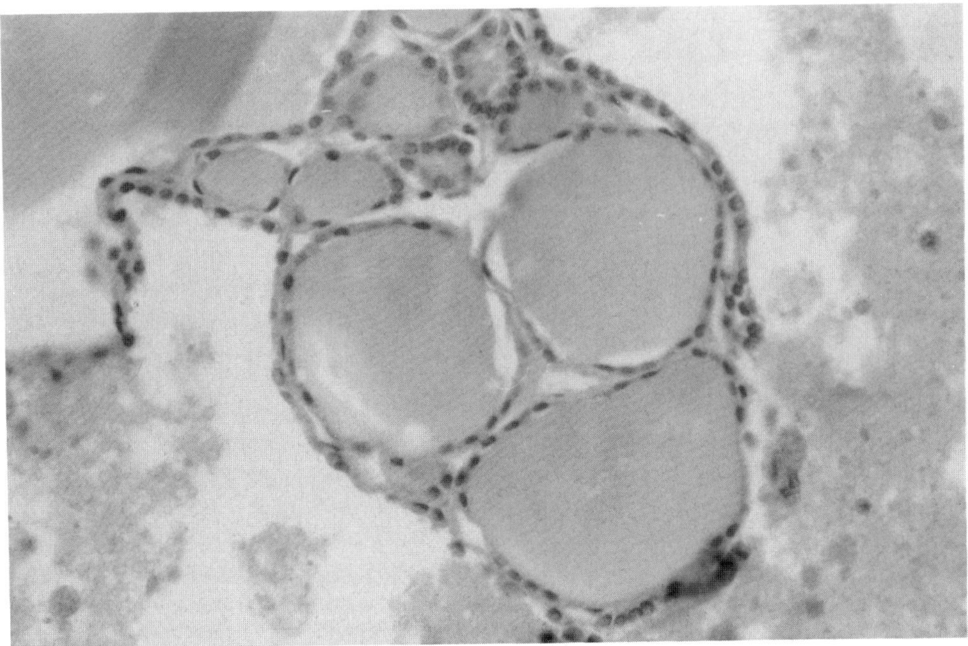

Fig. 8.4. Nodular goiter. In this cell block preparation there are follicles of varying size and shape including several large follicles. The colloid clump at the edge of the figure is quite large indicating that it came from a highly distended follicle. The nuclei are uniform and evenly spaced and have a slightly hyperchromatic appearance. In the most enlarged follicles the follicular cells are flattened rather than cuboidal in appearance [hematoxylin & eosin (H & E) stain, × 80].

important to recognize Hürthle cells since they occur in several diseases—nodular goiter, Hashimoto's thyroiditis, and benign and malignant Hürthle cell tumors. In nodular goiter Hürthle cells are typically intermixed with normal follicular epithelium. They may be intermixed in a single follicle or normal follicles may be intermixed with follicles composed of all Hürthle cells.

Faroux *et al.*[34] determined that the morphologic criteria best able to separate a nodular goiter aspirate from an atypical adenoma or carcinoma were organization of cellular clustering, nuclear hypertrophy, and the amount of colloid.[34] The quantity of colloid in the aspirate was the weakest criterion and, furthermore, if a nucleolus was present the diagnostic power of lack of colloid was further diminished.

Hashimoto's Thyroiditis

Lymphocytes are usually a very prominent component of an aspirate of Hashimoto's thyroiditis, but sometimes they are overlooked since the epithelial atypia may be so marked that this component overshadows the lymphocytes. The features of Hashimoto's thyroiditis have been previously described by Kini *et al.*[66] and Ravinsky and Safneck.[94] In FNA it is imperative that the lymphocytes in the background of the smear be evaluated. Since a thyroid FNA is often quite bloody, the relative proportion of lymphocytes to polymorphonuclear leukocytes

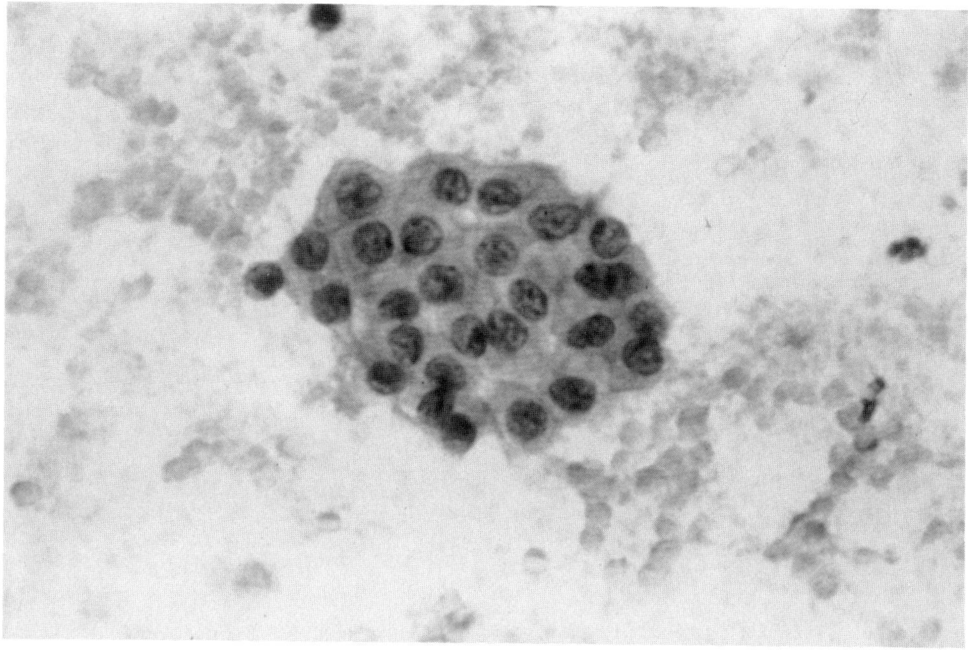

FIG. 8.5. Nodular goiter with Hürthle cell change. Notice that the structure seen here is more sheet-like than a typical follicle group. The nuclei are about the same size as in the previous figure; however, the cytoplasm is more dense and granular. Cytoplasmic margins are distinct. The nuclear to cytoplasmic ratio is typical of that seen in Hürthle cells. In Hürthle cells nuclei may have several different patterns as seen here. (Papanicolaou stain, ×400).

should be considered. If lymphocytes are more common than expected then Hashimoto's thyroiditis is a consideration. It is also important to determine whether there is a mixture of larger, activated lymphocytes with normal, small lymphocytes (Figs. 8.6 and 8.7). Immunoblasts and tingible body macrophages may sometimes be seen. Lymphocytes seen admixed within follicular epithelial groups are highly suggestive of thyroiditis (Fig. 8.8).

Whenever there is a question of a cytologic diagnosis of Hashimoto's thyroiditis, serum antibody titers should be requested although there are cases in which antibody levels cannot be detected.[87] As more becomes known about the genetic characteristics of patients with Hashimoto's thyroiditis,[26] it may be possible to develop more sensitive tests for this disease.

When Hashimoto's thyroiditis is present, there is often very significant epithelial atypia (Fig. 8.9). This atypia may be far worse in this benign disease than is seen in cells of a well-differentiated follicular carcinoma. Hürthle cells usually are also identified. It is difficult to diagnose a follicular lesion in a patient with known Hashimoto's thyroiditis; therefore, this diagnosis should be made with caution.

The two lesions that must be considered in the evaluation of a FNA from a patient with thyroiditis are papillary carcinoma and malignant lymphoma. Papillary carcinoma is diagnosed using the same criteria discussed in the following

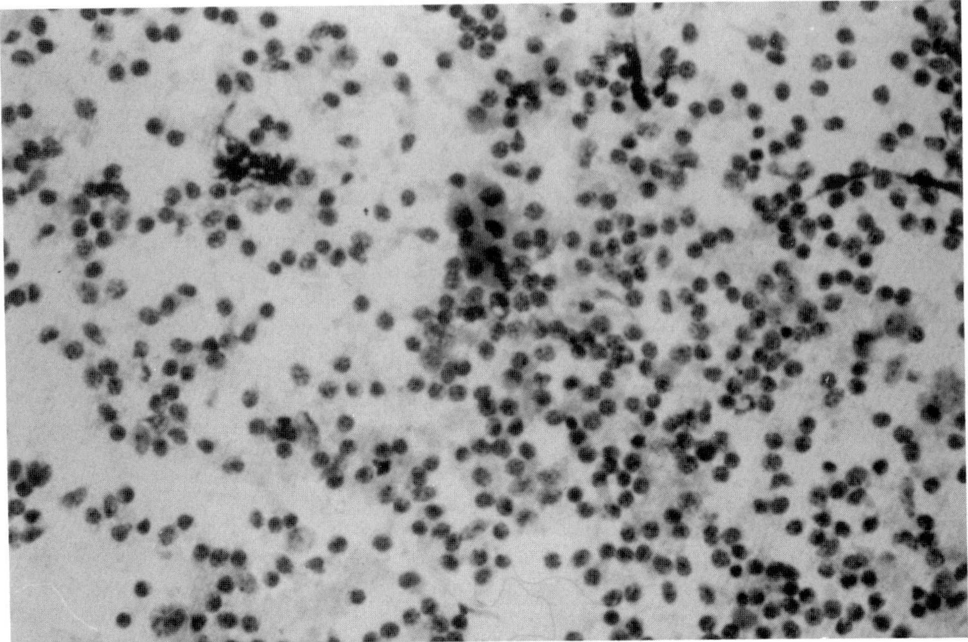

FIG. 8.6. Hashimoto's thyroiditis. Abundant lymphocytes are present which vary in size from normal, small lymphocytes to larger, activated lymphocytes. The predominant population is composed of medium-sized lymphocytes. Some nucleoli are present. There is one small group of follicular cells near the center of the field. These cells have abundant cytoplasm with distinct cell borders indicating Hürthle cell change (Papanicolaou stain, ×125).

section, although it is rare to be able to diagnose a follicular variant of papillary carcinoma. The epithelial atypia of Hashimoto's thyroiditis often has nuclear clearing as a prominent feature.

The presence of malignant lymphoma can also be very difficult to determine since there are numerous highly activated, germinal center lymphocytes present in Hashimoto's disease. The diagnosis of reactive hyperplasia is made the same way it would be made in a lymph node aspirate, which also has germinal centers. It is essential to establish whether there is a uniform population of lymphocytes present (as expected in a malignant lymphoma) or a mixture of lymphocytes of different maturation (as seen in a reactive population). A reactive pattern is best recognized as a combination of normal, small lymphocytes admixed with larger lymphocytes which have larger nuclei, nucleoli, and a more vesicular chromatin.

Another type of thyroiditis rarely seen in FNA is Reidel's thyroiditis. Cytologic findings from this entity have been described,[100] but cellularity is usually scant, so the specimen is often unsatisfactory. This is probably due to the marked fibrosis often associated with this disease.

Papillary Carcinoma

Thyroid FNA is particularly useful in making the diagnosis of papillary carcinoma. The major diagnostic features are nuclear clearing, grooves, intra-

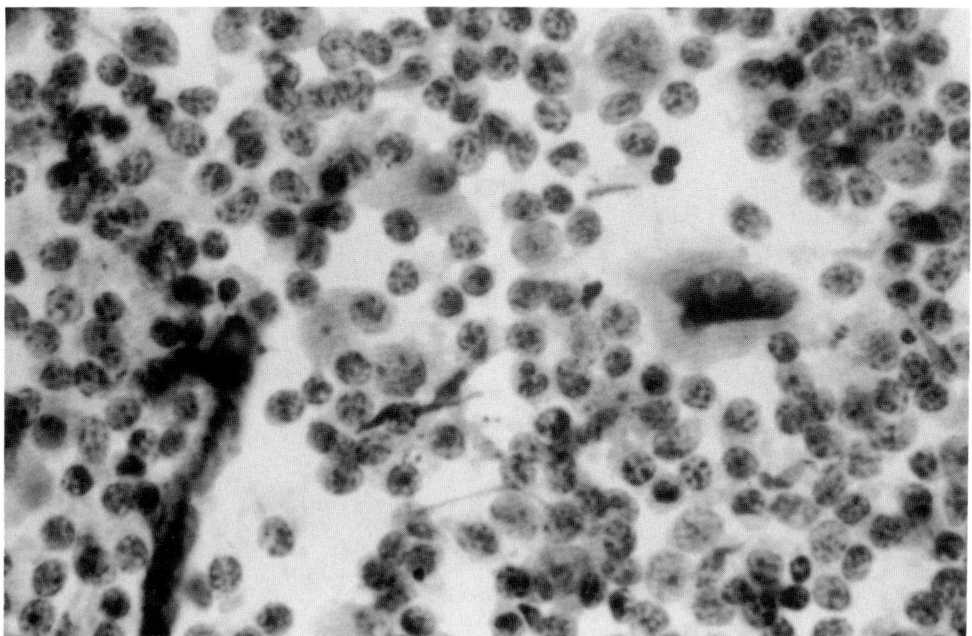

FIG. 8.7. Hashimoto's thyroiditis. This higher magnification demonstrates the range of lymphoid cells. Most are medium-sized, activated lymphocytes; however, several large lymphoid cells are also apparent. The largest cell, which has a hyperchromatic, multilobated nucleus, is a Hürthle cell (Papanicolaou stain, ×400).

nuclear cytoplasmic inclusions, papillary fragments, and psammoma bodies[65] (Figs. 8.10, 8.11, and 8.12). Nuclear clearing is one of the most common findings and should be found in nuclei throughout whole follicles (Figs. 8.13 and 8.14). The nuclei are usually slightly larger than normal. Nuclear grooves are seen particularly well in May-Grunwald-Giemsa and Diff Quik stained smears[11] (Fig. 8.15). Both nuclear chromatin clearing and grooved nuclei, however, can occasionally be seen in aspirates from benign thyroid lesions.

Whenever nuclear clearing or nuclear grooves are prominent but only a follicular growth pattern is present, the follicular variant of papillary carcinoma must be a consideration. In this entity there are no papillary groups, but the nuclear features are typical of papillary cancer. Hugh *et al.*[55] discuss cytologic findings in 3 cases of this entity.[55] The distinction of the follicular variant of papillary carcinoma from follicular tumor may be difficult (Fig. 8.16), so a differential diagnosis including both may need to be suggested. It is not essential to make this distinction prior to surgical excision.

Nuclear grooves have been studied in papillary carcinoma by several authors.[65,85,97,103] A recent study by Harach and Zusman[52] found nuclear grooves in cells of all 8 cases of the follicular variant of papillary carcinoma they examined. Six cases had grooves in 20–50% of cells on the smears. In addition, all 8 cases of typical papillary carcinoma had grooves, and 75% of these had grooves present in 20–50% of cells. In contrast, nuclear grooves were found in 1% of colloid

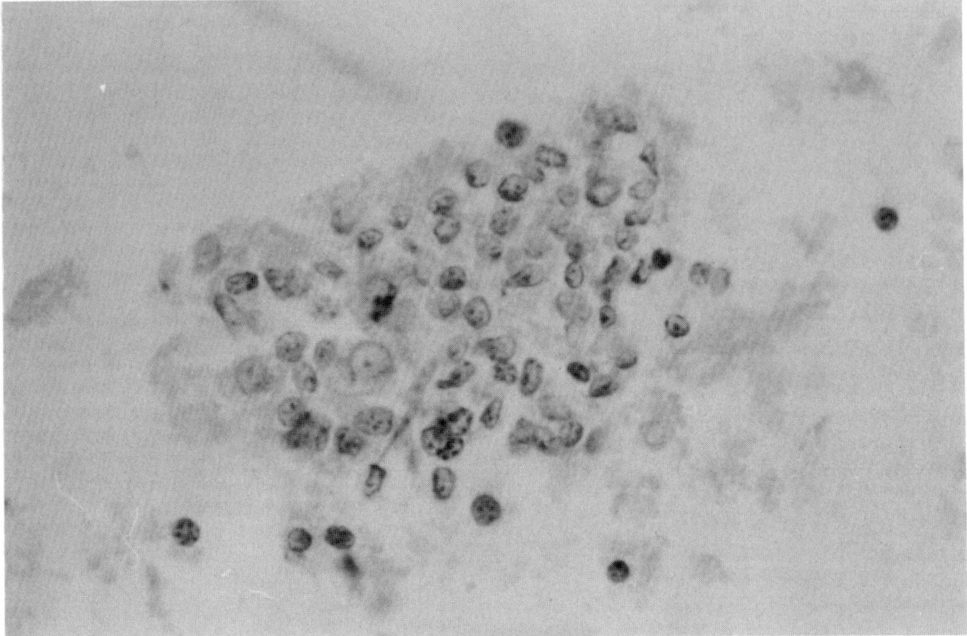

FIG. 8.8. Hashimoto's thyroiditis. This cell block preparation demonstrates a fragment of a germinal center. The lymphoid cells are medium- to large-sized. The nuclei have a vesicular chromatin pattern and prominent nucleoli. There are several normal, small lymphocytes and plasmacytoid cells for comparison (H & E stain ×250).

nodules, 26% of hyperplastic nodules, 40% of follicular adenoma cases, and 50% of follicular carcinoma cases, but they were never present in more than 5% of cells. While the finding of nuclear grooves is significant, particularly when present in a large number of cells, it is certainly not specific for papillary carcinoma.

Other features commonly found in the follicular variant of papillary carcinoma include nuclear-cytoplasmic inclusions (present in 7 of 8 cases) and colloid (present in 6 of 8 cases) reported by Harach and Zusman.[52] Nuclear-cytoplasmic inclusions were also present in all cases of typical papillary carcinoma, but only 1 of 8 cases had them in more than 20% of cells. They were also found in less than 7% of cases of colloid nodule, hyperplastic nodule, follicular adenoma, or follicular carcinoma. When present, they were always detected in less than 5% of cells.

While psammoma bodies are also excellent markers for typical papillary carcinoma, they are often not seen in an evaluation by FNA. Further, they may occasionally be seen in aspirates from nonmalignant entities such as nodular goiter and Hashimoto's thyroiditis.[21,32,96] Despite this, the finding of a psammoma body in a thyroid FNA is worrisome; depending on the clinical situation, it may warrant an excisional biopsy.

The diagnosis of papillary carcinoma is often made when the tumor is occult. Very small lesions are sometimes picked up by aspiration but they may also be missed. Tumors as small as 0.7 cm have been found by FNA,[48] but the need for

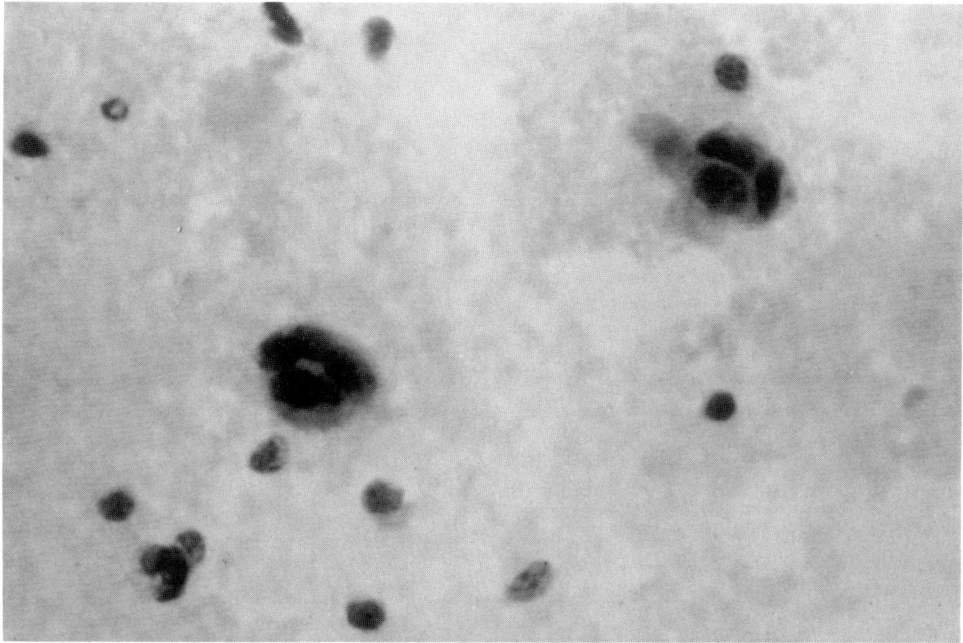

FIG. 8.9. Hashimoto's thyroiditis. Scattered lymphocytes are present in the background. They include rare small lymphocytes, several medium-sized lymphocytes, and one plasmacytoid cell. There are two epithelial groups. The nuclei in these groups are hyperchromatic and enlarged and demonstrate some atypia. Epithelial atypia is commonly seen in Hashimoto's thyroiditis (Papanicolaou stain, ×400).

surgical resection of all small papillary carcinomas is not clear since these tumors often progress very slowly.[4]

FOLLICULAR TUMORS

The most difficult diagnostic problem in thyroid FNA is differentiating nodular goiter, follicular adenoma, and follicular carcinoma. The major features to use to determine whether a follicular tumor is present are nuclear enlargement (Fig. 8.17), the presence of nucleoli, nuclear size and chromatin variability, vesicular or finely granular chromatin pattern, crowding and overlapping of cells (Figs. 8.18 and 8.19), or the presence of abundant cellular material with numerous follicular "balls."[68] Nodular goiters may have a few of these features, but usually only in scattered cells or groups. Hashimoto's thyroiditis is associated with more of these nuclear changes. Syncytial-type fragments are present in both nodular goiter and follicular tumors. In nodular goiter these are typically arranged in orderly sheets and fragments forming a regular honeycomb, while in follicular tumors there is often nuclear atypia and disorganization of arrangement as well.[95]

The atypical adenoma group of follicular lesions includes Hürthle cell tumors and tumors with microfollicular and trabecular growth patterns (Figs. 8.20 and 8.21). These all are relatively easy to recognize by FNA, and they are especially

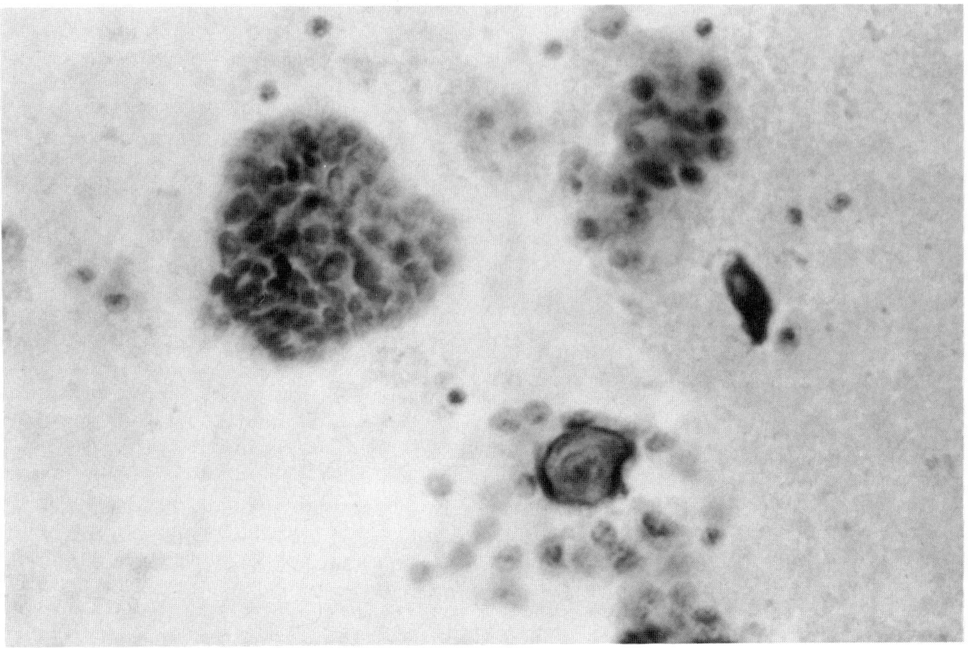

FIG. 8.10.   Papillary carcinoma. A papillary group with a psammoma body is seen. The psammoma body shows concentric lamellar rings. The nuclei are irregularly spaced around the psammoma body and the group has a smooth border typical of a papillary fragment. The nuclei in the other epithelial sheet also show some abnormality. There is variation in the size of the nuclei and a disordered appearance of the group. At least one nucleus in the center of the group shows a localized clearing of the chromatin (Papanicolaou stain, ×125).

easy to evaluate in a cell block fragment. When any of these atypical patterns is recognized, then a surgical resection is recommended. A microfollicular pattern is recognized by the presence of numerous small follicles without the intermixing of large- and medium-sized follicles. Often there is only a small amount of colloid which sometimes has only single cells wrapping around it. The trabecular or embryonal pattern has solid, cord-like columns of cells usually with little colloid or follicle structure seen.

The identification of Hürthle cells was discussed previously under "Nodular Goiter." A Hürthle cell neoplasm is suggested when there are large tissue fragments in which whole areas or all cells are of the Hürthle type (Figs. 8.22 and 8.23).

Hürthle cell tumors also often lack colloid and may not have a typical follicle structure.[64] Commonly, their growth pattern is trabecular. Papillary Hürthle cell tumors may also be seen. Their biologic behavior may more closely resemble that of a papillary carcinoma than a typical Hürthle cell tumor.[20]

Bronner *et al.*[15] have found that flow cytometry measurements of DNA content could not be used to separate cases of Hürthle cell adenoma from Hürthle cell carcinoma. Aneuploid populations were present in 55% of adenomas and 67% of carcinomas. There were no unfavorable prognostic implications related to aneu-

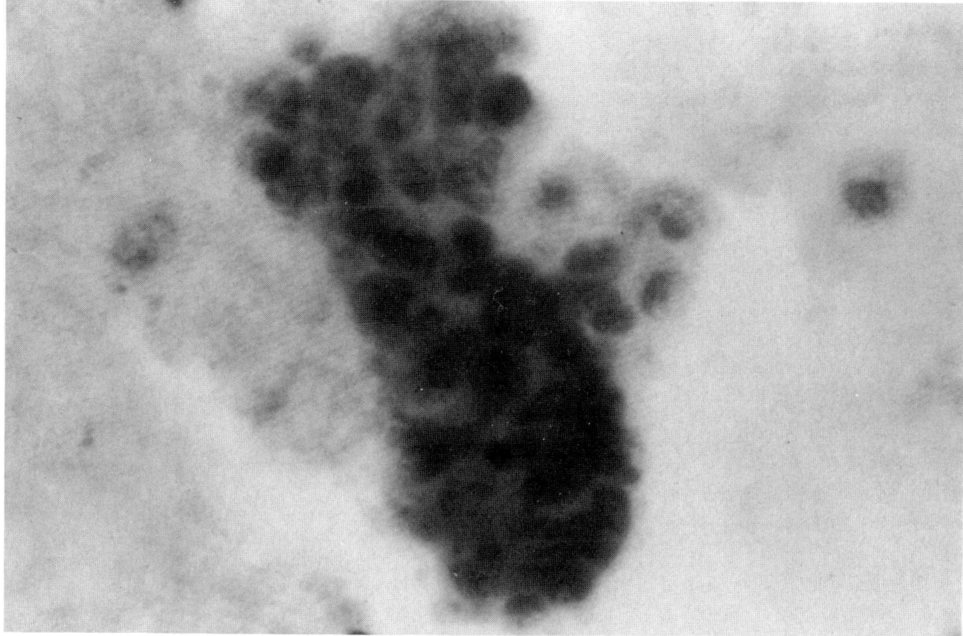

FIG. 8.11. Papillary carcinoma. Papillary groups in the thyroid often have the typical villus or finger-like shape seen here. There are multiple planes of focus within the papillary group. The most important papillary feature is the smooth border surrounding the whole structure. There is nuclear atypia and some crowding and overlapping of the nuclei. There is also minimal size and shape variation of the nuclei (Papanicolaou stain, ×400).

ploidy found in adenomas, but the only patient to die of tumor in this series had a Hürthle cell carcinoma that was aneuploid.

My personal bias at the present time is not to definitively distinguish follicular carcinoma from adenoma by FNA specimen.[7] I make a diagnosis of "suspicious for follicular tumor, suggest surgical biopsy" whenever any atypical growth pattern is present or if there is enough epithelial atypia to raise the possibility of a well-differentiated follicular carcinoma. The larger and more pleomorphic the follicular nuclei, the higher the likelihood that the lesion will ultimately prove to be a carcinoma; however, examination of the surgical specimen is necessary to determine whether vascular and/or capsular invasion is present.

A number of studies have examined the issue of whether there are valid criteria for the separation of proliferative follicular lesions. Results are mixed, although recent studies indicate that progress is being made. Sassi *et al.*[98] used morphometry to measure a variety of parameters and found that mean values of nuclear area, perimeter, and maximum diameter were significantly different between adenomas and carcinomas although there was some overlap. Nuclear area measurements had an accuracy of 77% in discriminating benign from malignant lesions.

A similar study by Cavallari *et al.*[19] also found mean nuclear area to be significantly higher in carcinomas as compared to adenomas, and also in adeno-

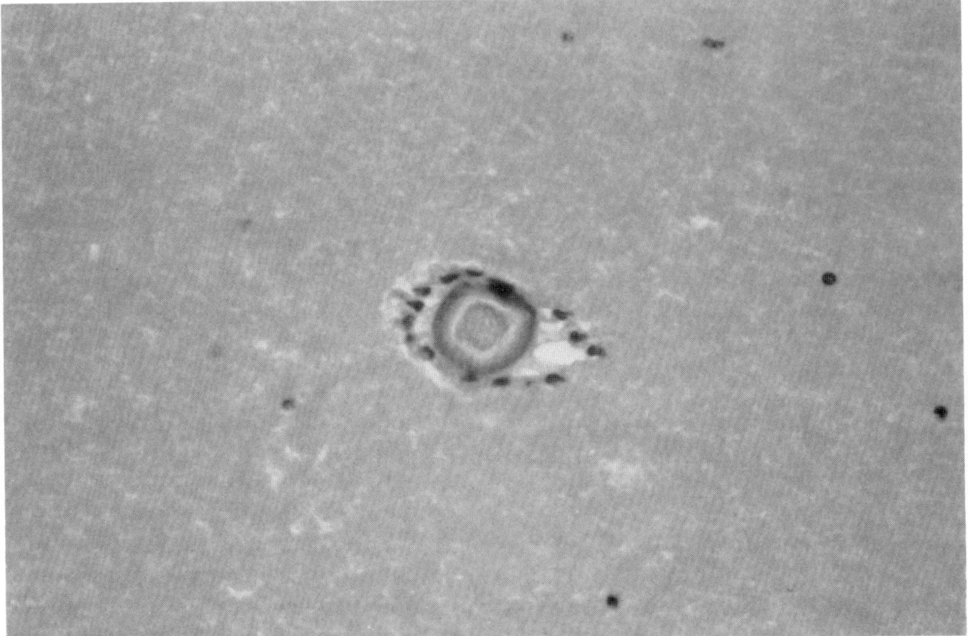

FIG. 8.12.   Papillary carcinoma. The psammoma body seen here has a characteristic lamellar structure. It is surrounded by very bland, slightly degenerate cells. In this case the patient had a papillary carcinoma, but occasionally psammoma bodies may be seen in benign lesions (H & E stain, ×125).

mas as compared to nontoxic goiters. They found, however, that using these data in linear discriminant analysis, they were unable to differentiate benign from malignant tumors or goiters from adenoma. They concluded that this technique was not able to differentiate these lesions.

LaRosa *et al.*[75] analyzed similar parameters and agreed that mean values of nuclear area showed significant differences between the three groups. They also found considerable overlap in size distribution of nuclei, and they concluded that it was not possible to categorize cases on the basis of nuclear size.

On a more positive note, Montironi *et al.*[88] correlated a variety of nuclear features including size with DNA content in a series of patients with adenomas and carcinomas. They first determined that there were two significant parameters and then they further validated these parameters in a new set of patients. They found that the combined evaluation of these two parameters (the mean of the major nuclear diameter and the percentage of nucleolated nuclei) allowed distinction between follicular adenoma and carcinoma. In their second test set they were able to determine that these parameters led to a diagnostic accuracy of 87%, a sensitivity of 86%, a specificity of 88%, a predictive value of adenoma of 88%, and a predictive value of carcinoma of 85%. They concluded that the mean of nuclear diameter and percentage of nucleolated nuclei are valuable diagnostic parameters in evaluation of follicular lesions.

Joint collaborations between investigators in Chicago and Spain have led to

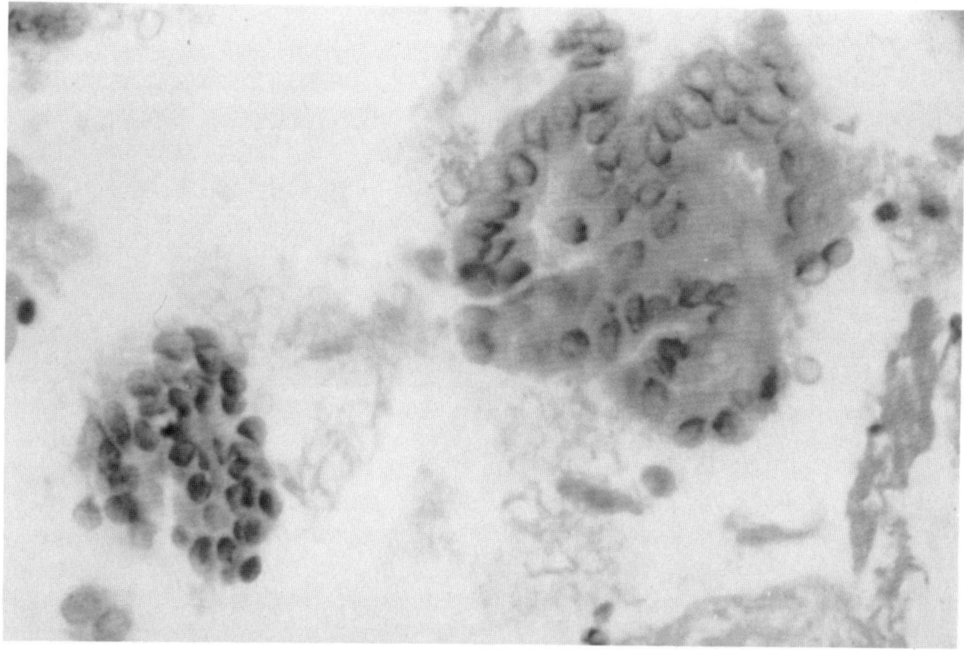

FIG. 8.13. Follicular variant of papillary cancer. The small cells with hyperchromatic nuclei are relatively normal. These may be compared to several acinar groups with enlarged nuclei and prominent clearing of the nuclear chromatin that is typical of papillary carcinoma. The nuclear membrane is distinct. This type of nuclear clearing is suggestive of papillary carcinoma, but may sometimes be seen in other entities such as Hashimoto's thyroiditis and follicular tumors (Papanicolaou stain, ×250).

reports on karyometric measurements of 95 nuclear features in several series of cases. They found that several features produce statistically significant discrimination of normal nuclei from adenoma nuclei,[78] invasive follicular carcinoma nuclei from normal nuclei,[38] and microinvasive follicular carcinoma nuclei from normal nuclei.[13]

All of these studies and the many others reported in the literature suggest that a discriminatory test for follicular lesions may be developed in the future. At present these techniques still appear to be in the research and development phase and have not yet become clinical, diagnostic tests.

MALIGNANT LYMPHOMA

Malignant lymphoma has already been mentioned under Hashimoto's thyroiditis and has been discussed by Matsuda *et al.*[84] A determination of monomorphism of the lymphoid population is the most helpful feature (Figs. 8.24 and 8.25). Malignant lymphoma in the thyroid is usually large cell type. The cells may be markedly enlarged and pleomorphic and may even be mistaken for anaplastic carcinoma. It is important to order immunoperoxidase markers such as leukocyte common antigen when lymphoma is a possibility. More specific markers can be used to classify the tumor as a B-cell type.[57] Two markers, CD45RO (UCHL1)

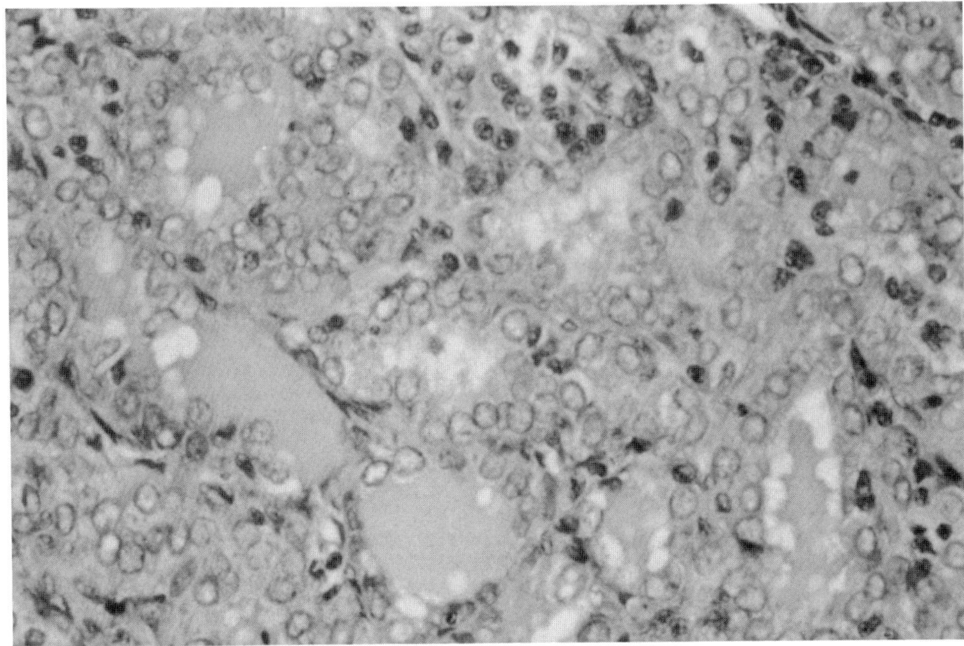

FIG. 8.14.   Follicular variant of papillary cancer. This cell block preparation demonstrates the uniform, monomorphic appearance of the nuclear clearing that is typical of papillary carcinoma. In this case the follicular organization is quite prominent and colloid is easily identified (H & E stain, ×250).

and CD20 (L26), may also be used on paraffin-embedded material. However, immunocytochemical studies are not usually helpful in a practical sense for distinguishing between lymphoma and Hashimoto's thyroiditis.[107]

MEDULLARY CARCINOMA

Cytologic features of medullary carcinoma have been described[67] as have the clinical and histopathologic manifestations of this disease.[108] Cells of medullary carcinoma can be relatively bland and may not be that different in cytologic appearance from normal follicular cells or cells of a follicular tumor. They are usually slightly larger and have somewhat more vesicular nuclei than typically seen in follicular cells from nodular goiter. In addition, the cells are often less cohesive than normal follicular cells (Figs. 8.26 and 8.27).

If spindle cells are seen, this is very helpful in suggesting medullary carcinoma, but many medullary carcinomas do not have a spindled component. Nuclei of the spindled component are often cigar-shaped and have slightly hyperchromatic chromatin. Some medullary carcinomas have cells that are very large and bizarre. True follicles are not seen and colloid is either not present or is sparse. Amyloid is rarely seen in FNA, but when it is present it may resemble colloid. Being denser than colloid, it can be differentiated. Rarely mucin may be seen in medullary carcinomas.[45]

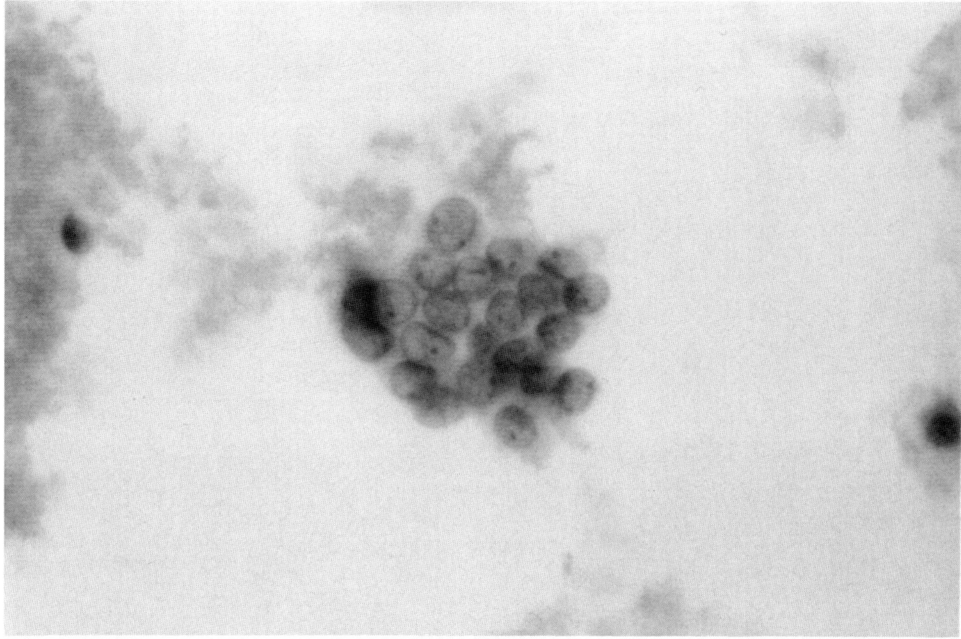

FIG. 8.15. Follicular variant of papillary cancer. In this follicular group the nuclear clearing is not as apparent as in the previous figures; however, nuclear grooves are identified. Nuclear grooves are common in papillary carcinoma but are not specific for this entity (Papanicolaou stain, ×400).

Calcitonin is an excellent immunocytochemical marker for medullary carcinoma and should be used whenever this diagnosis is a possibility. It is worthwhile to order this test whenever there are spindled cells, dense material suspicious for amyloid, or atypical, relatively uncohesive follicular-like cells present. Commercially available antibodies to calcitonin are highly sensitive, and the immunocytochemical reaction works very well on fixed cells. If no additional material on a suspicious sample is available, then the coverslip can be removed and the stain applied on slides previously Papanicolaou-stained. Carcinoembryonic antigen is also usually present in medullary carcinomas, so the use of calcitonin and carcinoembryonic antigen with thyroglobulin provide an effective panel to discriminate medullary versus follicular tumor. Serum calcitonin levels can also be measured if there is any question of the diagnosis.

Medullary carcinoma is an uncommon tumor, but it is an important diagnosis to make since a preoperative workup for multiple endocrine neoplasia syndrome can then be performed. Medullary carcinoma is an example of a tumor in which a cell product has provided a tool to further advance the understanding of the disease process.[27] Additional discussions of the diagnostic features of medullary carcinoma are found in several recent articles[2,31] and Chapter 4 of this volume.

ANAPLASTIC CARCINOMA

Anaplastic carcinoma is the only primary tumor of the thyroid that has the cytologic criteria of malignancy that are typical of these seen in other sites. Cells

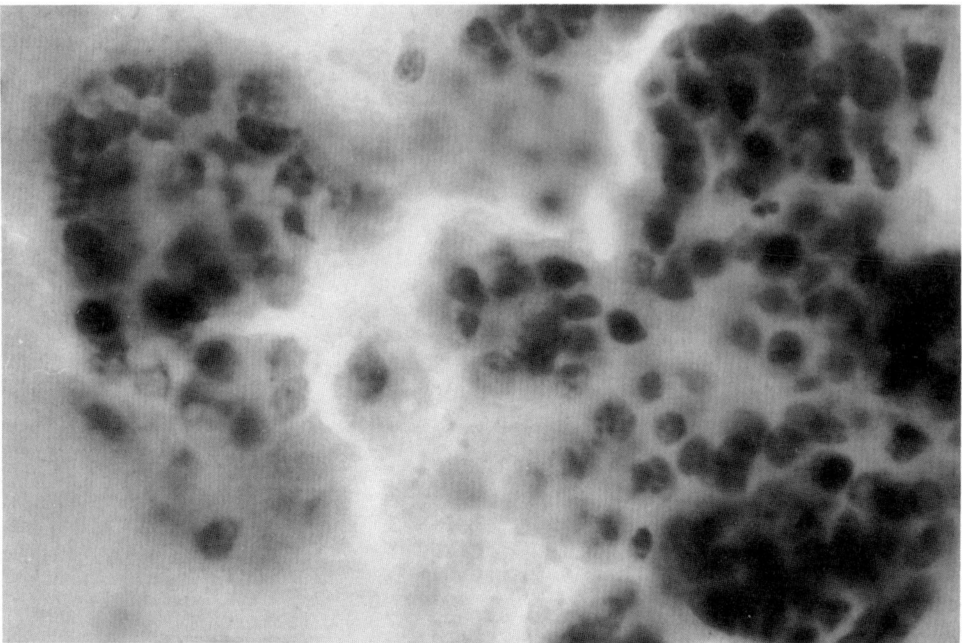

FIG. 8.16. Papillary carcinoma. There are no papillary groups present here; all the groups are follicular in appearance. Nuclear abnormalities are typical of papillary carcinoma and include variation in size and shape of the nuclei, variations in the density of the chromatin, and nucleoli. Occasional nuclei show chromatin clearing (Papanicolaou stain, ×250).

of anaplastic carcinoma are usually large and bizarre[16] (Figs. 8.28 and 8.29). Sometimes numerous giant cells are present.[9] Nuclei are often multilobated, and the chromatin is clumped with prominent parachromatin clearing and multiple prominent nucleoli.[43] There is usually no follicular growth pattern but rather sheets of cohesive and uncohesive malignant cells. The typical clinical setting is an elderly patient with a tumor that has enlarged rapidly. The mass is usually large, firm, and fixed to adjacent structures. There is often tracheal obstruction. If the clinical setting is not typical, the diagnosis is probably not anaplastic carcinoma. In these cases it is necessary to exclude malignant lymphoma and to consider a diagnosis of metastatic carcinoma. Immunocytochemical studies are useful to rule out other lesions, especially malignant lymphoma. A recent study found thyroglobulin to be positive in only 27% of cases of anaplastic carcinoma and calcitonin never positive.[82] In 30% of anaplastic carcinoma cases, there was no reactivity to any of a wide variety of markers.

When a diagnosis of anaplastic carcinoma is considered, the possibility of metastatic tumor must be raised. Panels of antibodies can be used to test and classify thyroid lesions. Since most primary thyroid tumors express either thyroglobulin or calcitonin, availability of appropriate antibodies is important. Leukocyte common antigen is used because malignant lymphoma can often resemble an epithelial tumor. Several groups have found that papillary carcinoma and follicular carcinoma express a variety of epithelial markers. In one study all

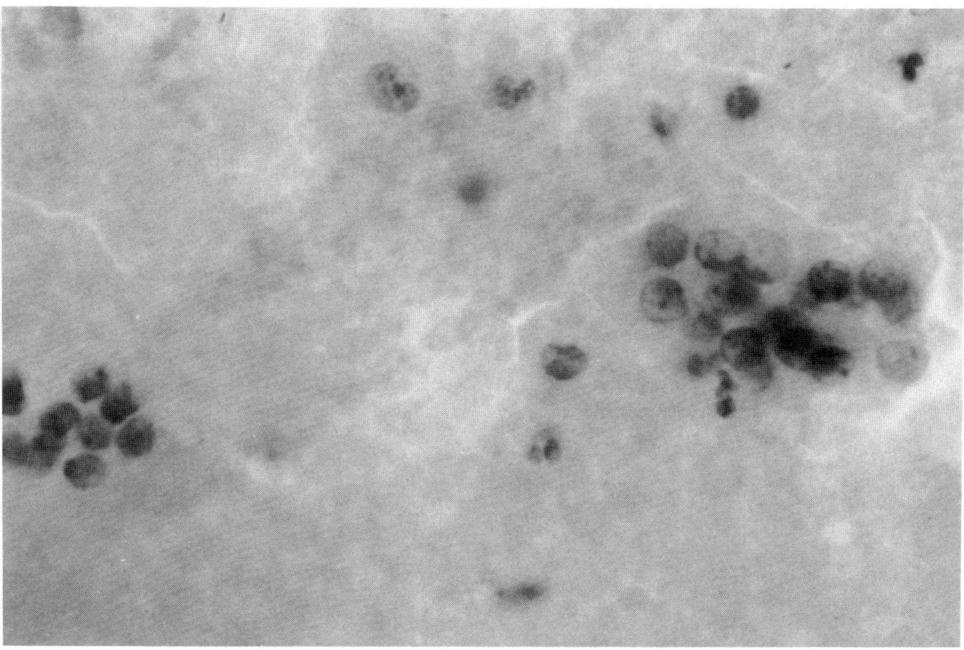

FIG. 8.17. Follicular neoplasia. A group of normal follicular cells is seen at one edge of the field which may be used for comparison to the cells of a follicular tumor. The increase in size of the nuclei is apparent, as is the more vesicular quality of the chromatin pattern. There is also an abnormal crowding and overlap of the nuclei (Papanicolaou stain, ×400).

cases of papillary carcinoma expressed thyroglobulin and cytokeratin and a high proportion also expressed estrogen receptor; however, the clinical significance of estrogen receptor positivity is unknown.[29]

UNUSUAL THYROID LESIONS

Cytologic appearance and diagnostic criteria of several unusual types of thyroid tumors have been recently reported including hyalanizing trabecular adenoma,[39,106] diffuse sclerosing carcinoma,[18] insular carcinoma,[92] and columnar carcinoma.[56] Any subtype of thyroid tumor that is described by histopathology should soon have an appearance reported by FNA.

METASTATIC CARCINOMA AND OTHER TUMORS

Although any tumor may metastasize to the thyroid, the more common tumors include renal cell carcinoma,[30,44] lung carcinoma (any type), breast carcinoma, other adenocarcinomas including colon carcinoma,[23] squamous carcinoma and melanoma.[72,83] Kini *et al.*[69] discussed diagnostic features of metastatic carcinoma to the thyroid. Sarcomas may also be metastatic[36,37] or may invade the thyroid by local extension of a neck primary. Metastasis should be suspected when there are obviously malignant cells which do not fit the pattern of any primary thyroid neoplasm. Immunocytochemical studies can sometimes be useful to distinguish

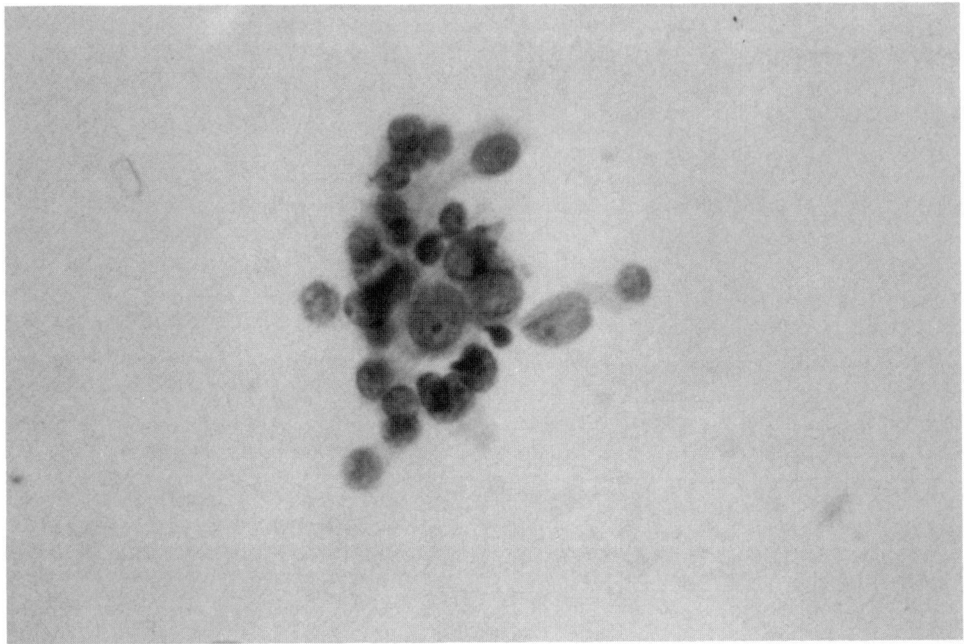

FIG. 8.18.   Follicular neoplasia. In this follicular group there is major variation in size of the nuclei within a single follicle group. There is also piling and crowding of the nuclei, as well as variation in chromatin pattern. Nucleoli are prominent in some of the cells (Papanicolaou stain, ×400).

such cases from primary thyroid tumors. Hodgkin's disease can rarely present as an enlarged thyroid[41] as can histiocytosis X.[40]

Occasionally, cervical lymph nodes, parathyroid glands,[25,86] and salivary gland tumors are mistaken for thyroid lesions. Cystic parathyroid lesions can be particularly difficult to differentiate from thyroid neoplasms.[76] Rarely a thymoma may extend into the neck and present as an apparent thyroid mass.[109]

When thyroid carcinoma presents as a metastasis, an aspirate of the lesion as well as of the thyroid is the most effective approach to confirm the diagnosis. Some diagnostic criteria for metastatic thyroid tumors have been presented.[93]

COMPLICATIONS

Complications of thyroid FNA are unusual. There is a recent report of one case of needle tract implantation of a papillary carcinoma of the thyroid following FNA.[46] A more common clinical problem is hemorrhage after aspiration. This rarely causes clinical problems, but it may cause internal hemorrhage into the aspirated lesion. At the time of surgical resection of such a nodule, there will be evidence of hemorrhage and there may be active granulation tissue, depending on the time interval since the FNA. Other histopathologic complications include infarction,[3] necrosis,[62,77] and papillary endothelial hyperplasia.[8] Artifacts related to prior aspiration must therefore be considered in evaluation of any surgically resected thyroid lesion, but they do not negate the usefulness of the aspiration.

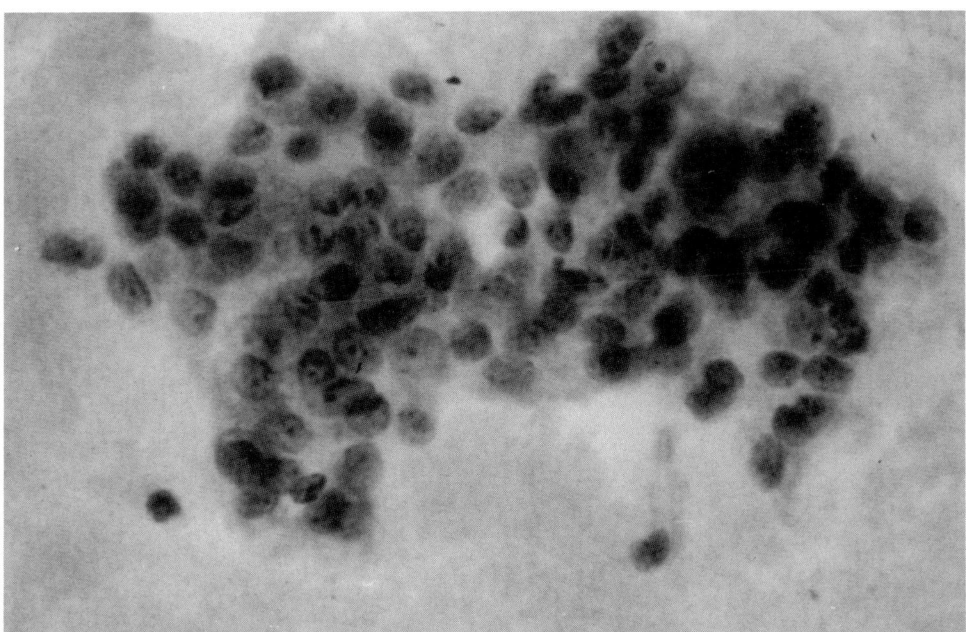

FIG. 8.19. Follicular neoplasia. In this sheet of cells there is no apparent follicular structure. There is disarray of the nuclei with evidence of piling and crowding. Nucleoli are particularly prominent. The size of nuclei is large compared to normal follicular nuclei (Papanicolaou stain, ×400).

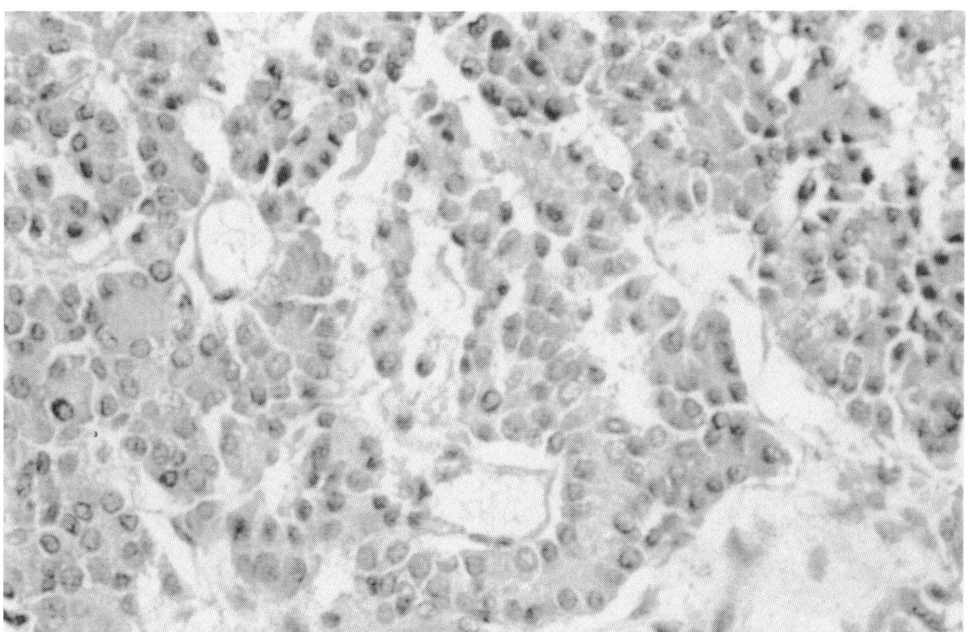

FIG. 8.20. Follicular neoplasia. In this cell block preparation there is a lack of normal follicular structure. At least one small follicle is present, but a trabecular pattern is more prominent. Note the relatively bland appearance of the nuclei although there is some variation in chromatin pattern and minimal architectural abnormality (H & E stain, ×125).

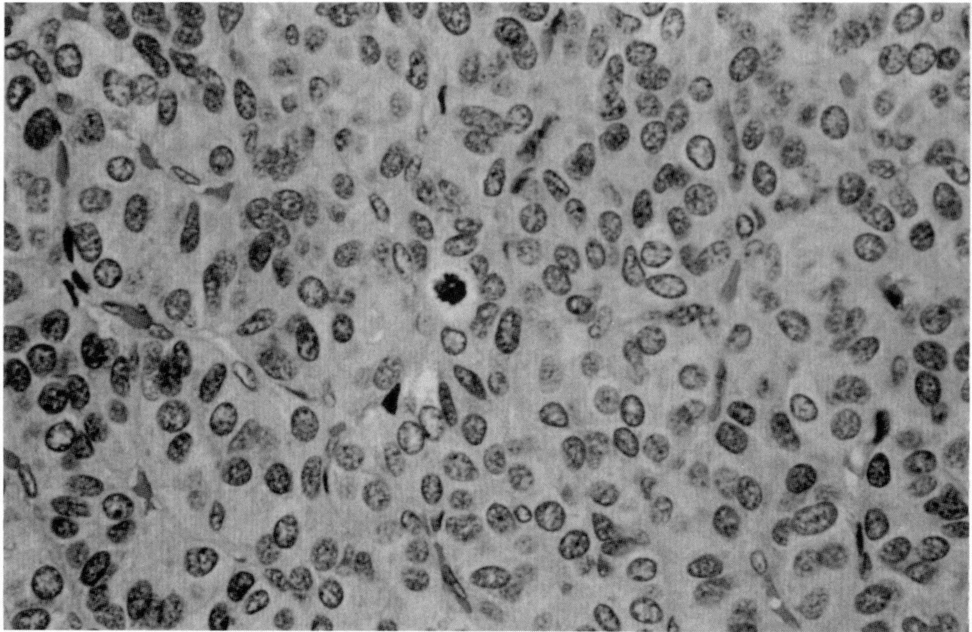

FIG. 8.21.   Follicular neoplasia. The architectural arrangement is solid and trabecular. A mitosis is prominent in the center of the field. A mitosis found in a follicular cell is a very worrisome feature (H & E stain, ×250).

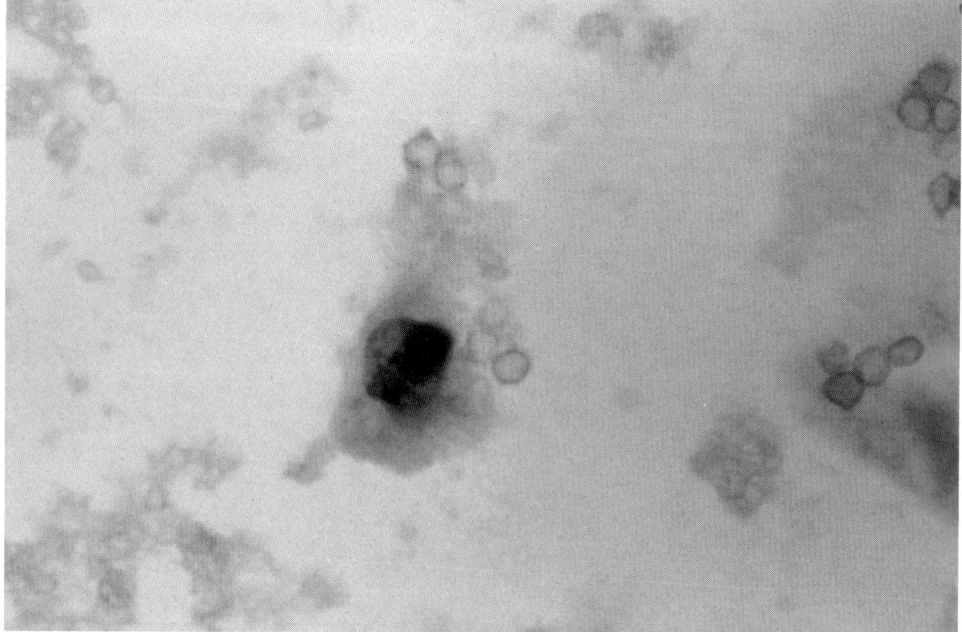

FIG. 8.22.   Hürthle cell tumor. This large cell can be identified as a Hürthle cell because of its abundant granular cytoplasm. The nucleus is enlarged, but the nuclear to cytoplasmic ratio is normal. Dark, angular nuclei such as these are sometimes seen in Hürthle cells (Papanicolaou stain, × 400).

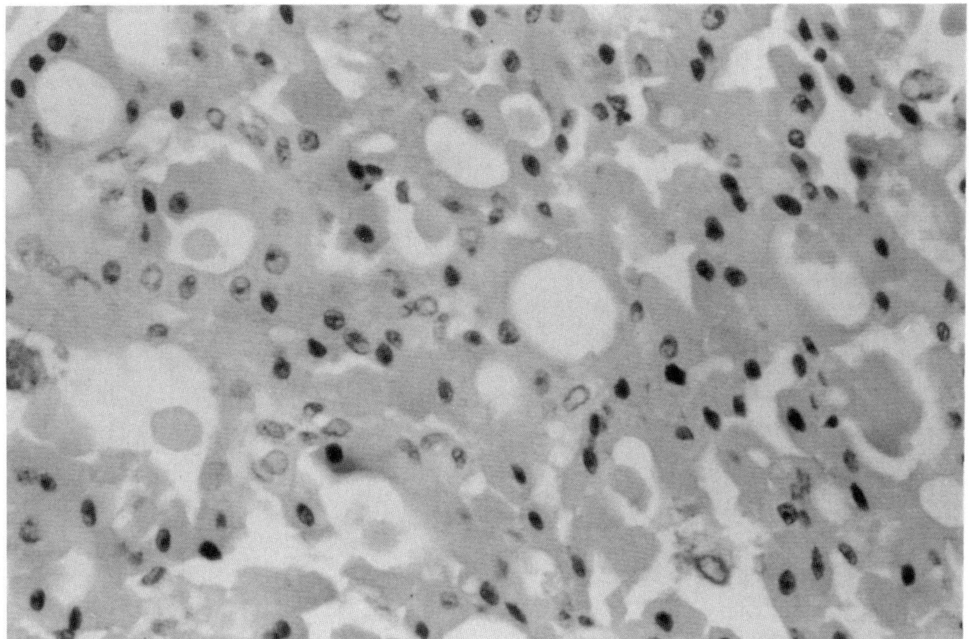

FIG. 8.23. Hürthle cell tumor. Numerous Hürthle cells are seen in this cell block and are organized in trabecular and follicular patterns. Some of the nuclei have the hyperchromatic, angular nuclei and others have a more normal appearance. Abundant cytoplasm is particularly apparent (H & E stain, ×250).

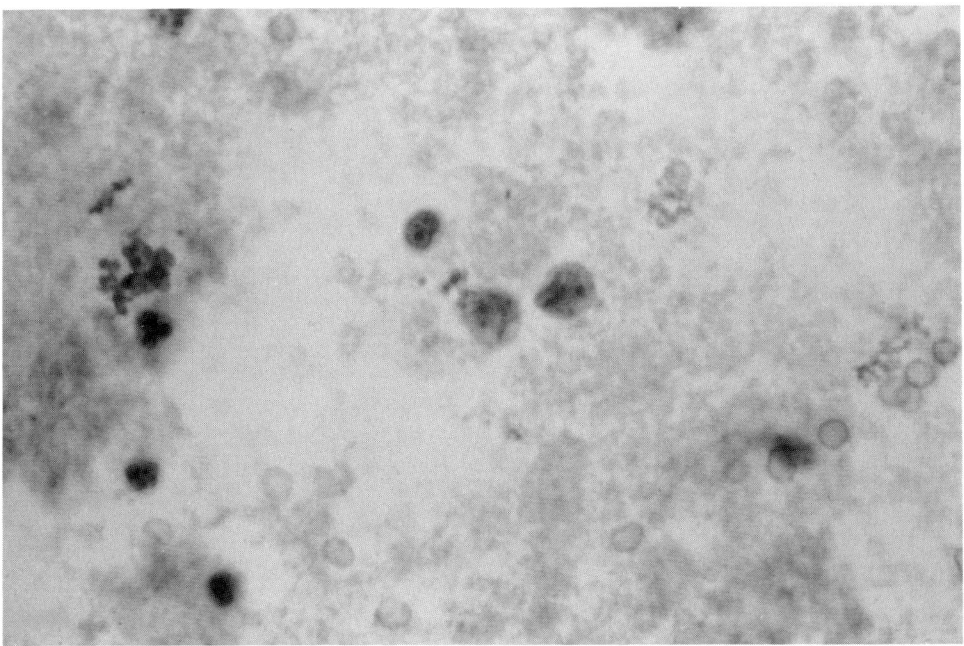

FIG. 8.24. Malignant lymphoma. Distinction of cells of malignant lymphoma from activated lymphocytes of Hashimoto's thyroiditis can be very difficult. It is necessary to see a uniform population of atypical lymphoid cells. This diagnosis should only be made with extreme care. The cells seen here are large lymphoid cells with irregular chromatin clumping. At least one cell has a prominent nucleolus (Papanicolaou stain, ×400).

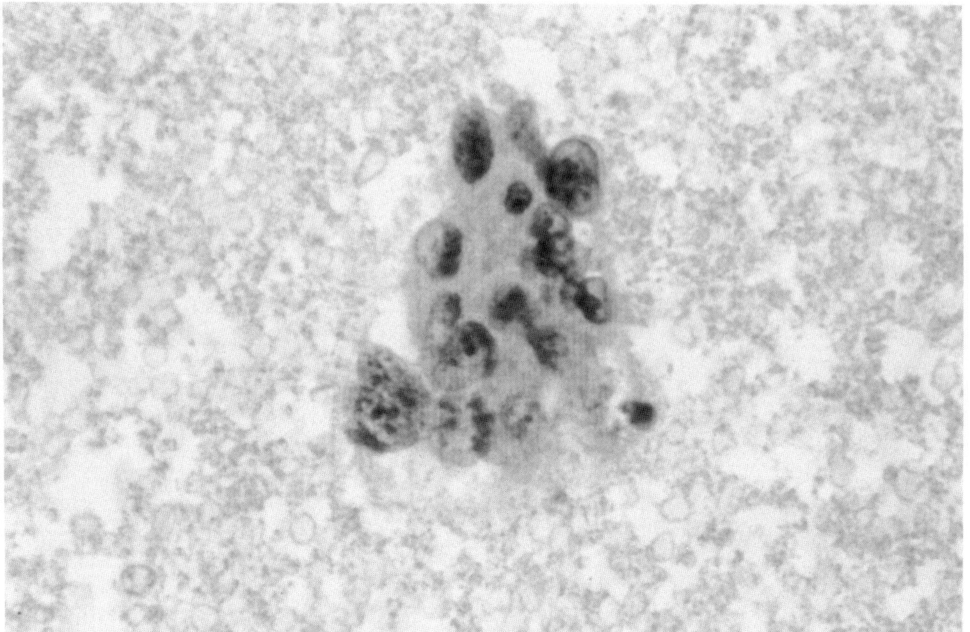

FIG. 8.25.   Malignant lymphoma. In this cell block preparation the malignant lymphoid cells appear to be clustered together in a group. This may sometimes be seen in a FNA from a lymphoma. The needle does a mini-biopsy of the tissue and cells may appear to be cohesive when they are not. Leukocyte common antigen can be used to distinguish these cells from epithelial cells (H & E stain, ×400).

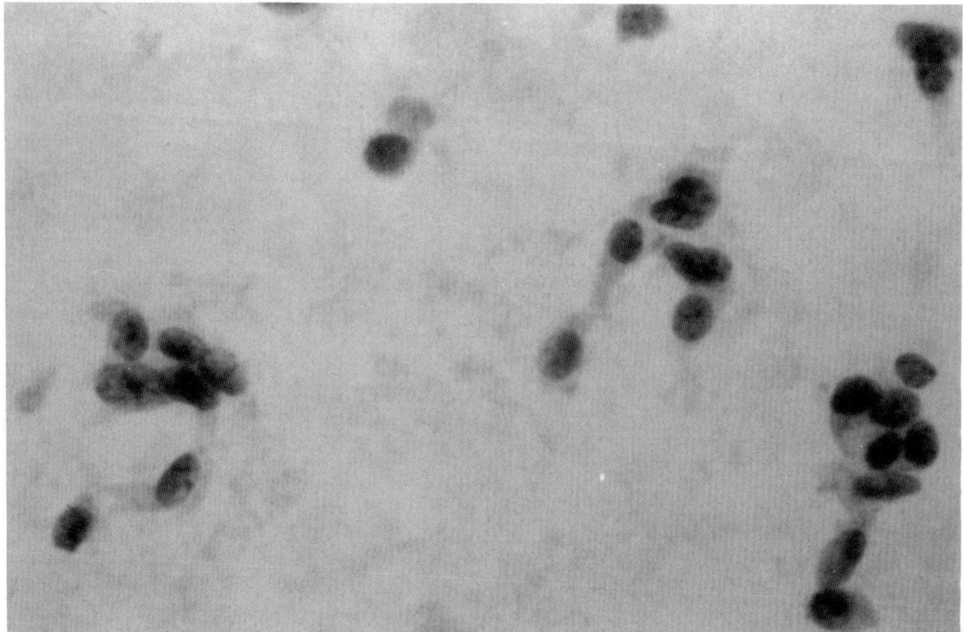

FIG. 8.26.   Medullary carcinoma. The cells seen here show lack of cohesion and follicular structure. The nuclei are about the same size as slightly enlarged follicular nuclei. Several of the cells have an elongated spindled cytoplasm. In order to confirm that this is a medullary carcinoma it is necessary to do immunoperoxidase stains for thyrocalcitonin (Papanicolaou stain, ×400).

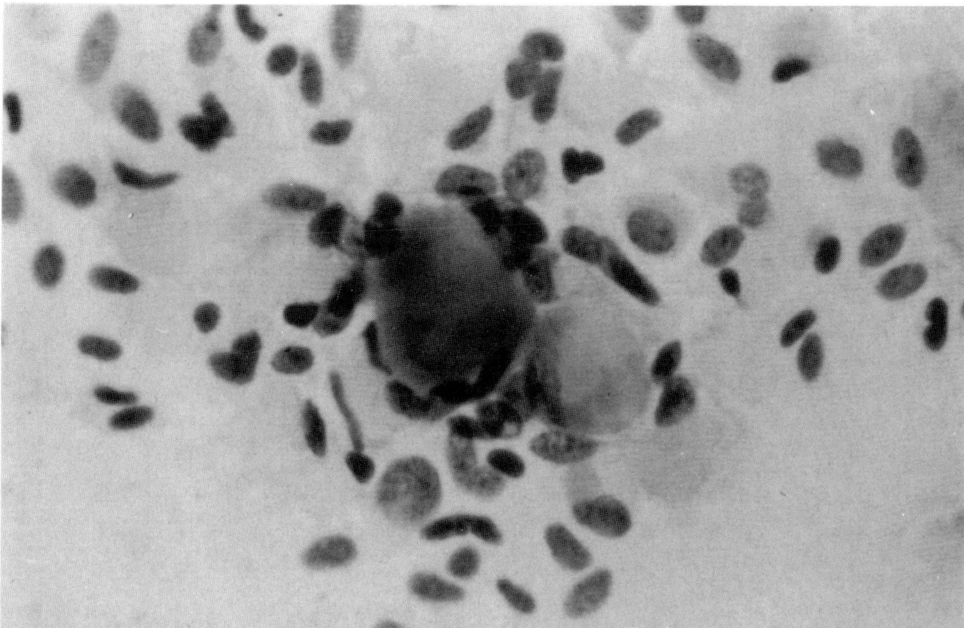

FIG. 8.27. Medullary carcinoma. Amyloid is present in the center of this field. It may be similar in appearance to colloid; however, it is usually more dense. Notice the variation in size and shape of the nuclei of the tumor cells and the spindled shape of many of these nuclei (Papanicolaou stain, ×400).

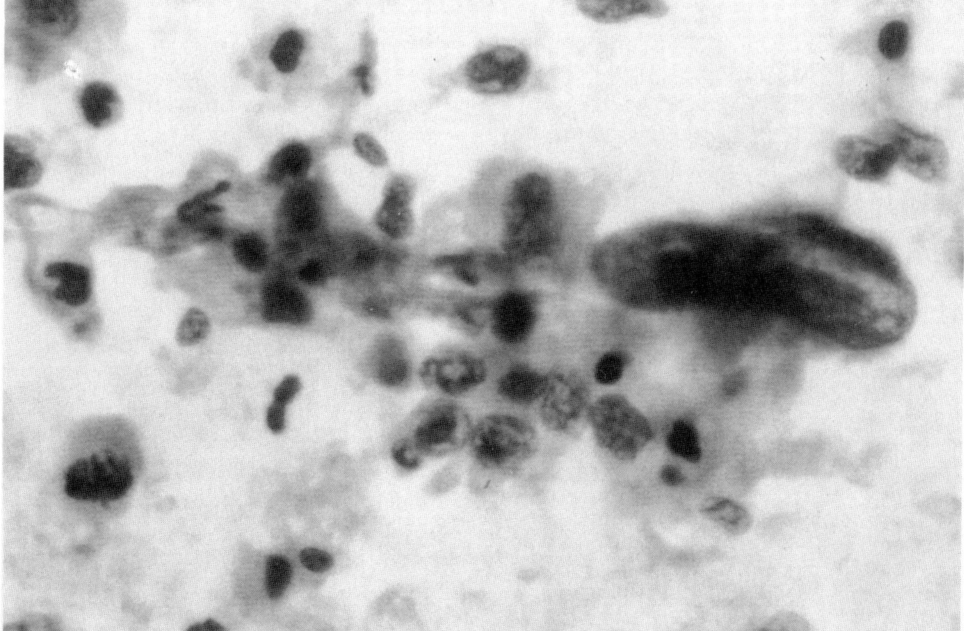

FIG. 8.28. Anaplastic carcinoma. The large size of the cells and this degree of pleomorphism are only seen with anaplastic carcinoma or metastatic tumor (Papanicolaou stain, ×400).

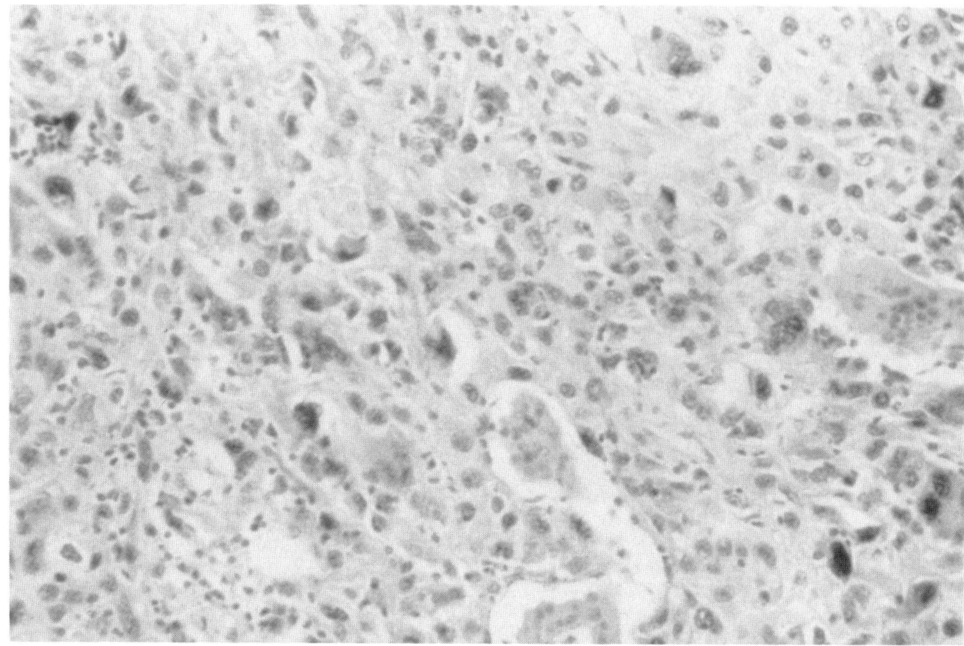

FIG. 8.29. Anaplastic carcinoma. This cell block preparation demonstrates the lack of architectural arrangement as well as the pleomorphism of the individual cells. This is typical of anaplastic carcinoma (H & E stain, ×125).

CONCLUSIONS

Thyroid FNA is now recognized as a reliable, safe, and effective test to determine which patients require surgical resection of a thyroid nodule. It is also prudent to reserve a diagnosis of definite malignancy for those unequivocal cases such as anaplastic carcinoma or papillary carcinoma with all the diagnostic criteria. If diagnostic pitfalls are avoided,[54] then a positive impact can be made on the care of patients with thyroid nodules.

ACKNOWLEDGMENTS

The author would like to thank and acknowledge Mary E. Dooney and Sheila Gillespie for secretarial assistance and Drs. Amy Llewelyn and Catherine R. Looby for critical review of the manuscript.

REFERENCES

1. Aggarawal, S. K., Jayaranm, G., Kakar, A., Goel, G. D., Prakash, R., and Pant, S. Fine needle aspiration in cytologic diagnosis of the solitary cold thyroid nodule. Comparison with ultrasonography radionuclide perfusion study and xeroradiography. *Acta Cytol. 33:*41–47, 1989.
2. Albores-Saavedra, J., LiVolsi, V. A., and Williams, E. D. Medullary carcinoma. *Semin. Diagn. Pathol. 2:*137–146, 1985.
3. Alejo, M., Matias-Cruiu, X., and delas Heras-Duran, P. Infarction of a papillary thyroid carcinoma after fine needle aspiration. *Acta Cytol. 35:*478–479, 1991.

4. Altavilla, G., Pascale, M., and Nenci, I. Fine needle aspiration cytology of thyroid gland diseases. *Acta Cytol. 34:*251–256, 1990.
5. Atkinson, B. F. Carbowax fixation of needle aspirates. *Diagn. Cytopathol. 2:*231–232, 1986.
6. Atkinson, B. F., ed. *Atlas of Diagnostic Cytopathology.* Philadephia, W. B. Saunders, 1992.
7. Atkinson, B. F., Grotkowski, C. S., and LiVolsi, V. A. Cytologic diagnoses of follicular tumors of the thyroid. *Diagn. Cytopathol. 2:*1–3, 1986.
8. Axiotis, C. A., Merino, M. J., Ain, K., and Norton, J. A. Papillary epithelial hyperplasia in the thyroid following fine-needle aspiration. *Arch. Pathol. Lab. Med. 115:*240–242, 1991.
9. Berry, B., MacFarlane, J., and Chan, N. Osteoclastomalike anaplastic carcinoma of the thyroid. Diagnosis by fine needle aspiration cytology. *Acta Cytol. 34:*248–250, 1990.
10. Betsil, W. Thyroid fine needle aspiration in pregnant women. *Diagn. Cytopathol. 1:*53–54, 1985.
11. Bhambhani, S., Kashyap, V., and Das, D. K. Nuclear grooves. Valuable diagnostic feature in May-Grunwald-Giemsa-stained fine needle aspirates of papillary carcinoma of the thyroid. *Acta Cytol. 34:*809–812, 1990.
12. Bibbo, M., ed. *Comprehensive Cytopathology.* Philadelphia, W. B. Saunders, 1991.
13. Bibbo, M., Bartels, P. H., Salguero, M., Dytch, H. E., Lerma-Puertas, E., and Galera-Davidson, H. Karyometric marker features in fine needle aspirates of microinvasive follicular carcinoma of the thyroid. *Anal. Quant. Cytol. Histol. 12:*42–47, 1990.
14. Block, M. A., Dailey, G. E., III, and Muchmore, D. Avoiding reoperation for indeterminate thyroid nodules identified as malignant after surgery. *Arch. Surg. 126:*598–602, 1991.
15. Bronner, M. P., Clevenger, C. V., Edmonds, P. R., Lowell, D. M., McFarland, M. M., and LiVolsi, V. A. Flow cytometric analysis of DNA content in Hürthle cell adenomas and carcinomas of the thyroid. *Am. J. Clin. Pathol. 89:*764–769, 1988.
16. Carcangiu, M. L., Steeper, T., Zampi, G., and Rosai, J. Anaplastic thyroid carcinoma: A study of 70 cases. *Am. J. Clin. Pathol. 83:*135–158, 1985.
17. Carpi, A., DiCoscio, G., and Toscano, S. Needle aspiration of thyroid nodule: Long-term control of its efficiency in preoperative selection. *Thyroidology 1:*35–39, 1988.
18. Caruso, G., Tabarri, B., Lucchi, I., and Tison, V. Fine needle aspiration cytology in a case of diffuse sclerosing carcinoma of the thyroid. *Acta Cytol. 34:*352–354, 1990.
19. Cavallari, V., Maiorana, A., LaRosa, G. L., Mairana, M. C., Scimone, S., and Fano, R. S. Morphometric studies on fine-needle aspirates from follicular proliferative lesions of the thyroid. *Pathologica 81:*441–446, 1989.
20. Chen, K. T. Fine-needle aspiration cytology of papillary Hürthle-cell tumors of thyroid: A report of three cases. *Diagn. Cytopathol. 7:*53–56, 1991.
21. Cooper, D. S., Tiamson, E., and Ladenson, P. W. Psammoma bodies in fine needle aspiration biopsies of benign thyroid nodules. *Thyroidology 1:*55–59, 1988.
22. Cristallini, E. G., and Bolis, G. B. Fine-needle aspiration biopsy in the preoperative diagnosis of solitary thyroid nodules. *Appl. Pathol. 7:*149–153, 1989.
23. Cristallini, E. G., Bolis, F. B., and Francucci, M. Diagnosis of thyroid metastasis of colonic adenocarcinoma by fine needle aspiration biopsy. *Acta Cytol. 34:*363–365, 1990.
24. Cusick, E. L., MacIntosh, C. A., Krukowski, Z. H., Williams, V. M., Ewen, S. W., and Matheson, N. A. Management of isolated thyroid swellings: A prospective six year study of fine needle aspiration cytology in diagnosis. *Br. Med. J. [Clin. Res.] 301:*318–321, 1990.
25. Davey, D. D., Glant, M. D., and Berger, E. K. Parathyroid cytopathology. *Diagn. Cytopathol. 2:*76–80, 1986.
26. Davies, T. F., Martin, S., Concepcion, E. S., Graves, P., Lahat, N., Cohen, W. L., and Ben-Nun, A. Evidence for selective accumulation of intrathyroid T lymphocytes in human autoimmune thyroid disease based on cell receptor V gene usage. *Clin. Invest. 89:*157–162, 1992.
27. DeLellis, R. A., and Wolfe, H. J. Contributions of immunohistochemical and molecular biological techniques to endocrine pathology. *Histochem. Cytochem. 35:*1347–1351, 1987.
28. Denmeure, M. J., and Clark, O. H. Surgery in the treatment of thyroid cancer. *Endocrinol. Metab. Clin. North Am. 19:*663–683, 1990.
29. Diaz, N. M., Mazoujian, G., and Wick, M. R. Estrogen-receptor protein in thyroid neoplasms. *Arch. Pathol. Lab. Med. 15:*1203–1207, 1991.

30. Domegala, W., Lasota, J., Wolska, H., Lubinski, J., Weber, K., and Osborn, M. Diagnosis of metastatic renal cell and thyroid carcinoma by intermediate filament typing and cytology of tumor cells in fine needle aspirates. *Acta Cytol. 32:*415–421, 1988.

31. Driman, D., Murray, D., Kovacs, K., Lucia, S., and Higgins, H. P. Encapsulated medullary carcinoma of the thyroid. *Am. J. Surg. Pathol. 15:*1089–1095, 1991.

32. Dugan, J. M., Atkinson, B. F., Avitabile, A., Schimmel, M., and LiVolsi, V. A. Psammoma bodies in fine needle aspirate of the thyroid in lymphocytic thyroiditis. *Acta Cytol. 31:*330–334, 1987.

33. Dwarakanathan, A. A., Ryan, W. G., Staren, E. D., Martirano, M., and Economou, S. G. Fine-needle aspiration biopsy of the thyroid. Diagnostic accuracy when performing a moderate number of such procedures. *Arch. Intern. Med. 149:*2007–2009, 1989.

34. Faroux, M. J., Pluot, M., Delisle, M. J., and Coninx, P. Evaluation of morphological criteria in the cytological diagnosis of thyroid cold nodules. *Pathol. Res. Pract. 186:*330-335, 1990.

35. Frable, W. J. *Thin-Needle Aspiration Biopsy.* San Francisco, W. B. Saunders, 1983.

36. Gattuso, P., Castelli, M. J., and Reyes, C. V. Fine needle aspiration cytology of metastatic sarcoma involving the thyroid. *South. Med. J. 82:*1158–1160, 1989.

37. Geisinger, K. R., Silverman, J. F., Cappellari, J. O., and Dabbs, D. J. Fine-needle aspiration cytology of malignant hemangiopericytomas with ultrastructural and flow cytometric analyses. *Arch. Pathol. Lab. Med. 114:*705–710, 1990.

38. Glaera-Davidson, H., Bartels, P. H., Fernandez-Rodriques, A., Dytch, H. E., Lerma-Puertas, E., and Bibbo, M. Karyometric marker features in fine needle aspirates of invasive follicular carcinoma of the thyroid. *Anal. Quant. Cytol. Histol. 12:*35–41, 1990.

39. Goellner, J. R., and Carney, J. A. Cytologic features of fine-needle aspirates of hyalinizing trabecular adenoma of the thyroid. *Am. J. Clin. Pathol. 91:*115–119, 1989.

40. Goldstein, N., and Layfield, L. J. Thyromegaly secondary to simultaneous papillary carcinoma and histiocytosis. X. Report of a case and review of the literature. *Acta Cytol. 35:*442–446, 1991.

41. Granados, R., Pinkus, G. S., West, P., and Cibas, E. S. Hodgkin's disease presenting as an enlarged thyroid gland. Report of a case diagnosed by fine needle aspiration. *Acta Cytol. 35:*439–442, 1991.

42. Grant, C. S., Hay, I. D., Gough, I. R., McCarthy, P. M., and Goellner, J. R. Long-term follow-up of patients with benign thyroid fine-needle aspiration cytologic diagnoses. *Surgery 106:*980–985, 1989.

43. Guardia, L. A., Peterson, C. E., Hall, W., and Baskin, H. J. Anaplastic thyroid carcinoma: Cytomorphology and clinical implications of fine-needle aspiration. *Diagn. Cytopathol. 7:*63–67, 1991.

44. Halbauer, M., Kardum-Skelin, I., Vrane, D., and Crepinko, I. Aspiration cytology of renal-cell carcinoma metastatic to the thyroid. *Acta Cytol. 35:*443–446, 1991.

45. Haleem, A., Aktar, M., Ali, M. A., and Iqbal, Z. Fine-needle aspiration biopsy of mucus-producing medullary carcinoma of thyroid: Report of a case with cytologic, histologic and ultrastructural correlations. *Diagn. Cytopathol. 6:*112–117, 1990.

46. Hales, M. S., and Hsu, F. S. Needle tract implantation of papillary carcinoma of the thyroid following aspiration biopsy. *Acta Cytol. 34:*801–804, 1990.

47. Hall, T. L., Layfield, L. J., Phillippe, A., and Rosenthal, D. L. Sources of diagnostic error in fine needle aspiration of the thyroid. *Cancer 63:*718–725, 1989.

48. Hamburger, J. I. Fine needle biopsy diagnosis of thyroid nodules: Perspective. *Thyroidology 1:*21–34, 1988.

49. Hamburger, J. I., and Husain, M. Contributions of intra-operative pathology evaluation to surgical management of thyroid nodules. *Endocrinol. Metab. Clin. North Am. 19:*509–522, 1990.

50. Hamburger, J. I., Husain, M., Nishiyama, R., Nunez, and Solomon, D. Increasing the accuracy of fine-needle biopsy for thyroid nodules. *Arch. Pathol. Lab. Med. 113:*1035–1041, 1989.

51. Hamming, J. F., Goslings, B. M., vanSteenis, G. J., vanRavenswaay Claasen, H., Hermans, J., and vandeVelde, C. J. The value of fine-needle aspiration biopsy in patients with nodular

thyroid disease divided into groups of suspicion of malignant neoplasm on clinical grounds. *Arch. Intern. Med. 150:*113–116, 1990.

52. Harach, H. R., and Zusman, S. B. Cytologic findings in the follicular variant of papillary carcinoma of the thyroid. *Acta Cytol. 36:*142–146, 1989.

53. Hedinger, C., Williams, E. D., and Sobin, L. H. Histological typing of thyroid tumors. *International Histological Classification of Tumors,* 2nd ed. Albany, New York, World Health Organization, 1988.

54. Hsu, C. H., and Boey, J. Diagnostic pitfalls in the fine needle aspiration of thyroid nodules. *Acta Cytol. 31:*699–704, 1987.

55. Hugh, J. C., Duggan, M. A., and Chang-Poon, V. The fine-needle aspiration appearance of the follicular variant of thyroid papillary carcinoma. A report of three cases. *Diagn. Cytopathol. 4:*196–210, 1988.

56. Hui, P. K., Chan, J. K., Cheung, P. S., and Gwi, E. Columnar cell carcinoma of the thyroid. Fine needle aspiration findings in a case. *Acta Cytol. 34:*355–358, 1990.

57. Jayaram, G., Raina, V., Singh, C. H., Chandra, M., and Marwaha, R. K. B cell lymphoma of the thyroid in Hashimoto's thyroiditis monitored by fine-needle aspiration cytology. *Diagn. Cytopathol. 6:*130–133, 1990.

58. Jayaram, G., Singh, B., and Marwaha, R. K. Graves disease. Appearance in cytologic smears from fine needle aspirates of the thyroid gland. *Acta Cytol. 33:*36–40, 1989.

59. Jones, A. J., Aitman, T. J., Edmonds, C. J., Burke, M., Hudson, E., and Tellez, M. Comparison of fine needle aspiration cytology, radioisotopic and ultrasound scanning in the management of thyroid nodules. *Postgrad. Med. J. 66:*914–917, 1990.

60. Julian, J. S., Pittman, C. E., Accettullo, L., Berg, T. A., and Albertson, D. A. Does fine-needle aspiration biopsy really spare patient thyroidectomy? *Am. Surgeon 55:*238–242, 1989.

61. Kendall, C. H. Fine needle aspiration of thyroid nodules: Three years' experience. *Clin. Pathol. 42:*23–27, 1989.

62. Keyhani-Rofagha, S., Kooner, D. S., Keyhani, M., and O'Toole, R. V. Necrosis of a Hürthle cell tumor of the thyroid following fine needle aspiration. *Acta Cytol. 34:*805–808, 1990.

63. Kini, S. R. *Guides to Clinical Aspiration Biopsy: Thyroid.* New York, Igaku-Shoin, 1987.

64. Kini, S. R., Miller, J. M., and Hamburger, J. I. Cytopathology of Hürthle cell lesions of the thyroid gland by fine needle aspiration. *Acta Cytol. 25:*647–652, 1981.

65. Kini, S. R., Miller, J. M., Hamburger, S. I., and Smith, M. J. Cytopathology of papillary carcinoma of the thyroid by fine needle aspiration. *Acta Cytol. 24:*511–521, 1980.

66. Kini, S. R., Miller, J. M., Hamburger, J. I., and Smith, M. J. Problems in the cytologic diagnosis of the "cold" thyroid nodule in patients with lymphocytic thyroiditis. *Acta Cytol. 25:*506–512, 1981.

67. Kini, S. R., Miller, J. M., Hamburger, J. I., and Smith, M. J. Cytopathologic features of medullary carcinoma of the thyroid. *Arch. Pathol. Lab Med. 108:*156–159, 1984.

68. Kini, S. R., Miller, J. M., Hamburger, S. I., and Smith, M. J. Cytopathology of follicular lesions of the thyroid. *Diagn. Cytopathol. 1:*123–132, 1985.

69. Kini, S. R., Smith, M. J., Miller, J. M., and Hamburger, J. I. Fine needle aspiration cytology of tumors metastatic to the thyroid gland. *Acta Cytol. 26:*743, 1982 (abstract).

70. Klemi, P. J., Joensuu, H., and Nylamo, E. Fine needle aspiration biopsy in the diagnosis of thyroid nodules. *Acta Cytol. 35:*434–438, 1991.

71. Kline, T. S., and Kannan, V. Aspiration biopsy cytology and melanoma. *Am. J. Clin. Pathol. 77:*597–601, 1982.

72. Kopald, K. H., Layfield, L. J., Mohrmann, R., Foshag, L. J., and Guiliano, A. E. Clarifying the role of fine-needle aspiration cytologic evaluation and frozen section examination in the operative management of thyroid cancer. *Arch. Surg. 124:*1202–1204, 1989.

73. Kung, I. T., and Yuen, R. W. Fine needle aspiration of the thyroid. Distinction between colloid nodules and follicular neoplasms using cell blocks and 21-gauge needles. *Acta Cytol. 33:*53–60, 1989.

74. LaRosa, G. L., Belfiore, A., Giuffrida, D., Sicurella, C., Ippolito, O., Russo, G., and Vigneri, R. Evaluation of the fine needle aspiration biopsy in the preoperative selection of cold thyroid nodules. *Cancer 67:*2137–2141, 1991.

75. LaRosa, G. L., Cavallari, V., Giuffrida, D., Scimone, S., LaPorta, G. A., Maiorana, M. C., Maiorana, A., and Belfiore, A. Morphometric analysis of cell nuclei from fine needle aspirates of thyroid follicular lesions does not improve the diagnostic accuracy of traditional cytologic examination. *J. Endocrinol. Invest. 13:*701–707, 1990.

76. Layfield, L. J. Fine needle aspiration cytology of cystic parathyroid lesions. A cytomorphologic overlap with cystic lesion of the thyroid. *Acta Cytol. 35:*447–450, 1991.

77. Layfield, L. J., and Lones, M. A. Necrosis in thyroid nodules after fine needle aspiration biopsy. Report of two cases. *Acta Cytol. 35:*427–430, 1991.

78. Lerma-Puertas, E., Glaera-Davidson, H., Bartels, P. H., Kim, D. H., Dytch, H. E., and Bibbo, M. Karyometric marker features in fine needle aspirates of follicular adenoma of the thyroid. *Anal. Quant. Cytol. Histol. 12:*223–228, 1990.

79. Liel, Y., Zirkin, H. J., and Sobel, R. Fine needle aspiration of the hot thyroid nodule. *Acta Cytol. 32:*866–867, 1988.

80. Linsk, J. A., and Lowhagen, T. Aspiration biopsy cytology of the thyroid gland. *Clinical Aspiration Cytology.* Philadelphia, PA, J. B. Lippincott, 1989.

81. LiVolsi, V. A. *Surgical Pathology of the Thyroid.* Philadelphia, W. B. Saunders, 1990.

82. LiVolsi, V. A., Brooks, J. J., and Arendash-Durand, B. Anaplastic thyroid tumors: Immunohistology. *Am. J. Clin. Pathol. 87:*434–442, 1987.

83. Marcus, J. N., Dise, C. A., and LiVolsi, V. A. Melanin production in a medullary thyroid carcinoma. *Cancer 49:*2518–2526, 1982.

84. Matsuda, M., Sone, H., Koyama, H., and Ishiguro, S. Fine needle aspiration cytology of malignant lymphoma of the thyroid. *Diagn. Cytopathol. 3:*244–249, 1987.

85. Miller, T. R., Bottles, K., Holly, E. A., Friend, N. F., and Abele, J. S. A step-wise logistic regression analysis of papillary carcinoma of the thyroid. *Acta Cytol. 30:*285–293, 1986.

86. Mincione, G. P., Borelli, D., Cicchi, P. Ipponi, P. L, and Fiornini, A. Fine needle aspiration cytology of parathyroid adenoma: A review of seven cases. *Acta Cytol. 30:*65–69, 1986.

87. Mizukami, Y., Michigishi, T. I., Hashimoto, T., Tonami, N., Hisaba, K., Matsubara, F., and Takazakura, E. Silent thyroiditis: A histologic and immunohistochemical study. *Hum. Pathol. 19:*423–431, 1988.

88. Montironi, R., Albert, R., Sisti, S., Braccishi, A., Scarpelli, M., and Mariuzzi, G. M. Discrimination between follicular adenoma and follicular carcinoma of the thyroid: Preoperative validity of cytometry on aspiration smears. *Appl. Pathol. 7:*367–374, 1989.

89. Muller, N., Cooperberg, P. L., Suen, K. C. H., and Thorson, S. C. Needle aspiration biopsy in cystic papillary carcinoma of the thyroid. *Am. J. Pathol. 144:*251–253, 1985.

90. Ng, E. H., Tan, S. K., and Nambiar, R. Impact of fine needle aspiration cytology on the management of solitary thyroid nodules. *Aust. N. Z. J. Surg. 60:*463–466, 1990.

91. Nunez, C., and Mendelsohn, G. Fine-needle aspiration and needle biopsy of the thyroid gland. *Pathol. Annu. 24:*161–198, 1989.

92. Pietribiasi, F., Sapino, A., Papotti, M., and Bussolati, G. Cytologic features of poorly differentiated "insular" carcinoma of the thyroid, as revealed by fine-needle aspiration biopsy. *Am. J. Clin. Pathol. 94:*687–692, 1990.

93. Pitts, W. C., and Berry, G. J. Marginal vacuoles in metastatic thyroid carcinoma. *Diagn. Cytopathol. 5:*200–202, 1989.

94. Ravinsky, E., and Safneck, J. R. Differentiation of Hashimoto's thyroiditis from thyroid neoplasms in fine needle aspirates. *Acta Cytol. 32:*854–861, 1988.

95. Ravinsky, E., and Safneck, J. R. Fine needle aspirates of follicular lesions of the thyroid gland. The intermediate-type smear. *Acta Cytol. 34:*813–820, 1990.

96. Riazmontazer, N., and Bedayat, G. Psammoma bodies in fine needle aspirates from thyroids containing nontoxic hyperplastic nodular goiters. *Acta Cytol. 35:*563–566, 1991.

97. Rupp, M., and Ehya, H. Nuclear grooves in the aspiration cytology of papillary carcinoma in the thyroid. *Acta Cytol. 33:*21–26, 1989.

98. Sassi, I., Mangili, F., Sironi, M., Freschi, M., and Cantaboni, A. Morphometric evaluation of fine needle biopsy of single thyroid nodules. *Pathol. Res. Pract. 1985:*722–725, 1989.

99. Schmid, K. W., Ladurner, D., Zechman, W., and Feichtinger, H. Clinicopathologic management

of tumors of the thyroid gland in an endemic goiter area. Combined use of preoperative fine needle aspiration biopsy and intraoperative frozen section. *Acta Cytol. 33:*27–30, 1989.

100. Schwaegerle, S. M., Bauer, T. W., and Esselstyn, C. B. Riedel's thyroiditis. *Am. J. Clin. Pathol. 90:*715–722, 1988.

101. Seya, A., Oeda, T., Terano, T., Omura, and Yoshida, S. Comparative studies on fine-needle aspiration cytology with ultrasound scanning in the assessment of thyroid nodule. *Jpn. J. Med. 29:*478–480, 1990.

102. Shaha, A. R., DiMaio, T., Webber, C., and Jaffe, B. M. Intraoperative decision making during thyroid surgery based on the results of preoperative needle biopsy and frozen section. *Surgery 108:*964–967, 1990.

103. Shurbaji, M. S., Gupta, P. K., and Frost, J. K. Nuclear grooves: A useful criterion in the cytopathological diagnosis of papillary thyroid carcinoma. *Diagn. Cytopathol. 4:*91–94, 1988.

104. Silverman, J. F., West, R. L., and Larkin, E. W. The role of fine-needle aspiration biopsy in the rapid diagnosis and management of thyroid neoplasm. *Cancer 57:*1164–1170, 1986.

105. Smejkal, V., Smejkolova, E., Rosa, M., Zeman, V., and Smetana, K. Cytologic changes simulating malignancy in thyrotoxic goiters with carbimazole. *Acta Cytol. 29:*173–178, 1985.

106. Strong, C. J., and Garcia, B. M. Fine needle aspiration cytologic characteristics of hyalinizing trabecular adenoma of the thyroid. *Acta Cytol. 34:*359–362, 1990.

107. Tani, E., and Skoog, L. Fine needle aspiration cytology and immunochemistry in the diagnosis of lymphoid lesions of the thyroid gland. *Acta Cytol. 33:*48–52, 1989.

108. Uribe, M., Fenoglio-Preiser, C. M., Grimes, M., and Fiend, C. Medullary carcinoma of the thyroid gland: Clinical, pathological and immunohistochemical features with review of the literature. *Am. J. Surg. Pathol. 9:*577–594, 1985.

109. Vengrove, M. A., Schimmel, M., Atkinson, B. F., Evans, D., and LiVolsi, V. A. Invasive cervical thymoma masquerading as a solitary thyroid nodule. Report of a case studied by fine needle aspiration. *Acta Cytol. 35:*431–433, 1991.

Index

Page numbers followed by italic "t" denote tables; those followed by italic "f" denote figures.